Polly,

I love that
you have made
so much

good from you

Pauly's influence

Jack

Cures vs. Profits

Successes in Translational Research

Cures vs. Profits

Successes in Translational Research

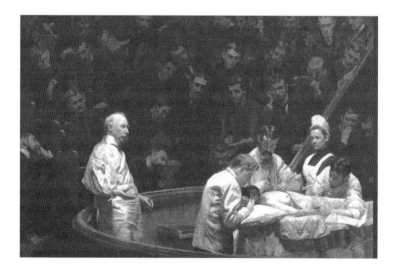

James Lyons-Weiler

Institute for Pure and Applied Knowledge, USA
ipaknowledge.org

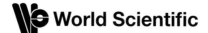 **World Scientific**

NEW JERSEY · LONDON · SINGAPORE · BEIJING · SHANGHAI · HONG KONG · TAIPEI · CHENNAI · TOKYO

Published by

World Scientific Publishing Co. Pte. Ltd.

5 Toh Tuck Link, Singapore 596224

USA office: 27 Warren Street, Suite 401-402, Hackensack, NJ 07601

UK office: 57 Shelton Street, Covent Garden, London WC2H 9HE

Library of Congress Cataloging-in-Publication Data
Names: Lyons-Weiler, James, author.
Title: Cures vs. profits : successes in translational research / James Lyons-Weiler,
    Institute for Pure and Applied Knowledge, USA.
Description: New Jersey : World Scientific, 2016. | Includes bibliographical references and index.
Identifiers: LCCN 2015038339| ISBN 9789814730136 (hardcover : alk. paper) |
    ISBN 9814730130 (hardcover : alk. paper) | ISBN 9789814730143 (paperback : alk. paper) |
    ISBN 9814730149 (paperback : alk. paper)
Subjects: LCSH: Medicine--Research--History. | Medicine--Research--Moral and ethical aspects. |
    Medical innovations--History.
Classification: LCC R852 .L96 2016 | DDC 610.72--dc23
LC record available at http://lccn.loc.gov/2015038339

British Library Cataloguing-in-Publication Data
A catalogue record for this book is available from the British Library.

Printed in Singapore

*It is no measure of health to be well adjusted
to a profoundly sick society.*

– Jiddu Krishnamurti

*The most dangerous man, to any government,
is the man who is able to think things out for himself,
without regard to the prevailing superstitions and taboos.
Almost invariably he comes to the conclusion
that the government he lives under is dishonest,
insane and intolerable, and so, if he is romantic,
he tries to change it. And if he is not romantic personally,
he is apt to spread discontent among those who are.*

— HL Mencken

The best doctor gives the least medicine.

— Benjamin Franklin

*It is the responsibility of intellectuals to speak
the truth and expose lies.*

— Noam Chomsky

Scientists will save us all.

— Johnny Gunther

Contents

Preface

An era of progressive, enlightened biomedical research is needed, and these changes must begin with each individual realizing the potential benefits to humanity first, and the bottom line second.

The history of medicine is filled with advances that have saved millions of lives and improved the outcome of diseases for millions more. From the invention of X-rays and the discovery of antibiotics to the creation of replacement organs in the lab from stem cells, these are translational successes. Someone had an idea, performed some type of research, and medical care was changed forever — to the betterment of humankind.

This not a book about alternative medicine. Alternative medicine, by its very nature, is *counterculture*. It poses itself against the mainstream, positioning itself in opposition to "Big Pharma." The positions in this book were formed as the result of my research on the history and recent events, including recent clinical studies, about topics which I thought important, not the other way around. While certain themes on that conflict emerge occasionally in this book, it is not a main theme, although it may prove informative to those on both "sides." This is a book about successes in translational biomedical research in the face of what I call profit pressures. For example, whether a compound is effective against cancer, or not, is a scientific, empirical question, and if sufficient observational data existed to suggest that certain compounds might kill cancer cells, the compounds therein should be studied, unless prior knowledge of severe toxicity exists.

The hurdles that might exist represent barriers to translation. Those hurdles may be found in the processes of science — or in the numerous biases of business interests. They may also be found in a given people's culture. If the compound exists naturally, it might face patent and exclusivity hurdles. If the compound is found in *Cannabis*, there may be additional cultural hurdles. Ethnobotanists often work with pharmaceutical companies to identify new compounds in plants; the popularity of *Cannabis* as a recreational drug, however, puts a spin on that plant as pro-*Cannabis* people want to popularize the drug as something that our government wants to keep from us. There may or may not be truth in such claims, but then, that kind of speculation is not the focus of this book.

I start, and end, with the premise that profit alone should never be the primary objective for developing health care options. However, this is also not a book (entirely) about the influence of profit motives on research in academia. That topic is adroitly (and thoroughly) examined by Sheldon Krimsky, who reviews the changes in the operations and cultures within universities in response to the profit motive in his book *Science in the Private Interest: Has the Lure of Profits Corrupted Biomedical Research?* (Rowman and Littlefield Publishers).

This book was written in response to my personal bouts of dread, grief and depression that resulted from my analysis of the international governmental, medical and scientific community's late, misguided, and awkward response to the 2014 Ebola epidemic. The international events and fiascos surrounding that event are chronicled in my first book, *Ebola: An Evolving Story* (World Scientific). I was appalled by how wrong we (the collective we) got it, such that it proved difficult to tease out any sensible logic of how ignorance (of the biology of the virus), fear, belief, reason, superstition, dogma, culture, science, and political agendas all played a role in determining public policy. The notable exceptions were, in my view, Dr. Gavin MacGregor-Skinner and Doctors Without Borders. I was dismayed by the unintentional use of *de facto* concentration camps to isolate diagnosed and suspected ebolavirus disease patients. As the Ebola Treatment Units filled up, the Ebola Triage Camps became isolation camps, dooming many who did not have Ebola to contract the disease, and dooming nearly everyone in those camps to either beat the disease on their own, without treatment, or to die.

My reaction was to write a second book, in search of silver lining in where we are and what we know in medicine as a result of (mostly) recent research. I started each chapter open-minded about the influences of profit pressures, competition vs. collaboration, remaining objective as long as possible with regard to the actors involved so as to discover, if possible, what some would call the truth. My goal was to provide a sober, logical look at any emergent issues. It did not take too long before I found the limits of knowledge imposing themselves, or, I should say, the limits we impose on what we think we can know via the ways we choose to go about the business of doing science in the name of medicine. In doing research on the very first chapter, I found myself deconstructing the gold standard of the design of the FDA's sacred randomized clinical trial. I found that a change in how results from RCTs are interpreted may be in order. I have a high standard for science: Knowledge claims must be based on solid assumptions, using robust and reproducible measurements. I will grant that sounds ostentatious; however, it is not the first time in my career that I have developed improvements to the most popular methodologies for doing data analysis for biological and medical sciences. My "hit list" has included advances in methods for:

understanding species diversity patterns;

phylogenetic data analysis;

studying molecular evolution;

survival analysis in clinical trials;

analysis of genomic data;

analysis of proteomic data;

identifying statistically significant prediction models using biomarkers;

identifying significant differences between clinical groups with respect to survival;

predicting the effects of integrating a diversity of methods into a coherent, cost-effective clinical diagnostic workflow;

Next-Generation Sequence (NGS) variant calling;
NGS gene expression studies;
NGS methylation studies;
Low-bias methods for identifying differentially expressed genes and proteins.

I have a personal policy, however, and I have followed this policy throughout my career: My understandings of the flaws of the methods involved are made public only once I have found what I believe to be a suitable, demonstrably superior alternative.

This was not the case for my assessments of progress in translational research in medicine. This time, I could remain biased, I allowed myself to seek the positive, but still analyze what I encountered with a cold, hard look at many topics in translational research with an open mind. By allowing myself a bias toward finding the silver linings, I would let the negative stories emerge in spite of my efforts to find good news in biomedical research.

To that end, any discussion of successes in translational research requires working definitions, both of "translational research (Fig. 1)" and of "successes." And any viable definition of the terms must capture

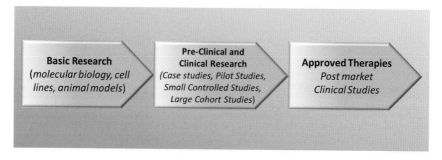

Fig. 1 Typical view of translational research overview. Knowledge at one phase informs the next. A common view is "Bench to bedside and back," with the effects in the clinical informing basic and pre-clinical phases. Translational research involves effort at each transition at overcoming pitfalls and hurdles that prevent movement from one phase to the next. Effort between Basic and Pre-clinical is considered T1 effort. Similarly, effort between clinical research and approved therapies is considered T2 effort.

activities involved in the movement of knowledge, i.e., degree of understanding, from one phase to a more advanced phase. It should also address the type of knowledge, and for our purposes, the application of knowledge toward clinical impact. In biomedical research, this may mean improved understanding of the mechanism of a drug, or the molecular basis of a disease.

Some measure of the degree of impact of scientific findings on personal and public health is necessary. Most of modern medicine is conducted in the reality of a climate of profit pressure — with significant opportunities for profit. I had to make a choice in setting out in this book: Do I look for examples of successes that include profit (win-win) or do I take an objective approach and provide an overall treatment regardless of, or in some cases, in spite of, profit pressures? Some advances, such as the allotransplantation of olfactory (bulbar) nerves to repair a man's severed spinal cord — allowing him to walk again (Tabakow *et al.*, 2014) — are easy to identify as successes, but even this clear example has its detractors (see Guest and Dietrich, 2015).

Any ethical definition of a measure of the utility in clinical translational research must include, as the majority component, consideration of the effects on the reduction of human pain and suffering via improvements in clinical practices. I leave it to the reader to decide where I landed on the balance of that score, chapter by chapter.

This book is meant to be a scholarly treatment that informs a conversation that has been going on in countries around the world, from people in all walks of life, regarding medicine, medical treatment, and medical research. Although medical doctors are at the core of that discussion, they are rarely overtly invited to participate. It would be impolitic to suggest to your physician that you suspect that their intentions are not to cure you of your diseases, but, rather, to keep you sick and on treatment so they may personally profit. The argument, more on point, goes something like this: Medical doctors and the pharmaceutical industry do not want cures for the diseases that afflict us; instead, they want treatments, because if there were cures, they could not profit.

Combined with this is the secondary topic of how doctors do not treat diseases, rather, they treat symptoms, often not really knowing what ailment they are treating, and that they perform "diagnosis by treatment" — that is, trying treatments until the patient feels better. In effect, they use the patient in an unregistered clinical trial. These are serious charges being leveled at the medical community; they are trusted with our care, and trusted to reduce our pain and suffering. They are trusted with our very lives. And yet no one has brought the issue forward in a manner that might lead to change within the institutions of medicine and medical research within the US if and when these charges are supported by the facts.

Books on closely related topics are often done to pitch so-called "alternative medicine," and while such books may be somewhat effective at promoting their specific alternative agendas, they are written with an agenda, and not with the objectivity of a scientist. Anyone can find confirming instances to support their claim of what is wrong with a particular brand of modern medicine, thus seemingly bolstering their own alternative treatment. This is not science. It is arguing with statistics. Lining up many confirming instances is not science (Popper).

By contrast, I have no particular agenda for this book other than to hopefully open up a dialog among all stakeholders in medicine with an eye on the positive. From the patient to the CEO, my goal is to help bring about changes in our practices and policies that might lead to a larger number of effective and safe medical treatment options for doctors and patients to choose from, thus reducing death due to disease. Most importantly to me personally, these options should reduce human pain and suffering.

For some authors, it may be tempting to partake in the non-scientific near hysteria of people questioning the validity of western medicine. A counterculture exists in which suspicion, rumor, and idle speculation fan the flames of discontent. If I were to write a book in that vein, I could expect disdain from my colleagues, whose esteem I hold dear... but I would expect to sell more books. No, this is no anti-medicine, anti-science book, either. It is instead an attempt to scrutinize objectively, and explain in simple, understandable terms, a number of important topics in medical research that I believe deserve a wider audience. For each topic, I began my research with an open mind. If, after my research, I have formulated an opinion, one way or the other, on a given topic, I say so. If I have reached a conclusion, I make it clear. Where I have not, I call for more research.

Each individual medical doctor has taken the Hippocratic Oath, by which they pledged to "First, do no harm." Violations of this oath occur on a regular basis. Via this oath and in our placing our lives, and our children's lives, in their hands, medical doctors share a sacred social contract with the rest of humanity. We place our esteem in them, we give them influence on social matters and public health matters, and we bestow upon them great wealth. While many doctors deserve the respect, social status, and wealth that come with their position, those guilty of egregious instances of abuse should be tried, and if convicted, sentenced.

Many Americans believe that for some doctors, the Hippocratic Oath is often made with some qualifiers in fine print, such as "First, do not harm (to profit)." It is not hard to see why; medicine is projected to become a trillion-dollar industry worldwide (Perkowski, 2014). The US is one of only two countries that permit, by law, direct-to-consumer marketing of pharmaceuticals (the other is New Zealand).

This book is not about heroes in medicine. That said, some rough estimates of lives saved by advances in specific medical practices and procedures paint the picture of medicine in a more beautiful palette. The website Science Heroes, for example (www.scienceheroes.com) reports that blood transfusions are estimated to have saved over one billion people. Their list goes on to report 109 medical heroes, estimated to have saved billions of lives. (The website is a companion to the book *Scientists Greater than Einstein* (Woodward *et al.*, 2009; Quill Driver Books).

So where does the concern over undue profits fit in? While it is true that we are all treated with options that, from a pharmaceutical corporation's standpoint, were deemed potentially profitable, is this a mere fact of reality, or something else? Regardless of the nuances of motive, it means that many potentially effective drugs have not been brought to market. Why? Profitability is certainly a filter that has a homogenizing effect on medicine — our treatment options are much more limited than they could be. This seems to be a perfectly acceptable norm to many.

On April 1, 2015, Anne De Groot, CEO of EpiVax, testified before the Blue Ribbon Study Panel on Biodefense at the Hudson Institute in Washington, D.C. Her focus was the need to prioritize innovative, nimble, responsive ways for dealing with existing and new biothreats.

Former HHS Secretary Donna Shalala commented on the problems of balancing innovation and manufacturing at large capacities:

> Sec. Shalala: *It's one of those fundamental questions of what should government be doing, and when does it profit share. We're talking about vaccines where the margins are smaller than other drugs.*

> De Groot: *We have also been able to look at existing vaccines and say 'Wait a minute, we don't think this is a good idea.' There should be a place for us to say that where it's going to be heard. And really, there's no one I can talk to. My experience during H1N1 and during H7N9 is that the CDC doesn't want to hear that. People do not want to hear that the vaccines that they are going to make (are not going to work). The H7N9 vaccine that we have today is the least effective vaccine that's ever been made... We told you that in 2013 when sequence (of the virus) was published. We published a paper that the virus was a stealth virus, that new vaccines would be ineffective. Less than 10 months later, we were proven right.*

C-SPAN2 recorded a stream of the proceedings. Another CEO, Daniel Abdun-Nabi, of Emergent BioSolutions, also testified for the need to find a way to fund small companies like De Groot's to be innovative, but offered that *"she's not going to manufacture."* According to a report in American Progress, Emergent BioSolutions received some $1.3 billion from the US government to produce an anthrax vaccine, when it cost them only $250 million to manufacture the vaccine doses.

The contrast between EpiVax's focus and the focus of Emergent BioSolutions at the Blue Ribbon Panel was stark. EpiVax wants to reduce roadblocks and costs so the overall approach can be safe and effective. They are extremely good at predicting whether specific vaccines will likely be effective on emerging infectious diseases. In some ways, they are way ahead of the pack. In reality, they are one step behind. By the time they complete their analyses in response to a threat, the big wheel of the *status quo* has already started turning, and their input is seen as a distraction. This does not need to be so, of course. The big wheel could easily absorb *a priori* checks on the computed fit between antigen and antibodies, given the sequence, as first-step screen for existing vaccines likely to (or not to) work. The panel seemed focused on the status quo; Gov. Ridge discussed how government has "always worked this way," and both he and Sec. Shalala acknowledge the need for some type of reform. They seemed to want somehow to keep the old system in place and add EpiVax's ideas to the established large-contract process.

After the testimony concluded, while the Blue Ribbon panelists were not aware, a microphone was left on which captured the conversation between former HHS Secretary Donna Shalala and Gov. Tom Ridge.

> Secretary Shalala: *He (Daniel Abdun-Nabi) is making a fortune over there (at Emergent BioSolutions CEO). He's figured out how to do it. She has not figured out a way to do that yet.*
>
> Gov. Ridge: *That was my take-away exactly.*

Whatever profit model is in play that would transform $250 million in investment into over $1 billion in profit seems par for the course. For others, such outcomes appear to be a necessary evil, but this is partly because we lack an obvious alternative means by which corporations can bring effective products forward. As health care costs skyrocket and Americans are asked to pay for their mandatory health insurance or face a fee, one wonders how the Ebola crisis might have been handled if even half of that $1 billion went into the development of a vaccine.

The design of clinical trials is a key to success in medical research. As dry as that topic may be, it also part of the answer to why so few drugs are available to us. It is how medical research is done. Thus, the public should learn some details of how clinical trials are conducted. They should also learn of the limitations that are inherent to clinical trials, and find out whether alternatives to the gold standard might improve rates of discovery and translation, and if so, how. I, and many of my colleagues in research, would like to know that we are treated with options that are considered to be most effective, and safe, for each individual patient. There is, therefore, a movement afoot toward "personalized medicine," which attempts to secure, based on information gleaned from individual patients, the best possible clinical route for that patient. Personalized medicine is juxtaposed as an alternative to population-based medicine, and yet the entire biomedical research paradigm is centered on population science. Seeing the tree for the forest can be challenging. But individualized medicine is a key to the success of the effective treatment of many of our most deadly diseases.

There are thousands of promising pharmaceutical compounds on the shelves at pharmaceutical companies. These are known as "orphan drugs," and they exist at a loss for companies. In fact, they are often pointed to as justification for the high cost of successful drugs. The argument goes like this: For every drug that actually makes it to market, there are a large number of other drugs that do not; we need to recoup the cost of those investments, too. While it is certainly true that pharma spends billions on R&D, they also spend billions on salaries and bonuses for executives. Also, it is not altogether clear that companies who experience losses due to poor or ineffective exploratory R&D are entitled to recoup their losses. Imagine an ice cream business stating that their high prices were due to all of the flavors they tried out while developing their blockbuster flavors. The difference is the presumed added value in doing failed research because it could have benefited humanity. However, exactly how much of this failed effort is due to poor practices, or inefficiencies that resulted in profit-taking instead of re-investment, is unknown.

Another complicating factor is a trend toward homogenization of health care options. While the capitalist in me appreciates an honestly earned financial incentive just like anyone else, there seems to be a missing financial mechanism that uses consumer demand; consumers are often not free to choose directly (they are rarely told all of the options), and this places the medical community as an arbiter in the economic cycle. On top of that sits a regulatory body that by its very nature restricts treatment options and has moved aggressively to restrict health claims for food products, even when studies strongly support those health claims.

While idealists call for collaborative medical research on tough problems, there is a paradox of translation. The more valuable a new approach to medicine is, the more likely a research institution is to keep it a secret. This means that fewer people around the world can study the problem, and increase knowledge. The more ubiquitous a technique or new drug is, the less valuable it is to a single corporate entity, and while many more people can study it, it is less likely it is to be brought forward as a product. Further, as research is a massively parallelized endeavor, it seems likely that some parts of a solution to a medical issue may be known and owned by one entity, while another critical part may be known by others. I have been told by CEOs of some companies that these parts of knowledge often cannot be brought together thanks to the network of lawyers who protect their companies' intellectual property.

At the height of the Great Recession, I proposed an Intellectual Property Share Market (Lyons-Weiler, 2009) to allow investors to drive forward good ideas in biomedicine and other areas allowing the dollars to vote for the IP that might be brought forward. This idea exists in a less formal way via crowdsourced funding; however that approach lacks the financial payoff to investors, as crowdsourced funding is usually a gift.

Some point out the fact that people can live with HIV as evidence of success at the level of the FDA, specifically in terms of being able to expedite turn-around times on treatments. However, given that so much is known about the biology of HIV, and that it remains endemic in the human population, AIDS due to HIV infection can hardly be called a translational success. In 2015, estimates are that one in eight people who are infected with HIV do not know they are infected. Approximate one in four new HIV infections are in youth aged 13–24, and most of them are not aware of their infection, and that they can pass it on to uninfected persons. Between 1.5–1.9 million people die every year from HIV/AIDS. Over 39 million people have died from HIV/AIDS since the transfer to humans occurred. While the number of deaths due to HIV/AIDS is decreasing, the number of new infections in 2013 was 2.3 million. Overall, there have been 75 million infections worldwide, with around 35 million deaths thus far. That's a kill rate of around 46%. There are currently around 6,300 new infections per *day*.

How can the US government agency responses be lauded as a "success?" Where is the vaccine? Where is the cure?

HIV is now highly profitable for the pharmaceutical industry, as it produces patients who require lifelong treatment. And yet with a kill rate that rivals that of the deadly Ebolavirus disease, HIV/AIDS is accepted by the public as a fact of life. While we all hope for a cure, the fact is, the disease is endemic to our species until further notice of cure.

Is this necessary? Or is there a cure, and the HIV drugs are more profitable? This type of conspiracy thinking occurs in large part due to the lack of leadership. Key individuals in positions could have, for example, protested against the US's solitary negative vote in 2003 against a United Nations resolution on access to drugs in global epidemics such as HIV/AIDS, tuberculosis and malaria. The resolution would have made low-cost, generic versions of drugs available worldwide. When one realizes that the massive profits the pharmaceutical companies make from treating HIV/AIDS in developed countries come at a cost of lives in less developed countries, it is easy to see why some proportion of people find those profits ill-gotten. In matters of public health, profit should come as a secondary, not a primary consideration.

Cost effective analysis is usually conducted from an institutions' point of view, and includes consideration of the cost of adopting a new drug relative to the cost of existing practice, compared to the increase in clinical effectiveness upon adoption of the new drug, i.e.,

$$CE = (C1-C0)/(E1-E0)$$

This conceptual analysis is made challenging due to the different units (effectiveness must be monetized to appear in the same units (dollars) as cost), and this makes analysis not at all straightforward. Profit models nearly always result in the determination of charging what the market will bear. There are some circumstances, at a fixed production cost, in which the increase in the number of units sold due to lowering prices is a major factor in clinical adoption. The larger the percentage of the clinical population that can afford a treatment, the more widespread its use may be. Thus, price models of drugs (something that pharmaceutical companies rarely share) may have two or more optimal price points when price can make adoption less likely. Classic break-even analysis does not apply in these situations, because if no one in a clinical population opts for a new treatment due to cost, no price will allow cost recovery.

Not all profits from disease share moral equivalence. Profits gleaned from the prevention of the spread of the disease seem morally sound. Take, for example the case of HIV/AIDs. The FDA approved, in July 2012, the drug Truvada (Gilead, Inc.), which reduces HIV infections in people at high risk of HIV infection when used in combination with condoms and counseling (Grant *et al.*, 2010). Truvada, a fixed-dose combination of Tenofovir/emtricitabine, has minimal side effects. Truvada is not indicated for general use, and HIV/AIDS is on the rise in the poorest parts of the world. Whether cheap generic versions of Truvada may be made available to people with HIV-positive partners in less-developed countries or not remains to be seen. A vaccine for HIV/AIDs always seems to be just around the corner; I hope that research using Virus-Like Particles (VLPs), such as those used in the Ebola outbreak to screen thousands of potentially effective approved drugs (Kouznetsova *et al.*, 2014) may provide carriers of multivalent vaccination against all major clades of HIV strains. I will explore the translational successes of cures for HIV/AIDS in another book.

As ugly as the truth about the preference of profits over treatment options exposed by HIV/AIDS may appear, it would be terribly naïve and a great disservice to my biomedical and pharma executive colleagues to represent their mindset considering economic dimensions alone. They, and insurance companies, and health care consumers are stakeholders with very distinct — and often contrasting — perspectives and interests. Many prefer to think also in terms of benefits and utility to society. Measures such as quality of life years (QALY) are often considered, and are occasionally monetized for inclusion in cost models. Some models are fairly sophisticated, using statistical resampling methods and Monte Carlo simulations. Nevertheless, the definition of QALY still contains a high degree of subjectivity. However, the concept allows the consideration of the valuation of the clinical benefits of the cost of new treatments compared to existing treatments. A common method is Incremental Cost-Effectiveness Ratio (ICER). Bang and Zhao (2012) advocate for using of the median, not the mean, in ICER analysis due in part to the potential for highly skewed distributions when the cost of care of a few patients is very high. They have also worked out median-based ICER for use with censored data (Bang and Zhao, 2015).

Total costs and total benefits within a given area of clinical practice would capture the entire distribution for an institution, however, and there is no reason not to consider them. From an institutional point of view, and from the producers' point of view, few factor in the lost income and loss of benefit due to non-adoption caused by price (declined treatments), and therefore cost effectiveness considerations need updating to consider expected partial adoption in the consideration of relative gain.

Price gouging takes place when the seller can set any price, knowing the buyer will pay — or at least try to pay — any price for the product. There are approximately 2.6 million hepatitis C patients in the US. Imagine a drug that could cure hepatitis C — nearly any price above production cost would be a blockbuster and generate remarkable revenue for the company that produced the treatment. Imagine a company that priced that drug to the point where a mere 30,000 patients and their insurers could afford the treatment in the first year. At high enough prices, with even 30,000 patients the drug is a moneymaker, and on the books, projections are that at least that many if not more cases among the wealthy are expected. Thus, massive profits are expected, and the disease will continue to flourish among the (relatively) poor, generating sufficient numbers of paying patient to keep those profits coming.

Express Scripts (2015) produced a report that summarized the trend succinctly, identifying compounded therapies, hepatitis C and cancer medications as the major drivers of increases in health care costs in the US. In 2014, these three types of treatments made up two-thirds of pharmaceutical drug spending in patients whose care cost exceeded $100,000. This is due in part to the number of patients receiving medication treatment for hepatitis C jumping 733% in 2014. Many had delayed other treatment, waiting for a breakthrough. The trends involved increase in use and cost.

Gilead Sciences acquired and manufactures and sells a drug called Harvoni, which completely cures most people with the most prevalent hepatitis C subtype. A three-month regime costs $94,500, over $1,000 a pill. According to a Bloomberg report, that is more than double the expected cost for the treatment when Gilead acquired the drug from another company (at a reported cost of $11 billion). The drug generated over $10 billion in sales in 2014; thus, Gilead has by now (June 2015) easily recouped the cost of the investment. There are alternatives to Gilead's one pill per day treatment that are nearly as effective, and insurers are recommending those options to patients.

All of these formal considerations of price and value assessment would be nice if there were evidence that these factors actually are considered in setting a price for new drugs. In June 2015, in an analysis of 51 cancer drugs approved over five years, Mailankody and Prasad (2015) of the NIH's Medical Oncology Service, National Cancer Institute found that the average cost of new drugs was over $100,000. They failed to find any difference in the cost of drugs approved on the basis of progression-free survival and overall survival; they found no difference between new drugs with a novel mechanism of action and next-in-line drugs. In fact, there was no discernable relation between the overall improvement in endpoints and cost. The authors concluded that Pharma set the cost at "what the market would bear."

The tendency to price medicines based on what the market will bear has placed many treatments out of the reach of the masses, and causes payees — including Medicare and insurance companies — to refuse treatments based on cost. This leads to lower than possible consumption, and also to artificially-justified inflated prices for similar, even pre-existing options, spiraling health care costs — and profits — into the stratosphere. Competition is supposed to keep prices down. In the case of effective treatments, however, Pharma seems to believe that patients will pay nearly any price. As long as competitors raise prices to maintain projected revenues for investors, the practice will continue until some unseen ceiling is hit. The practice has increased the cost of treatment of multiple sclerosis from about $10,000 a year in the 1990s to over $50,000 a year or higher (Hartung *et al.*, 2015).

The copays add a significant financial burden to patients. All of the major drug companies have patient-assistance programs that help cover the cost of medication when patients have insufficient insurance, or no coverage and cannot otherwise afford it. However, the cost to the government-insured, especially those with fixed annual budgets, means refusal of coverage to other patients, placing effective treatments out of reach for many doctors and patients.

Insurers have long complained about the skyrocketing costs of treatments, and doctors are joining in. The study by Hartung *et al.* (2015) was motivated in part by the inability of doctor co-authors to provide treatments to their patients.

This practice is anti-capitalist, inhumane, and unsustainable. *Bloomberg Business* (Tozzi, 2015) called these market trends "Bizarro," providing an analogy of the first iPhone being manufactured and sold alongside its newer versions at ever increasing prices. The percent increase in the cost of drugs was compiled for Table A1.

The prices for these drugs are about half those in Table A1 in Canada, Australia, and the UK (Hartung *et al.*, 2015). These patterns reflect a trend not restricted to MS drugs.

Table A1   Percent Increase in Cost in Key Drugs by Pharma

DRUG	DATE APPROVED	INITIAL COST (IN 2013 DOLLARS)	2013 COST	**INCREASE**
Interferon-β-1b (Betaseron)	7/23/1993	$18,591	$61,529	**231.00%**
Interferon-β-1a IM (Avonex)	5/17/1996	$12,951	$62,394	**381.80%**
Glatiramer acetate (Copaxone)	12/20/1996	$12,312	$59,158	**380.50%**
Interferon-β-1a SC (Rebif)	3/7/2002	$19,763	$66,394	**236.00%**
Natalizumab (Tysabri)	11/23/2004	$31,879	$64,233	**101.50%**
Interferon-β-1b (Extavia)	8/14/2009	$35,644	$51,427	**44.30%**
Fingolimod (Gilenya)	9/21/2010	$54,245	$63,806	**17.60%**
Teriflunomide (Aubagio)	9/12/2012	$48,349	$57,553	**19.00%**
Dimethyl fumarate (Tecfidera)	3/27/2013	$57,816	$63,315	**9.50%**

Notes: All costs are annual.
2013 costs were sampled in December of that year.
Interferon-β-1b is marketed as Betaseron by Bayer and Extavia by Novartis.
Source: Hartung *et al.*, 2015.

The tendency for old, competing drugs to be priced higher due to overpricing by the latest approved drug is bizarre; it is hard to understand in terms of standard supply-side driven competitive market dynamics.

Under normative free market supply and demand dynamics, producers will provide increased supply as prices rise because all firms will look to maximize profits. Under this model, supply is a function of price and quantity. A positive correlation usually exists between price and quantity. Typically, demand increases when prices are low, consumers tend to purchase a larger quantity of the product. When prices are high, consumers tend to purchase a lower quantity. Supply and demand influence each other differently depending on availability of the product — that is, it is usually seen that producers control the specific conditions that drive supply, and therefore, demand. Surpluses and shortages due to changes in production cause fluctuation until the product reaches a fair market value.

There are myriad oddities about pharmaceutical economics (pharma economics) that do not fit this typical model. Factors that increase demand (in addition to decreased prices due to surplus and competition) include increased incidence of disease, greater consumer awareness, and advocacy for purchase via clinicians. Direct-to-consumer marketing can increase demand for a specific treatment. DTC marketing tends to make consumers believe that the drug being advertised is as the latest-breaking treatment, and they assume that it is also the most effective. Neither of these assumptions are safe assumptions, and thus patients rely heavily on the advice of their doctors.

In market force economics, price is usually negatively responsive to competition. In pharma economics, this dynamic is missing because producers of older options find that the average market value of treatments same in class increases. The result is a positive feedback loop with negative consequences: Price increases become a runaway process, leaving some consumers out. A main difference here is that in medicine, consumers may be left out of the selection of offerings on the market by many intermediary stakeholders.

In pharma economics, individual patients do not consume more than the prescription requires; theirs is a fixed consumption schedule, and, for many conditions, for a short duration. The demand curve is not only flat, as some have decried. In normal market economics, a flat demand curve makes it difficult for producers to effectively vary their production output in a manner that allows them to take advantage of the principles of supply and demand. This usually drives innovation.

In pharma economics, the flat (but steady) demand curve is of little significance because the majority of consumers have less control over their consumption decisions. It is as if the markets for some drugs are stuck on a single point of demand (high) when in fact, demand is inflated by the existence of payors other than the consumer: Medicare, Medicaid, insurance companies, and even the producers will pay into the cost of the medicine for a patient as a free subsidy of their entire copay.

When the drugs are life-saving, this comes across to the public as philanthropy. A pure cynic would view this strategy as a shrewd investment with a handsome profit and a PR boost. After all, copays are often a mere fraction of the total price of a drug, and the cost of the product is much lower than the price. Thus, the idea goes, pharmaceutical companies manipulate both the supply and demand side of the market, driving the runaway price increases.

Some in business will see this as an ultimate expression of free market capitalism, and will celebrate pharma's successes unapologetically.

Others (mostly consumers) will see this as a perversion of free market capitalism; they will feel manipulated, and they will experience a sort of buyer's regret for not having received a better deal — not knowing the details of the imagined better deal. They will know that they (as a class) will have been bilked somehow, in some way (perhaps via higher insurance premiums, or higher overall copays).

Even when some patients are left out due to cost, the fact that some consumers cannot afford the treatments is irrelevant because the loss in potential profit from those consumers is hidden by the artificial increase in drug prices. This inflation is boon for everyone except low-income consumers.

This outcome is similar to a phenomenon in market science in which one producer is strong and is faced with weak competitors; providers facing weak competition are likely to apply high mark-ups and set prices above the competitive level.

This unhooking of the relationship between supply and demand replaces the free market with an economic oligarchy. The process is not identical to price fixing, because companies that are competing are not communicating with each other directly. They pay less attention to the normative factors that cause them to set a price (units sold) and more attention to the price range of similar options for health care, even when those options are not same-in-class. The competitors are, however, communicating with each other via their pricing.

Society objects to exorbitant profits when it means that the price will place the product out of reach of some of the patients. However, when society values a product to the extent that our society values drugs that either save our lives or dramatically improve or maintain our quality of life, the potential for market-independent pricing is high.

Such an outcome can have dire consequences, especially in terms of limited supply for deadly infectious diseases and in seasonally fluctuating diseases. These factors conspired to lead to a serious shortage of availability of effective malaria drugs in Cambodia (Patouillard *et al.*, 2015).

In the US, key voices have described pricing as "chaotic," citing immense and unpredictable pricing from provider to provider, and high regional variation (Shanley, 2011).

In a large market where company value is measured in terms of stock values (which are in principle determined by dividends), the pressure to stay competitive is immense. At some point, the absolute value of a product loses meaning, and the relative value becomes paramount. That is, the dollar value of your product only makes sense in terms of the value of your competitor's product because as they stand to profit more than you, the value of their company stands to increase faster than yours. They stand to benefit at a compounded rate, and thus will be able to outcompete you directly on the product in question, and also in other areas of competition (better investment in R&D, more marketing, etc.). Thus, to stay relevant, the pressure to keep your price up with others is immense: Prices begin to drift higher and higher away from commodity value as each company checks the value of their offerings against the market.

The resulting runaway increase in pricing brings to mind the statement by the Red Queen to Alice in Lewis Carroll's *Through the Looking Glass*:

> *"Now, here, you see, it takes all the running you can do, to keep in the same place."*

Go/No Go decisions also influence the scope of health care options. Such was the case for vaccine development in Ebola. The pharmaceutical company's profit filter is one of many that determine which options for care are even available to our doctors. But it is not the only factor. At question is not whether doctors are willing to treat patients, or cure them. The action of choosing a particular route of medical care is often a result of consultations with peers, dependent on protocols, approved by associations, limited by the FDA regulatory process and dependent on approval by health care insurance providers. Sometimes, small changes in health care practices are so easy, practical, and inexpensive, that it makes one wonder why all improvements don't come that easy. An example of this kind of translation is the observation by one doctor that patients who were acquiring pneumonia infections after surgery and dying while being treated for other diseases needed to have the head of their beds raised. Patients at risk of developing pneumonia are now also advised to breathe deeply and cough four to five times an hour to prevent the illness — a no-cost, life-saving practice that can never be put on the stock market.

Health care spending on prescription medications accounts for 1.6% of gross domestic product in the US (Centers for Medicare and Medicaid, 2014). The use of, and constant increase in the price of brand-name prescription medications is the primary driver of this growth, increasing 15% in price in 2014 alone (Silverman, 2015).

Use of comparatively lower priced generic drugs now accounts for 86% of all prescriptions. Generics have cost US consumers nearly $1.5 trillion in the past decade (GPHA Online, 2014).

One might suspect that some doctors may offer name-brand drugs over less expensive generics; to a degree, those suspicions are correct. Patients are evidently complicit in this; Campbell *et al.* found that patient demand for name-brand drugs is one factor that in part explains why doctors tend to prescribe more expensive name-brand options over generics. Other factors include type of doctor, and years of clinical experience: Older doctors were more likely to acquiesce to patient requests for name-brand drugs (Campbell *et al.*, 2013). Some doctors may write "Dispense as Written," or check a box, which then mandates that the pharmacist use only name-brand versions of a drug. They do so at the risk that some patients will be less likely to use the medication as directed: They may skip doses to extend the time between filling expensive scripts, leading to less efficacy. Patients receiving less expensive generics showed a 12% increase in compliance (Shrank *et al.*, 2006).

To stem the rising tide in cost, substitution laws have been passed in every state. These laws either authorize or mandate pharmacists to fill most prescriptions for a brand-name drug with its generic counterpart. Similarly, tiered insurance formularies are used to impose higher cost-sharing obligations on patients for brand-name drugs. Paying clinicians to prescribe generics is legal for some, but not all payors (Sarpatwari *et al.*, 2015).

With all of the regulatory hurdles, and the profit pressures, sometimes it seems a wonder that any improvements in medicine occur at all. In this book, I explore the pitfalls of modern medical research and point to instances that seem to confirm the American public's suspicion of cure vs. treatment decisions. I also try to provide a balanced view by interviewing experts on specific topics, and highlight where more information via research is needed. A book on those topics alone would do nothing more than stir discontentment and suspicion. I use this book also as an opportunity to explore the many successes in a type of medical research called translational research. As I researched each topic and dove deep into the published records of scientific publications, articles, prospectuses from corporations, and interviews with the researchers behind the translational successes, my journey was open-ended. However, I sought to identify the key characteristics of the researchers, the medical problems, and the research studies themselves that contributed to their translational successes.

My questions included practical questions such as:

At the time of your research, what was the standard of care for the clinical problem you chose to study? What were its limitations?

What regulatory hurdles did you face?

What improvements in health care practices can be expected by your findings?

If you had to do it all over again, and had more money for research, how would you have changed your study?

Which are the most important aspects of your topic of research that you would like the public to know?

In considering successes, I wanted to find treatments, therapies, approaches to diagnostics that, first and foremost, were successful at the superior goal of medicine: to reduce human pain and suffering. If, secondarily, they were found profitable by the discoverers and their partners, that would be fine, but I wanted to balance the stories told irrespective of profitability to provide the reader with models of pathways to success for the well-being of patients. I wanted to focus on the processes of effective translational research practices, not exclusively on their outcomes. Successes do not have to be expensive. An example of a relatively inexpensive therapy is Eye Movement Desensitization and Reprocessing (EMDR), an effective treatment of post-traumatic stress disorder. This approach involves a therapist asking a client to recall a traumatic experience, and to move their eyes back and forth for sessions that can last 90 minutes. The data supporting the effectiveness of EMDR is compelling, and it is used in some practices.

I had to decide how I would go about choosing those studies that were worthy of the title "success." Some advances in medicine are rarely seen or come to the patient's attention. For example, it is now commonplace for surgeons and pathologists to use *in vivo* visualization systems designed to enable real-time study of tissue images during surgeries and biopsies. These more or less obvious applications of advances in technologies, such as macroscopic fluorescent imaging, are subjected to study and achieve FDA approval, as they impact clinical inferences. While a visualization component is FDA-approved (i.e., fluorescein), the impact of overall changes to surgical workflows associated with changes in imaging and visualization are measured in technical terms (within meristic (measurement) performance specification). But the contributed impact of changes to such systems on clinical outcomes (e.g., progression-free survival, overall survival) is rarely, if ever measured, and thus, their contribution to translational success is not known in those terms.

Naturally, it would be easy to prioritize research on those diseases that contributed to the largest percentage of mortality, and estimate their impact on the reduction in terms of number of deaths; however, I also wanted to balance the consideration to advances in approaches to diseases that horribly afflict a minority with pain and suffering. Thus, my filters on prioritization for inclusion included both absolute numbers and my understanding of the degree of severity of suffering by patients. At the onset of this project, these successes included some of my personal "favorites," ones that I had come to know about as a direct result of my participation in research. I am not in any way highlighting my own research — on the contrary, many of my favorites are those by colleagues whom I have come to know simply by virtue of being involved in biomedical and translational research. These became my favorites because they seemed to transcend the many pitfalls of translation in biomedical research; they seemed to be able to tell a complete story representing a specific stage in the knowledge acquisition via excellent research practices. Naturally, I wondered what other types of successes may exist beyond those that I happened to be most familiar with. More importantly, I wanted to know how these researchers were able to achieve their successes. Knowing these things might help others recognize the important value of getting the processes of research right in the face of profit pressures.

I include in the first chapter a litany of egregious abuses of modern medical practice for profit, as a reminder of the stains on the soul of medicine, in hope that contemplative meditation of those abuses might serve as a reminder to all to seek to do the best possible good they can do in all settings. I hope that by recounting these tales, the pain and suffering of those who endured bad medicine at the hands of criminal doctors should not be for nothing. My second chapter is reserved for the sins of those practicing biomedical research. These two first chapters are the sour medicine, so to speak. They should help put the rest of the actors mentioned in the book in context on each reader's abstract moral dimension.

I begin the book with optimism and hope for a much brighter future. This book is therefore dedicated to those behind the scenes who make real science possible in the face of unseemly pressures to do otherwise. It is written for the researcher, in hopes that they might glean characteristics of successful research studies. There are heroes in biomedicine, to be sure, and they are not always the best-paid people in the room, nor are they always the people in the front of the line awaiting receipt of their Nobel Prizes.

This book would not have been possible without the generosity of input from the following key people: Dr. David Sclar, Dr. Katrin Bruchmüller, Dr. Peter Strick, Dr. Steve Snyder, Dr. Andrew Vickers, Dr. J. Gregory Rosenthal, Dr. Peter Bonate, my beloved son Ben

Lyons-Weiler, Maria Reyes, Dr. Gretchen Watson, Dr. Cynthia Thompson, Dr. Caitlyn Dow, my friend, the resilient Dr. Kunwar Shailubhai, Dr. Ingolf Tuerk, Paul Reilly, Finula McCaul, Elli Kaplan, Dr. John Kirkwood, Dr. Lisa Butterfield, and Dr. Gerhard Leinenga. Thank you, Alex Ruggirello Sr., Alex Ruggirello, Jr., and Barbara Ruggirello for all of the interesting questions and discussions that led to the idea for this book. Grace, as always, thank you for the challenging questions and perspective. I love you.

The book is dedicated to the patients who enroll in clinical trials, past, present and future, because they lay their lives in the hands of their doctors for the benefit of humankind, in hope that their fight to survive and get well helps society learn how to reduce pain and suffering. This knowledge is especially precious, and the patients' sacrifice helps define what society can expect their doctors to know.

It is also dedicated to the late Dr. John McParlane, whose practice never once diagnosed a single case of ADHD.

References

Bang H, Zhao H. (2012) Median-based incremental cost-effectiveness ratio (ICER). *J Stat Theory Pract* **6(3)**: 428–42.

Bang H, Zhao H. (2015) Median-based incremental cost-effectiveness ratios with censored data. *J Biopharm Stat.* [http://dx.doi.org/10.1080/10543406.2015.1052482]

Campbell EG, *et al.* (2013) Physician acquiescence to patient demands for brand-name drugs: results of a national survey of physicians. *JAMA Intern Med* **173(3)**: 237–39. [doi: 10.1001/jamainternmed.2013.1539]

Centers for Medicare and Medicaid. (2014) NHE Factsheet. http://www.cms.gov/Research-Statistics-Data-and-Systems/Statistics-Trends-and-Reports/NationalHealthExpendData/NHE-Fact-Sheet.html

Express Scripts. (2015) Super spending: US trends in high-cost medication use. http://lab.express-scripts.com/insights/drug-options/super-spending-us-trends-in-high-cost-medication-use

GPHA Online (Generic Pharmaceutical Association & IMS Institute for Health-care Informatics). (2013) Generic drug savings in the U.S. http://www.gphaonline.org/media/cms/GPhA_Generic_Cost_Savings_2014_IMS_presentation.pdf

Grant RM, *et al.* (2010) Preexposure chemoprophylaxis for HIV prevention in men who have sex with men. *N Engl J Med* **363(27):** 2587–99.

Guest J, Dietrich WD. (2015) Commentary regarding the recent publication by Tabakow *et al.*, "Functional regeneration of supraspinal connections in a patient with transected spinal cord following transplantation of bulbar olfactory ensheathing cells with peripheral nerve bridging." *J Neurotrauma*, March 31, 2015. [Epub ahead of print]

Hartung DM, *et al.* (2015) The cost of multiple sclerosis drugs in the US and the pharmaceutical industry: too big to fail? *Neurology* **84(21):** 2185–92. [doi: 10.1212/WNL.0000000000001608]

Kouznetsova J, *et al.* (2014) Identification of 53 compounds that block Ebola virus-like particle entry via a repurposing screen of approved drugs. *Emerging Microbes and Infections* **3:** e84. [doi:10.1038/emi.2014.88]

Lyons-Weiler J. (2009) Time for an IP Share Market? *The Scientist.* To view online: http://www.the-scientist.com/?articles.view/articleNo/27084/title/Time-for-an-IP-Share-Market-/

Mailankody S, Prasad V. (2015) Five years of cancer drug approvals innova-tion, efficacy, and costs. *JAMA Oncology*, published online April 2, 2015. [doi:10.1001/jamaoncol.2015.0373] http://oncology.jamanetwork.com/article.aspx?articleid=2212206

Patouillard E. (2015) Determinants of price setting decisions on anti-malarial drugs at retail shops in Cambodia. *Malar J* **14:** 224. [doi: 10.1186/s12936-015-0737-9]

Perkowski J. (2014) Health care: a trillion dollar industry in the making. *Forbes Magazine*, November 12, 2014. [http:www.forbes.com/sites/jackperkowski/2014/11/12/health-care-a-trillion-dollar-industry-in-the-making]

Sarpatwari A, *et al.* (2015) Paying physicians to prescribe generic drugs and follow-on biologics in the United States. *PLoS Med* **12(3):** e1001802. [doi: 10.1371/journal.pmed.1001802]

Shanley A. (2011) From the Editor: Drug prices? Eenie meenie miney mo. *Pharmaceutical Manufacturing*, June 14, 2001. http://www.pharmamanufacturing.com/articles/2011/091/

Shrank WH, *et al.* (2006) The implications of choice: prescribing generic or preferred pharmaceuticals improves medication adherence for chronic conditions. *Arch Intern Med* **166:** 332–37.

Silverman E. (2015) Prices for prescription medicines rose how much last year? *WSJ Pharmalot*, January 26, 2015. http://blogs.wsj.com/pharmalot/2015/01/26/prices-for-prescription-medicines-rose-how-much-last-year/

Tabakow P, *et al.* (2014) Functional regeneration of supraspinal connections in a patient with transected spinal cord following transplantation of bulbar olfactory ensheathing cells with peripheral nerve bridging. *Cell Transplant* **23(12):** 1631–55. [doi: 10.3727/096368914X685131]

Tozzi J. (2015) How much would you pay for an old drug? If you have MS, a fortune. *Bloomberg Business*, April 25, 2015.

1 Abuses in Medicine

Imagine that you're visiting your doctor, and you hear the words: "We need to do more tests. The cells look unusual, it could be cancer."

Who would think of? Family? Your children? Your parents? Your friends?

Some follow-up tests are ordered, and your doctor tells you: "I'm sorry, it's cancer. We'll need to start chemotherapy right away."

You begin treatments. You have suffered through weeks or months of debilitating treatments; you have used your sick time. Maybe you have lost your job. Your family has seen you lose your hair; you've lost fat and muscle. You're in for the fight of your life. The side effects and emotional turmoil are so bad, you've thought about quitting the chemo, and giving in. You search for inspiration, and try to muster every ounce of strength and perseverance you can find.

And then you're given even more devastating news:

The doctor lied.

Meet Dr. Farid Fata, a doctor from Michigan, who pled guilty to 16 charges: money laundering, conspiracy to receive kickbacks, and 13 counts of health care fraud. Some of Fata's actions likely caused the deaths of patients.

Fata, who lived in Oakland Township north of Detroit, had offices in Clarkston, Bloomfield Hills, Lapeer, Oak Park, Sterling Heights, and Troy, Michigan. He was popular with his patients; some protested on his behalf with signs stating "We Love Him." Over the course of five years, Fata bilked patients of their lives and Medicare of at least $35 million, and perhaps as much as $91 million.

■ 1

Now meet Angela Swantek, the nurse who, in 2010, worked for Fata for about 1½ hours. When she figured out what Fata was doing, she quit her job, and wrote a letter to the State of Michigan. Swantek is a hero, and although that letter should have ultimately led to Fata's arrest and conviction, it didn't. The state investigated, and told her that they found no evidence of wrong doing. He wasn't arrested until August 2013. It took a male employee's report to the FBI and the Department of Health and Human Services to bring Fata to justice.

Fata spent $9 million of his ill-gotten spoils defending himself. After the federal government seized his assets, Fata pleaded guilty to 13 counts of Medicare fraud, one count of conspiracy to pay or receive kickbacks and two counts of money laundering. But he was never charged with murder. No assault and battery charges were filed. He saw over 1,200 patients from 2009 until he was ordered to stop practicing medicine.

Why the prosecutors did not push for assault charges and investigate whether any of the patients involved most likely died from chemotherapy may never be known. Some of Fata's patients have filed civil suits against him. In July 2015, Fata was sentenced to 45 years in prison. Prosecutors quipped: "Patients are people, not profit centers."

Thinking back to my own early childhood, I recall the suffering of my own mother during her fight with breast cancer. She loved her life. She never showed us any fear. The pain medication helped, but it wasn't always enough. I remember that part too well.

Fata is not the only evil doctor to practice medicine in the US. A doctor in Florida was found guilty of fraud after performing laser surgery on the skin of patients after false diagnosis of cancer. From 1996–2004, Dr. Michael A. Rosin had a perfect record of identifying cancer in every slide he was handed. In two cases, the slides did not even contain human tissue: Suspicious employees handed him a slide with chewing gum. His diagnosis? Cancer. Another test slide was of a slice of Styrofoam. He found more cancer. When over 4,000 slides were seized from his offices, over half were determined by independent pathologists as not being identifiable as human tissue because they were so poorly prepared. His unnecessary treatments led to fear, suffering and permanent scars in his patients.

He lived a lavish life in an $850,000 3500-square-foot home. He pleaded not guilty, only to then say he was "Very, very sorry" at his sentencing trial. He is serving a mere 22 years in prison.

Neither of these so-called doctors were ever charged with assault, attempted murder, or any crime related to harm inflicted on the bodies of their patients.

The FBI estimates that up to 10% of all Medicare billing is fraudulent. In 2011, that amounted to up to $57 billion. Looking at the top 2012 billers in Medicare, three of the top 10 are under close scrutiny and one has drawn an indictment. Fata had ranked #7 among the top billers.

Another example is an ophthalmologist who prefers to use the more expensive of two clinically equivalent drugs for age-related macular degeneration (AMD) in spite of six clinical trials that show that the much less expensive alternative is equally effective. AMD is the leading cause of vision loss in older Americans. Without treatment, AMD patients lose their ability to read, recognize people, drive, and perform many of the important but mundane tasks in life that most of us take for granted.

A single injection of Lucentis costs $2,000; the equally effective drug, Avastin, which has only minor molecular differences to Lucentis, costs $50–$60 per injection. Either treatment is required to prevent vision loss in patients diagnosed with AMD, and the results of both drugs are equally impressive. A number of other conditions that can lead to blood vessel growths that threaten sight and eye health can also be treated just as effectively with Avastin, including diabetes. Avastin works by inhibiting vascular endothelial growth factor A (VEGF-A), and is used routinely in metastatic colon cancer and numerous other cancers (including glioblastoma multiforme of the brain, lung cancer, ovarian cancer, and renal cancer). It is not indicated for use in breast cancer.

The choice to continue to use the more expensive option in eye care enrages doctors like Dr. J. Gregory Rosenthal, Director of the Retinal Service of Vision Associates in Toledo, Ohio and Chief of Ophthalmology at The Toledo Hospital and Toledo Children's Hospital. Dr. Rosenthal is a remarkable person — he donates time each year in the Dominican Republic providing much-needed retinal care to local communities, and training and working with his colleague Dr. Sebastian Guzman. These efforts are underwritten by the not-for-profit Jairus Foundation (www.jairusfoundation.org/).

Dr. Rosenthal also founded Physicians for Clinical Responsibility, or PCR (http://clinicalresponsibility.org/). He has testified to the Senate Select Committee on aging over egregious behaviors of retinal specialists who, according to his colleagues, have "sold out" and appear to have become "shills" of "Big Pharma." He reports that the differences between the two drugs, which are manufactured by the same company, are merely cosmetic.

Via PCR, Dr. Rosenthal has a finger on the pulse of the retina community, and he says that the good news is that the majority of the 20,000 ophthalmologists in the US are doing the right thing — using Avastin — while 800–900 of them use Lucentis. This is where the story gets interesting. He says that Genentech pays practices so-called "rebates" of $160,000 *each* to these 800–900 ophthalmologists to incentivize them to use Lucentis or the similarly priced Eylea. Dr. Rosenthal likens this to racketeering, and he points out that if this were truly a rebate, the money would go back to the payor — often Medicare — not the practice. In a careful study published in 2011 in the *New England Journal of Medicine*, Lucentis and Avastin were found to have no significant clinical differences in safety or effectiveness in the treatment of age-related macular degeneration (CATT Research Group, 2011), and while a meta-analysis of seven studies found Lucentis to be superior to Avastin at the end of year 1 in terms of both safety and efficacy, the differences in efficacy disappeared at year 2, and the two drugs were found to be clinically identical and just as effective (with fewer side effects) when used monthly, instead of "as-needed" (Wang *et al.*, 2015).

One of the biggest concerns for PCR, and eye doctors in general, is that the high cost of Lucentis would eat US$2 billion of the US$5 billion allocated within Medicare annually for eye medicine. They are similarly concerned over the much higher copays for (usually) mature (older and elderly) patients, and of the erosive effect of conflicts of interest on the objectivity of the bulk of science presented at national meetings.

Dr. Rosenthal is far from anti-capitalist. In fact, he celebrates that his volunteering in the Dominican Republic is both opening markets and meeting needs. He points to the position and the book by CK Prahalad, *The Fortune at the Bottom of the Pyramid*, as a good model for how developed countries should view venturing into needy areas. By increasing volume, the argument goes, drug companies and medical practices can reduce the margin and still come out way ahead. The key, says Dr. Rosenthal, is to actually be there to help the locals, not to be there to do things for them. That sounded very familiar to me — I had come to the same conclusion re: the West's potential responses to the Ebola crisis just months before our chat.

Physicians for Clinical Responsibility also reports a number of other concerns, including what they label a "scam" for unnecessary treatments for glaucoma — especially in elderly patients who show no sign of the disease.

There are incentives for people to come forward and report clear violations of medical ethics, but they are few and far between. The Centers for Medicare & Medicaid Services (CMS) currently incentivizes whistleblowers with a $1,000 reward. They have recovered less than $5 million since 1998, with a total of around $20,000 to whistleblowers. In 2013, CMS proposed offering up to 15% of monies recovered from successfully prosecuted Medicare fraud cases (up to a maximum of $9.9 million per case). This proposal has not yet led to legislation, and the bulk of the monies recovered from whistleblower activities are gained via civil suits for damages to patients.

Medicine is big money. The opportunity for fraud is rampant. If people cannot trust their doctors, they will not seek proper care. The purpose of this book is to help the American people sort through the complexities of particular kinds of care and the real challenges facing clinical researchers as they seek new cures and treatments. The doctors I have met and worked with over the last 16 years of my life are, to a person, deeply concerned about the well-being of their patients. I have seen some shady characters in my travels, and have personally come to know via the grapevine of alleged distasteful acts by some doctors designed to maximize their profit with minimal effort. I have overtly refused to work with such doctors. As far as I know, I have never worked with any doctors as evil and depraved as Fata and Rosin. Others have won my heart, and my admiration, for their passion, their long hours, for their work in reducing human pain and suffering, and for the many lives they try to save. To me, the best doctors are those who throw all they have into their clinical practice, and try very hard to push for advances in clinical practice.

Many of the researching physicians I have worked with are under immense pressure to perform as much clinical service as possible; not for their own bottom line but, instead, to meet the demands of their institutions. They find it difficult to find the time necessary to establish and maintain research programs. Some have been hired to run research programs only to be told within a year that the clinical expectations have been updated. One doctor quit when she was told this, and she felt cheated. She had relocated, set up her labs, hired her research staff, and was told point blank that the only effort that would matter was her clinical practice. She had tears in her eyes when she told me of her planned departure. She said her decision was, in part, due to the pain associated with telling her patients that they would not make it. I was part of her research enterprise, and we had a close professional relationship; she knew about my mom, and my own passion for getting to the bottom of how to improve research practices in cancer. This is the type of corrosive effect that bad actors in medicine can have; the profit motive is power-ful, but it does little to foster true passion toward curing patients.

The US NIH budget has stagnated; when adjusted for the value of the dollar, levels of funding in between 2010 and 2014 are roughly the same as funding levels in 2003. Due to inflation, the cost of doing bio-medical research has increased each year. Sequestration has strangled research institutions and is hampering their ability to capitalize on the hard-won knowledge of the past 30 years of molecular medicine. There is waste, for sure. We could never afford the parasitic cost of immense wages, charlatans, thieves and cheats on the biomedical research sys-tem. With the effective relative cuts in the NIH budget (adjusting for inflation), these debits on the account of the public trust do much more harm than can measured directly. Hopefully this book will help sort out the complexities of biomedical research and show the people behind the successes. If, in this book, the public learns something about both the positive and negative influences that exist in biomedicine and biomed-ical research, so much the better. I have seen some of both in my time; they can be extremely charismatic and snuff the very life out of any real hope for improvements in medicine. Institutions should purge them-selves of these abusive people — tenured or not — and replace them with honest, hard-working individuals who are about translation in terms of lives, not dollars. Others can inspire their mentees and peers to do great things, and support them in their career paths even if their own direction threatens to overturn or replace the *status quo*. Were it that higher ideals could lead the way over profit each and every time. That would lead to much benefit, and would be pretty wonderful.

I hope to inspire the public to continue to invest in biomedical research so future generations can experience less pain and suffering due to an abundance of effective treatments and cures, and challenge Pharma to re-think their cost and pricing models not just worldwide, but in the US as well.

References

CATT Research Group. (2011) Ranibizumab and revacizumab for neovascular age-related macular degeneration. *New England Journal of Medicine* **64:** 1897–1908.

Wang WJ, *et al.* (2015) Bevacizumab versus ranibizumab for neovascular age-related macular degeneration: a meta-analysis. *Int J Ophthalmol* **8(1):** 138–47. [doi: 10.3980/j.issn.2222-3959.2015.01.26]

Chapter 2

Outrageous Acts of Pseudoscience

The esteemed doctor-scientist in his (or her) white coat walks, no, strides confidently across a campus, with the stereotypical clipboard in their hand, ready to tackle the next most important meeting, to the sound of lively, upbeat music reassuring the viewer of the commercial that the deadly side effects being spoken of are not the only dimension of information about this new drug, which may or may not help them with their ailment.

This is the typical direct-to-consumer marketing commercial in the US by which drug companies lend credence to their presentation of their wares to the consumer. After all, the sun is shining, the doctor is smiling, why worry about side effects?

The American public spends over $250 billion on medicine per year. And drug companies, like anyone else, are entitled to communicate good news about their treatments. They must, by law, also provide key information on the potential negative effects. They are restricted from making unwarranted claims about their drugs' curative properties. They cannot, for, example, make the claim that their treatment for headaches also protects against heart disease — unless the FDA has provided a clear green light for labeling their drug for that purpose. The television commercials naturally portray their products in the best possible light. However, hearing the terrible side effects — risk of suicide, depression, etc. — during the "best possible light" portrayal is often surreal and can, at times, seem rather disingenuous.

Most Americans do not know that they are nearly alone in the world as being citizens of one of two countries where the governments permit direct-to-consumer advertising by pharmaceutical companies. The other country is New Zealand. The US Food and Drug Administration issued a "Draft Guidance" on DTC advertising, which was last updated in 2009. Each page of the Draft Guidance is labeled "Contains Nonbinding Recommendations" and "Draft — Not for Implementation." In the Draft Guidance, the FDA gives itself 45 days to review any televised advertising, after which time advertisers may still be subject to penalty, even if the FDA did not act within the 45-day period. It is seen by many people, and consumer advocacy groups, as toothless. These groups also see DTC as creating demand, instead of helping patients deal with the risk factors and stressors, especially for medicines such as a sleep aids and antidepressants.

The pharmaceutical industry has argued repeatedly that the benefits of DTC advertising include providing an opportunity to educate the public. An objective study of televised prescription drug ad samples over a four-week period captured 24 advertisements (Frosch *et al.*, 2007). The analysis shed damaging light on these claims. After scoring the televised ads using a standardized set of criteria, the authors found:

> *Most ads (82%) made some factual claims and made rational arguments (86%) for product use, but few described condition causes (26%), risk factors (26%), or prevalence (25%). Emotional appeals were almost universal (95%). No ads mentioned lifestyle change as an alternative to products, though some (19%) portrayed it as an adjunct to medication. Some ads (18%) portrayed lifestyle changes as insufficient for controlling a condition. The ads often framed medication use in terms of losing (58%) and regaining control (85%) over some aspect of life and as engendering social approval (78%). Products were frequently (58%) portrayed as a medical breakthrough.*

They went on to conclude:

> *Despite claims that ads serve an educational purpose, they provide limited information about the causes of a disease or who may be at risk;*

they show characters that have lost control over their social, emotional, or physical lives without the medication; and they minimize the value of health promotion through lifestyle changes. The ads have limited educational value and may oversell the benefits of drugs in ways that might conflict with promoting population health.

A more recent study, Faerber and Kreling (2014), found similar egregious facts about televised prescription drug ads:

Of the most emphasized claims in prescription (n = 84) and nonprescription (n = 84) drug advertisements, 33% were objectively true, 57% were potentially misleading and 10% were false. In prescription drug ads, there were more objectively true claims (43%) and fewer false claims (2%) than in nonprescription drug ads (23% objectively true, 7% false). There were similar numbers of potentially misleading claims in prescription (55%) and nonprescription (61%) drug ads.

The author of this study concluded:

Potentially misleading claims are prevalent throughout consumer-targeted prescription and nonprescription drug advertising on television. These results are in conflict with proponents who argue the social value of drug advertising is found in informing consumers about drugs.

A similar Harvard study, published in 2004, concluded:

Most gave consumers somewhat more time to absorb facts about benefits than those about risks, which could have implications for the "fair balance" requirement. Complete references to additional product information were given only in text, casting doubt on whether these ads are making "adequate provision" for dissemination of detailed product information. Overall, our results call into question the potential of these ads to educate consumers.

One example of misleading claims appeared in advertisements of Lunesta, a sleep aid manufactured and sold by Glaxo. The televised ads claimed that Lunesta could provide a full night's sleep, and the ad defines a full night's sleep as eight hours. In fact, the sleep study used to demonstrate efficacy of Lunesta showed on average only six hours of sleep per night among participants.

The American public, therefore, is being willfully misled by drug companies as they attempt to convince them to use pills to solve many of life's problems. Pharma spends billions each year on DTC ($36.1 billion in 2004, accounting for over 13% of all televised ad sales; Kornfield *et al.*, 2013). Upon reflection on these studies, one cannot help but think of a barker selling snake oil at a carnival. The ads are outrageous and flaunt the spirit and the letter of the law, and they use the social currency of the doctor, or scientist, in a white coat to sell pills to the public with dubious and exaggerated claims of efficacy.

Outrageous Acts of Medical Research Practices

Outrageous acts of breaches of ethics in medical practice are easy to recognize. Harder to pick out are those instances in which breaches of ethics have occurred during a research study. From falsifying data to cherry picking results, violations of ethical practice of research are, unfortunately, fairly commonplace in the US and elsewhere. The pressure to perform (publish or perish, secure grants) can be immense both in academia and in the corporate world, and some fall into temptation with astounding apparent ease in spite of the potential consequences. Penalties for defrauding the US National Institutes of Health via fraudulent research can range from retraction of the corresponding published research and a three-year ban on conducting NIH-funded research to hefty fines and prison sentences. In one infamous case, a researcher, Dr. Eric Poehlman, defrauded the NIH for over $3 million dollars. He pled guilty to felony crime, and was sentenced to prison for one year for falsifying data on the effects of menopause on obesity and was given a lifetime ban on conducting NIH-funded research. The prison sentence was a first for the US, and was supposed to provide deterrent against fraudulent research and to encourage researchers to act in an ethical manner.

In spite of the message these cases should send to the research community on the importance of ethics (as if an external threat should be needed!), still, somewhere in the US, or abroad, a scientist is, at this very time, likely working in secret, tweaking some data to reduce the error bars, using Photoshop to accentuate the color-stained differences on an image of a sample from a microscope slide, and perhaps cloning part of the image to better get their point across. Somewhere, someone is analyzing their data with multiple statistical methods and choosing the results that seem most compelling, with no intention of reporting their methods exploration, and with no paradigm of objective measures for favoring one result over the other. This is called "results shopping." In another place, someone is padding a colleague's resume by adding their name as author to a paper for publication of the results of a study to which they contributed little or nothing. Somewhere else, someone is not reporting the negative results of a study that would impede their sponsor's attempts to bring a drug to market because they had accepted terms of a research contract that gave the company the go/no go veto power over publication. Just down the road, another researcher is taking an idea from a paper or grant proposal from a competitor/colleague to which they have just given a bad review, and is planning a study inspired by those results with no intention of crediting the idea or its originator.

And nearby, a junior faculty member is learning that he has been lied to: He's being told that although he used his valuable time to procure funding on a major, multi-million dollar, multi-institutional grant, which was submitted in a senior faculty member's name, the credit for that success will not be given to him as originally promised. Although he did his job exceedingly well — he succeeded in securing four to five years' worth of funding — he is now being told that the plan to make him the principal investigator was canceled because, as young as he appears, he managed to do something else for his own career at the same time (let's say, hypothetically of course, that he managed to create an open-access peer-reviewed research journal for studies in cancer informatics, and is serving as the Founding Editor-in-Chief). And the senior faculty member is professing anger at this success because, he claims, even he does not have a journal of his own, and he's a fully tenured professor. Of course, there are no witnesses to this revelation, and the up-and-coming young scientist is realizing that his career is all but over; he has no one to go to bat for him for tenure, in spite of having done everything right. He is told he did too much, and that he just does not understand how "the system" works.

Later, the senior faculty member attempts to sabotage the objective peer-review system put into place by the junior faculty member, changing it to one in which the authors manage their own peer review with colleagues and submit their paper along with the reviews to lessen the burden of the publisher. His ploy does not work, as the junior faculty member leads a revolt and threatens to resign with nearly half of the editorial board if the publisher waters down the rigorous peer-review system. The publisher decides to keep the correct type of review system, and goes on to see the journal listed in Pubmed due in large part to the rigorous peer-review system that the junior faculty member had in place. This example is, of course, purely hypothetical.

Examples of this type of abuse are, unfortunately, not rare in academia. News of their occurrence can leave the most optimistic among us (including me) rattled, and perhaps a little more jaded about the scientific enterprise than we ever wanted to become. To me, they have served as opportunities to teach students (and on occasion, colleagues) about the unethical and criminal nature of such acts. Discussions of ethical considerations during a study almost never occur openly in academic settings during active research studies; one may be afraid to offend a colleague by seeming to draw their integrity into question. These examples are, fortunately, taught in courses like the popular course I enjoyed teaching on Research Study Design, with a healthy ethics component, at the University of Pittsburgh in the mid-2000s.

Bias

Sources of bias in research can either be intentional (fraud) or unintentional. Examples of unintentional bias would be the accidental allocation of all smokers to a treatment group, and all (or most) non-smokers to a control group. This type of bias can be eliminated by collecting patient demographic and clinical data, and using matching algorithms to assign close pairs of patients to either the control or treatment groups.

Intentional sources of bias can include controlling access to data from trials, charging enrollment fees for inclusion to treatment groups, offering financial incentives to patients to participate in trials (which does not represent real-life use of a treatment or drug), selective reporting of results, including failing to register trials and not reporting evidence that does not support the efficacy of a drug or that indicates adverse events, exclusion of subgroups after an analysis fails to indicate efficacy and safety followed by re-analysis of the data and, of course, willful non-randomization of patients already likely to have better outcomes or tolerate a drug better to a treatment arm. Another type of bias is self-deception — I have seen instances in which a researcher values their data so much that they have asked six or more statisticians to independently analyze the data, and then cherry-pick the "best-looking" result. I was once one of those data analysts — and when it came to my attention, I told the investigator that they had an obligation to report the full set of analysis results from all analysts. My then-supervisor "reassigned" the PI's data to yet another analyst, who of course got the same treatment. That PI's research still has yet to have made an impact on the clinical care of patients, due in large part to self-deception.

Researchers of course have a responsibility to society to not engage in such activities so as to bias the results. They also have a responsibility to their employers to avoid such practices, and to themselves, for if they are even suspected of participating in such unlawful behavior, their careers could be damaged permanently — even if they are innocent.

I understand that people are people. But scientists, especially medical researchers, represent themselves as — and we hold them up as — standard bearers in society, armed with special knowledge, able to defend the public from the evils scourges of suffering and death due to disease. They are to do-gooders, and deserve the additional pay and the social current of respect and authority that comes with working on behalf of our health. So when one or more of them cheats the system, it casts a grey pall, as thick as smoke from a coal stack, over the entire enterprise. And unless one aspires to play the game at all costs, they are unlikely to stay in the game, and the best people can be lost from academia.

Pharmaceutical companies — and other companies that market treatments of all kinds — have an obligation to place the safety of patients above profits. Cheating in medical research demonstrates a depravity and callousness for individuals who might be harmed by the adverse effects. It also shows a disturbing lack of concern for the poor outcomes associated with low effectiveness — and the patient's loss of opportunity to seek more effective treatments.

Down the road, cheating in medical science can ultimately cost investors, government agencies, and tax payers money and, in the worst-case scenario, lead directly at best to inefficient research, lost time on the part of participants (patients and scientists), lost talent, lost opportunity for real discovery and understanding, destroyed careers (guilt by association), stagnation in medicine, and patient deaths. And some people are very, very good at cheating.

References

Faerber AE and Kreling. (2014) Content analysis of false and misleading claims in television advertising for prescription and nonprescription drugs. *J Gen Intern Med* **29(1):** 110–18. [doi: 10.1007/s11606-013-2604-0]

Frosch DL, *et al.* (2007) Creating demand for prescription drugs: a content analysis of television direct-to-consumer advertising. *Ann Fam Med* **5(1):** 6–13.

Kaphingst KA, DeJong W, Rudd RE, Daltroy LH. (2004) A content analysis of direct-to-consumer television prescription drug advertisements. *J Health Commun* **9(6):** 515–28.

Kornfield R, *et al.* (2013) Promotion of Prescription Drugs to Consumers and Providers, 2001–2010. *PLoS ONE* **8(3):** e55504. [doi:10.1371/journal.pone.0055504]

3 Wait… Grapefruit is Bad for You?

If you are currently taking medicine for high blood pressure, and if you ask your doctor if you should eat grapefruit, chances are, they will tell you either no, you should not eat it due to interactions with your medicine, or that you should restrict consumption to one or two a week. The doctor is concerned that the grapefruit may exaggerate the effects of, or act synergistically, with the blood pressure medicine, and that you might pass out due to low blood pressure.

Then you ask them: "Well, should I take grapefruit instead of this medicine?"

Your doctor may not have an answer to this question. The best doctors will look into the question of, and may conclude that it's easier to dose-control the blood pressure treatment. They will find studies that show interactions between red grapefruit juice and blood pressure medicines. Grapefruit juice is described as prolonging the duration of the drugs in the blood stream by inhibiting an enzyme called CYP34A. CYP34A is an enzyme found in the tissues of the small intestine (and elsewhere, presumably). This enzyme metabolizes (breaks down) the hypertensive drugs, so the increased bioavailability and increased survival in the blood stream can cause blood pressure medication doses to interact with each other. Those same studies concluded that the best route was to remove grapefruit juice from the diet because in patients taking anti-hypertensives, grapefruit may cause hypotension (low blood pressure).

It may seem odd that the conclusion is not: "In people who eat grapefruit, the anti-hypertensives may cause hypotension."

It is, after all, the build-up of the drug that causes hypotension. Eating grapefruit has been shown to have health benefits such as reducing cholesterol in patients with high blood pressure and coronary atherosclerosis (Gorinstein *et al.*, 2006), and weight loss (de la Garza *et al.*, 2015; Fujioka *et al.*, 2006; Silver *et al.*, 2011).

However, the effects of grapefruit juice are also known to lead to toxicities in other drugs not related to hypertension, and grapefruit juice has been shown to affect the bioavailability of other drugs as well, including statins, which are designed to reduced cholesterol levels. It can interfere with drugs that treat arrhythmia in the heart.

Hypertension is a symptom often caused by atherosclerosis (hardening of the arteries) and thrombosis (clogging of the arteries). When considering the heart, atherosclerosis is called coronary artery disease. Narrowing or clogging to the blood vessels can lead to increased blood pressure. Anti-hypertensive drugs are a multi-billion dollar business. Is this why our doctors tell us to avoid grapefruit and olive oil if we are on blood pressure medication?

Given the fact that there seems to be a choice between either drugs or grapefruit, there are numerous reasons why doctors may prefer drugs over grapefruit. The dosages are more easily controlled, for example, and a patient might see grapefruit as part of their diet, and not part of a medical treatment. Nevertheless, I wondered if any clinical trials had been conducted that demonstrated a reduction in blood pressure due to grapefruit consumption.

That's when I learned about the work of a research team led by Dr. Cynthia Thompson. She was a mentor to her colleague, Dr. Caitlyn Dow. This duo, and the rest of their team, used a classical study design called a randomized clinical trial to determine whether eating grapefruit could be shown to effect obesity. Obesity is a plague that affects Americans and others worldwide that brings with it a host of other diseases and conditions that require medical intervention.

I was curious if the studies of grapefruit by Dr. Dow and colleagues led to a reduction blood pressure. The story of their study, it turns out, has immensely important insights for all of clinical research.

When considering a new drug, therapy, or diagnostic for medical use, the US FDA has a specific study design that they prefer. "Prefer" is actually too weak of a word: They require its use, considering it the "Gold Standard." The requirement of the use of randomized clinical trials is applied dogmatically in all areas of biomedicine. In fact, promising results from hundreds of clinical trials of promising treatments, therapies and diagnostics have been rejected by the FDA because the scientists conducting the study had to waver from the specific study design. The type of study that the FDA rather adamantly requires is called a Randomized Clinical Trial (RCT). In the case of drugs, they require a placebo controlled RCT (PC-RCT). In an RCT, the drug of interest is administered to a group of patients, while another group of patients receives a placebo (e.g., a sugar pill). In a double-blinded study design, neither the participants, nor the doctors, know whether a patient is being given the treatment or the placebo.

This type of study is considered superior to observational studies, in which experimentation using various options is conducted, and the effectiveness gauged based on direct observation of the patient's responses over time. The goal of medical research is to identify treatments and procedures that are effective on the relevant clinical populations and, therefore, comparisons of outcomes between or among groups treated differently is conducted in a more systematic manner. There are some instances in which many believe that repeated clinical course reversals under treatment may have to be sufficient due to the unethical lack of care for a randomized control group (for example, antibody-based Ebola treatments). Some interventions are obviously necessary and would not require prospective testing; the use of parachutes, for example, is based exclusively on observational data (see Smith and Pell, 2003, for a more thorough treatment of the lack of evidence that parachutes are safe and efficacious in preventing deaths due to risks of death associated with "gravitational challenge").

At the time of Dr. Dow's research, the current standard of care for obese patients was to promote weight loss via diet, physical activity and behavioral changes (eating habits). In their study, they randomly assigned one-half of their patients to a simple intervention: They asked the participants to eat half of a peeled Rio Red grapefruit before each meal, for six weeks. The control group was not told to eat grapefruit. Both groups had undergone a three-week "washout" diet (low in fruits and vegetables). At the end of six weeks, a variety of measurements were taken, such as weight, waist size, and blood pressure. Compared to the measurements before the addition of grapefruit to their diet, the control group had lost a significant amount of weight and saw a reduction in waist size. Importantly, they also experienced a reduction cholesterol, and in systolic blood pressure. Compared to their earlier versions of themselves, these patients seemed on the road to better overall health. The control group did not show a reduction in weight, or other measurements, compared to their former, baseline selves.

Oddly, when the two groups were compared after six weeks, as is the norm in clinical trial studies, the differences in weight, in cholesterol, and in systolic blood pressure disappeared. This paradox shows a weakness in the use of the so-called gold standard of Randomized Clinical Trials: The search for significant differences between groups can mask differences that are quite apparent within groups before and after treatment. So which design is superior, and which design is correct?

Inclusion of grapefruit in the diet had been previously shown to lead to a reduction in weight, so the finding by Dow *et al.* of weight loss within the treatment group seems to confirm that the baseline to treatment comparison was capable of finding a real, known effect of eating grapefruit. This would seem to suggest that the other results (reduction in waistline, total cholesterol, and systolic blood pressure) that can be expected to co-occur with weight loss are also real effects.

I asked Drs. Dow and Thompson to chat with me about their study.

I asked them if they had encountered any hurdles in the interpretation of the results; Caitlyn (Dow) mentioned that some reviewers of the study had pointed out that the publication of the results showing that grapefruit can reduce blood pressure and were concerned that some people might interpret the results to mean that grapefruit should replace blood pressure medication, and that grapefruit is contraindicated for people on certain blood pressure medications. "Well," I thought, "isn't that the reason why the study is so interesting?"

Right off the bat, Dr. Dow and Thompson said they had some notions that they wanted to be sure to share. First, they wanted to point out that the results of their study should not be taken to mean that grapefruit should replace statins. Statins are used to treat cholesterol, and grapefruit can interfere with the effectiveness of statins. However, they noted that the potential health benefits of grapefruit should be considered for people on diuretic-type blood pressure medications. People taking beta-blocker type blood pressure medicines, however, should avoid eating grapefruit due the known effects of grapefruit on their metabolism. So it seems that our doctors should be specific about their recommendations on eating grapefruit; people who are on drugs to reduce their cholesterol and people taking beta-blocker type blood pressure medicines should avoid it. The additional benefits of grapefruit are, by contrast, available to people not taking cholesterol drugs and to people taking diuretic-type blood pressure medicines.

Grapefruit is recognized by the American Heart Association as a healthy option for heart-healthy diets. It is a source of vitamins (A and C) and a good source of dietary fiber. It is naturally fat- and cholesterol-free, and low in calories. The first drug interaction with grapefruit was discovered in a study of the effects of alcohol — grapefruit masked an interaction between ethanol and felodipine, a calcium-channel blocker (Bailey *et al.*, 1989). Grapefruit is now known to interact with beta-blockers, statins and with at least 50 drugs, including Fexofenadine (Allegra), a popular antihistamine, felodipine (Plendil) and atorvastatin (Lipitor).

In spite of these interactions, the question remains: Is grapefruit itself effective at controlling blood pressure? The Dow *et al.* study suggests that yes, it can reduce blood pressure. This is a major finding as the drugs used to control blood pressure and cholesterol can have strong side effects for some patients. I asked Drs. Dow and Thompson if they could do the study over again, and if funds were not an issue, would they have done anything differently? Dr. Dow said that because human populations are heterogeneous, there was a lot of variation between the two groups during the six weeks. She pointed out that the grapefruit eating group happened to show a reduction in the number of vegetables in their diet, and that the control group somehow ended up with an increase in the amount of fruit in their diet (all compared to baseline). "If we had better control of the diet, we could have reduced the variability within and between groups for these factors, and perhaps the intervention vs. control group would have also been made apparent."

Both Drs. Thompson and Dow emphasized that proper control groups are useful and necessary. Dr. Dow in particular advocated for more use of cross-over randomized design, in which patients are first on one arm of a study (e.g., grapefruit) and then re-assigned to the placebo group in search for a reversal or discontinuation of the positive effects of grapefruit. These designs, also known as reversal designs, have numerous advantages over single baseline designs. For example, the causal relation of a significant main effect (grapefruit) can be established; the effect size can be better quantified, and they can also establish whether a particular treatment requires a maintenance schedule for continuing effectiveness. According to Dr. Dow, such studies, because they are primarily baseline to outcome comparisons, are also effective at removing the effects of heterogeneity in the population, including genetic diversity, which can make results difficult to interpret.

Is there more to learn about the health effects of grapefruit on its own merit? Dr. Thompson added that funding for studies is scarce, and that, in her opinion, the number one problem with biomedical research is that all studies are expected to be conducted over five years. "If we had more time, perhaps we could have performed more in-depth follow-up on the patients, to find out, for example, which patients needed to go on statins, and which patients could go without." It is remarkable to consider that perhaps one day we could know which patients would benefit from eating grapefruit and not have to take statins.

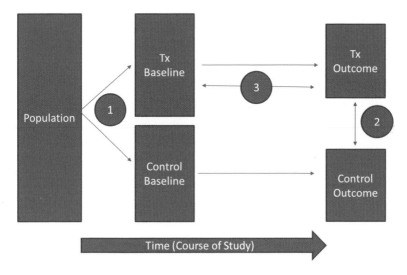

Fig. 3.1 Schematic of typical clinical study design elements, and the design used in the grapefruit study. After random allocation to Treatment (Tx) or Control groups, most frequent (and FDA "gold standard" comparisons use Treament (Tx) vs. Control comparisons (2). Fewer studies employ the within Treatment group comparison of the outcome after treatment to before (Tx Baseline), even though the statistical power of analysis at (3) is inherently higher than that at (2) due to isolation of variation from the main effect of treatment from variation resulting from random allocation of study participants at (1). Variation specific to Treatment or Control over time can occur under either analysis (2) or (3), but it can only be seen if analysis at (3) is conducted.

There are additional steps to the design of studies that can be used to improve those of Dow *et al.* (2012). These can be considered using Fig. 3.1. Fortunately, Dow *et al.* were wise enough to collect baseline data, allowing outcomes vs. baseline analysis. Baseline data are most often usually collected as auxiliary data to make sure that the two treatment arms in a clinical trial are about the same at the start of the trial.

Origins of the Mistaken Focus on Groupwise Comparisons Alone

Confusion over the handling of covariates and the analysis of adjusted or non-adjusted treatment effects has been a long-term, persistent issue in clinical research (Assmann *et al.*, 2000; Austin *et al.*, 2010; Rosenberger and Sverdlov, 2008; Egbewale *et al.*, 2014). Egbewale *et al.* (2014)

used extensive clinical trial simulations and reported that ANOVA and "Change Score Analysis" (CSA) were biased in the presence of baseline covariate differences, and that ANCOVA using baseline measurements as a covariate in a linear comparison of post-treatment measurements was unbiased.

For many, CSA is the most intuitive type of analysis, and apparently the easiest to interpret. Change scores, also known as "Difference Scores," are simply the difference in the dependent variable of interest at two time points, so

$$CHANGE = DS = \Delta_{X,Y} = Y_1 - Y_0,$$

where Y_0 is the baseline measurement and Y_1 is the outcome measurement after treatment or intervention.

The use of this type of analysis has, historically, been eschewed due to early works of Cronbach and Furby (1970) and Lord and Novick (1968). These papers focused on the worst-case scenario in which difference scores were unreliable. The history of the unfortunate overdrawn conclusions from these papers is reviewed thoroughly by Bonate (2000). After having a massively stagnating influence on the field of statistics, these early views have become, in Bonate's words, "dogma"; the fallacy has been perpetuated and oft-repeated (Linn and Slinde, 1977; Gupta, Srivastava & Sharma, 1988).

It seems that Cronbach and Furby (1970) and Lord and Novick (1968) fumbled in considering only what we see as a condition applicable only to the control case. Lord (1956), Cronbach and Furby (1970) and Lord and Novick (1968) concluded that when the reliability of a pretest and posttest is the same, their difference is equal to their reliability. This is true only in theory: When measurement errors are zero, and the variables of interest show no change over time (no within-individual differences). This is clearly not realistic. Rogosa (1988) demonstrated that the use of difference scores (in his application, 'gain scores') can provide unbiased estimator of "true change."

Frison and Pocock (1992) also referenced the futility of CHANGE due to correlation between outcome and baseline, which is a fumble when either the empirical loss of correlation relative to baseline is the statistic of interest (change of slope) or the shift in the magnitude of the intercept remains, as the correlation can be increased or decreased in response to the treatment with no change in correlation. For these early treatments, the existence of correlation is seen as a loss of information; whether they recognized the attendant increase in the power of the test due to paired sample analyses is unclear. For Frison and Pocock (1992), the inferiority of CHANGE was obvious: For repeated measures, the variance of ANCOVA was lowest, and the larger the number of repeated measures, the greater the superiority of ANCOVA. Clinical trials often proceed with multiple measurements over time. It seems to me that the statistic of interest with respect to CHANGE for multiple measures would be, in many instances, integrated (cumulative) change over time (area under the curve); in others instances, the efficacy of the treatment might wear off over time, and thus the single endpoint relative to baseline would be relative. Nevertheless, CHANGE does not measure the mere consistency of the test; it measures any and all variation over time between measurements and baseline.

The empirically unlikely, rare "expected" case of no difference between time points given the same assay applied to the same people at different time points has seriously hindered progress and limited clinical research. The mistake of early thinkers was to generalize from this unlikely "expected" the theoretical instance to all cases. They failed to note that differences before and after treatment are due to something other than the instrument of measure, the within-arm covariance of which they assumed was perfect (hence no reliability). Those factors, such as an intervention or treatment, are the "main effect" — the entire point of measuring differences. They failed to consider that when covariance was low, the power within arm was higher, and they attributed all of the significance found in comparison to baseline to measured covariate, or unknown, possible confounders. The purpose of the control arm is to represent a similar group within to control for such confounders. The number of false negative findings in clinical trials due to this mistake is unknown.

The influence of the conclusion that groupwise comparisons alone are relevant, specifically that the covariance of the measurement is the same as any measured difference of the "same" people at different time points, confuses the theoretical assumptions of a test under the null condition with that of the alternative hypothesis. If the treatment is effective, the group is the same people, yes, but if the treatment is effective, they are not the same due to treatment, so the measurement error of the device cannot be zero. The effect size will be measured with variance due to random error. And, more importantly, the effect size itself will contribute to differences in measurement with the same device between time points. The conclusion that has led the community to conclude that groupwise difference alone are valid, and that within-arm comparisons are invalid, is an absurd fallacy.

In plain terms, early on in determining rigorous clinical trials, some statisticians showed that if you measure a group of patients at time point 0, and then again at time point 1, with the same instrument, they would be highly correlated. No problem. But if you had an infinite number of patients, there would be no difference in the two measures and, the argument went, the instrument applied in that setting would unreliable because it would contain no information. As absurd as that logic seems, this argument has been the basis of the reason for the preference of using outcomes comparison (across treatment and control group). The position forms the basis of the FDA's "gold standard" position on clinical trials.

A succinct way of saying part of this is that before and after measures with the same instrument may have zero theoretical error (complete reliability in any application), whether the null hypothesis is true or not. It now seems obvious that the reliability can be the same before and after intervention, but the entire outcome of drug treatment, or surgical procedure, or the performance of the student in the classroom can increase (or decrease) as a direct result of the intervention. The existence of a control arm that shows no change from baseline merits interest in the significant change in the treatment arm.

The early theoretical treatments missed two points. First, within each arm, the observations at t_0 and t_1 are *paired* (they are same patients). The paired t-test, with variance

$$\text{Total Var} = \text{Var}(A) + \text{Var}(B) - 2\text{Covar}(A,B) \tag{1}$$

is more powerful than the independent sample t-test, with total variance

$$\text{Total Var} = \text{Var}(A) + \text{Var}(B). \tag{2}$$

Equation (1) applies to the within-arm (outcome vs. baseline) analyses. Equation (2) applies to the between-arm analysis (treatment vs. control). The subtraction of the term $2\text{Covar}(A,B)$ in Equation (1) necessarily increases the power of the statistical analysis in the analysis of the data; this point seems to have escaped most of the community involved in the analysis of data from randomized clinical trials.

From this, we can see that this small change in focus might reveal the efficacy of more drugs, while focus on the groupwise comparison may hide their efficacy. The use of within-arm comparisons might also help reveal hard-to-detect harmful side effects for drug safety studies.

Combined Baseline Groups

It should also be noted that before any treatment or sham (placebo) is given, both baseline groups (prior to any treatment) are still one sample from one population, and that combining them into one group to which both the treatment and control outcome groups can be compared later would seem an appropriate way to reduce baseline differences for arm-specific analyses. However, there would be an attendant loss of power as the samples would then be partially unpaired. ANCOVA does this, to a degree, but we are left with a less powerful between-group comparison, or an interaction to choose from, depending on which is significant.

The superiority of the outcomes vs. baseline analysis over the treatment vs. control analysis in clinical studies when covariance is low cannot be understated. Moreover, and equally important, covariate-outcome correlation, ρ, must be relatively large ($-0.7 < \rho < 0.7$) for

ANCOVA to be more powerful. This cut-off value of ρ is derived from extensive simulations by Egbewale *et al.* (2014) that under most conditions (independent of bias), CHANGE score analysis is more powerful than ANOVA. Specifically, ANCOVA was only more powerful than CHANGE score analysis when $-0.7 > \rho > 0.7$.

In any RCT, treatment vs. control risks a false negative discovery (missed significance) due to a low degree of control over unwanted variability that a random control group provides. This problem is exacerbated by low sample sizes (too few patients in a study; in the field, this is called "low N"). These sources of variability reduce the ability of the investigators to detect a significant effect of a treatment when an effect does, in fact, exist (power). Such unwanted sources of variation might even mask the result of the main effect, and mislead researchers to believe that a drug, intervention, therapy or diagnostic is not effective, when in reality it is. They can also have the opposite effect of making it appear that a given treatment is effective, when in reality it is not. Treatment vs. control comparisons, the gold standard of the FDA, are relatively messy comparisons, and they are less powerful.

An excellent review full of excellent counterpoints to the claim that gain scores are unreliable for both randomized clinical trials and for observational studies is provided by Smolmolski (2015).

Confounding Effects Both Types of Comparisons

Intrusions may occur during an outcome vs. baseline study, such as changes over time that are unique to the treatment group or unique to the control group. In fact, this is a common complaint used by the FDA to bring into question the outcome vs. baseline comparison, and is the reason they give for their preference of treatment vs. control outcome group comparisons. However, such intrusions are just as likely in the randomized allocation treatment vs. control group, and the lower power of unpaired between group comparison may make the confounding variable more confusing. Worse, if no baseline data are available in an RCT, these intrusive effects are hidden. At least with baseline vs. outcome studies, the possible sources of unwanted variation can be detected, as in the case of the grapefruit study, and limitations on the knowledge claims can be made explicit, and improvements on the next round of studies can be made.

Implications for Grapefruit and Drug Studies

If incidentally confounding variables add variation that looks like a main effect in the treatment arm, but not the control arm, that variance may be misleading in the groupwise comparison as well. The FDA's gold standard prospective RCT design allows the intrusion of accidental variation unique to either the treatment group (grapefruit) or the control group (no grapefruit) by virtue of the random allocation process, and given that within arm the two groups share a common trait (the treatment, or the lack thereof). However, any derivative influence due to the treatment (eating fewer vegetables, for example) should be attributed to the grapefruit, and are not "incidental covariates." Causal analysis would reveal that these attendant consequences are important as they may then, in turn, modify the main effect. Therefore (importantly) not all variation shared by covariates should be removed (as in ANCOVA) and the overall outcome to baseline result becomes even more important.

The current gold standard hinders findings of efficacy and safety due to relatively lower power than the within-arm outcomes to baseline comparisons. Moreover, universal use of pure randomization guarantees that some studies will be forever confused due to this type of unwanted variation as the clinical population is arbitrarily split into two groups. This confusion can be minimized via matched sample covariate balancing methods during randomization. The FDA typically requires at least two consistently positive results (so-called "pivotal" trials, usually Phase II); however, at sample sizes typically used in Phase I and Phase I/ II trials, many misses can be expected if significant outcomes to baseline difference are ignored. In their guidance, the FDA allows that in some cases a single efficacy trial with promising results may be sufficient (US FDA, 2015).

The use of baseline vs. outcome, within-arm comparison is intrinsically more powerful because the patients in the outcome group are matched perfectly with those in the treatment group — they are, after all, themselves! This is mathematically so, and not a matter of opinion. Better yet, if the patients are assigned as matched pairs to the two groups based on their individual characteristics (like smoking history, clinical history, age, gender, etc.), this dramatically reduces the possibility for intrusion of arbitrary variation via covariates among the groups being compared. The value of these reductions in unwanted variation would be shared by thousands of researchers if they could convince the FDA that baseline vs. outcome is an improvement on the RCT design, and that patients should always be matched during allocation. Significant covariation should be checked for secondarily, and between-group ANCOVA is always available as a secondary, less desirable back-up analysis. Under these conditions, the lesson is that if you need ANCOVA, the results may not be as reliable, the opposite of the last 30 years of understanding.

I have had conversations with statisticians about the issue of using baseline vs. outcomes results. Some seem reluctant to see, or to discuss, that the within-arm treatment comparisons are more powerful than the between-arm treatments. They seem more focused on the strictures that tell them that the two within-group comparisons are actually two "observational" studies and thus miss the opportunities that exist in the within-group analyses due to increased power.

They have been trained to think that the before-and-after comparisons are baseless and risky, and that nothing can be learned from focusing on them. This is a dire and costly mistake; these are not observational studies, in the sense that no control is provided. They are controlled experiments, and the comparison of the outcome groups to baseline uses all of the information from the control (or alternative treatment) in a direct manner.

Even when the disease condition (outcomes variable) in the treatment group is improved compared to itself before treatment but the disease condition in the control group has not changed, they simply shrug their shoulders and say "so what?" Unless the treatment outcome group is improved relative to control outcome, they say, the other analysis has no information, and they do not give full consideration to the relative power of the two analyses.

Alternatively Randomized Clinical Trials

Considering the principle of statistical power, other improvements over the FDA gold standard RCTs are possible under certain (not uncommon) conditions. These techniques are known, but they are rarely used, in large part due to the FDA's long-held insistence on pure randomization. First, during the allocation of patients to treatment groups, random pairs of patients can be selected that match in most of their demographics (gender, age, waistline, height, smoking history, etc.) to reduce variability between the groups, potentially making the control group a better control for the treatment group. This computational matching mimics the outcome group vs. baseline group by reducing variation between a participant in the study and that participant's control person. While not the same people, many factors are better controlled. Because they are matched on the basis of so many characteristics, they are not independent, and thus the paired t-test (or repeated sample ANOVA) may be applied.

These study designs fall into a category that I like to call "Alternatively Randomized Clinical Trials" (ARCTs). They dramatically increase the power of the test for the main effect (grapefruit) by removing variance not associated with the specific treatment under study. Larger sample sizes are nearly universally called for, because the intrusion of confounding factors is less likely at large N. While the Dow *et al.* study was sufficiently powered (had enough patients), and they found a significant effect in their baseline analysis, computational matching methods can homogenize the groups for variables that might otherwise impose themselves on the interpretation: They may have found a positive effect of grapefruit if their patient allocation process included matching.

How often are good findings masked by such factors because the FDA restricts consideration to "purely" randomized clinical trials? The FDA indemnifies itself on this issue by stating that they consider each clinical study independently. My impression, from speaking with many trialists, is that the answer is probably very, very frequently. The American public is often confused by reports in the media that first say that a particular food or medical practice is helpful only to be followed by reports that the results could not be reproduced or, even more confusingly, that the food or treatment is bad for you. The flaws in the strict adherence to RCTs without computational matching, and the failure of the understanding of the superiority of studies that collect baseline data are likely a main cause of inconsistent findings in science.

People doing good translational research like Drs. Dow and Thompson are limited in their abilities by competitive funding, by study design restrictions, and by time. The FDA should consider ARCTs as valid as purely randomized studies because they are equivalently randomized. They should also consider baseline vs. final study results as first-order results that may in fact be superior to treatment vs. control results due to heterogeneity between groups. Investigators would do well to plan randomized cross-over designs, as suggested by Dr. Dow, to really nail down the causal inferences in support of an intervention or treatment. And the US population should request increases in funding to the NIH for studies aimed at improving our health, reducing death rates, and reducing human pain and suffering.

It should be noted that the story told in this chapter is not restricted to grapefruit. Other foods may be effective at reversing indicators of ill health as well. Olive oil helps to keep the tissues of our blood vessels elastic, thus reducing the likelihood of developing high blood pressure. Olive oil has been given similar treatment by the medical community as grapefruit; its use should be considered in the pharmacological context of a given patient. It may have the same effects as some diabetes medicines. The fact that many doctors tend to not prescribe exercise, lower sodium, olive oil in your diet, an aspirin and a grapefruit a day for high blood pressure has many Americans suspicious that they are being fed medicines to treat a disease rather than being given a route to cures to reverse a disease. In the case of grapefruit, I think it is important to be specific about the types of blood pressure medication that might be avoided by grapefruit eaters, not the other way around. Anything a patient can do to improve their own health without medicines should be encouraged. Changes in the diet and behavior can reverse chronic inflammation, reduce weight, bring down bad cholesterol levels, and can reduce blood pressure. Such interventions can have the same effects as drugs, without the side-effects, and can especially be seen as a preventative step rather than a medical treatment. Your doctor should discuss these options with you first, before prescribing pills for blood pressure. These lifestyle changes have been shown to reverse disease, and thus they can be considered by the American public to be curative treatments.

The strict adherence to the outdated purely randomized clinical trials condemns clinical to being limited in their power to identify useful treatments. Because the outcome of these studies forms the basis upon which future health care practice options are based, the FDA's continued insistence on their use can be said to be impacting public health in a woefully negative manner. Unless they change their ways, successes in translational research will continue to be few and far between.

Given the strong evidence for the positive effects of grapefruit on weight loss (Fujioka *et al.*, 2006; Silver *et al.*, 2011; Dow *et al.*, 2012; de la Garza *et al.*, 2015), and on blood pressure (Dow *et al.*, 2012), medical doctors should carefully consider their advice to patients already and not yet eating grapefruit. Some blood pressure medications such as the beta blockers atenolol (Tenormin) and metoprolol (Lopressor, Toprol-XL) can cause weight gain and/or increases in triglycerides and cholesterol. In clinical studies, Carvedilol (Coreg) showed less weight gain than other beta blockers (Messerli *et al.*, 2007), and not significantly more than placebo controls. If the patients are also overweight, the best doctors might consider prescribing grapefruit and exercise first, or lowering the dose of the blood pressure meds for regular consumers of grapefruit, keeping their patient's entire pharmacopeia in mind, of course.

It should be noted that the results from some past clinical trial results may be worth re-examination in light of the increased power of the within-arm (outcomes to baseline) comparisons.

References

Bailey DG, *et al.* (1989) Ethanol enhances the hemodynamic effects of felodipine. *Clin Invest Med* **12**: 357–62.

de la Garza AL, *et al.* (2015) Helichrysum and grapefruit extracts boost weight loss in overweight rats reducing inflammation. *J Med Food*. [doi:10.1089/jmf.2014.0088]

Dow CA, *et al.* (2012) The effects of daily consumption of grapefruit on body weight, lipids, and blood pressure in healthy, overweight adults. *Metabolism* **61(7)**: 1026–35. [doi: 10.1016/j.metabol.2011.12.004]

Egbewale BE, Lewis M, Sim J. (2014) Bias, precision and statistical power of analysis of covariance in the analysis of randomized trials with baseline imbalance: a simulation study. *BMC Med Res Methodol* **14**: 49. [doi: 10.1186/1471-2288-14-49]

Fujioka K, *et al.* (2006) The effects of grapefruit on weight and insulin resistance: relationship to the metabolic syndrome. *J Med Food* **9(1)**: 49–54.

Gorinstein S, *et al.* (2006) Red grapefruit positively influences serum triglyceride level in patients suffering from coronary atherosclerosis: studies *in vitro* and in humans. *J Agric Food Chem* **54(5)**: 1887–92.

Messerli FH, *et al.* (2007) Body weight changes with beta-blocker use: results from GEMINI. *Am J Med* **120(7)**: 610–15.

Silver HJ, Dietrich MS, Niswender KD. (2011) Effects of grapefruit, grapefruit juice and water preloads on energy balance, weight loss, body composition, and cardiometabolic risk in free-living obese adults. *Nutr Metab (Lond)* **8(1)**: 8. [doi: 10.1186/1743-7075-8-8]

Smith GC, Pell JP. (2003) Parachute use to prevent death and major trauma related to gravitational challenge: systematic review of randomised controlled trials. *BMJ* **327(7429):** 1459–61.

US Food and Drug Administration (FDA). (2015) Guidance for Industry: Providing Clinical Evidence of Effectiveness for Human Drugs and Biological Products. FDA website. http://www.fda.gov/downloads/Drugs/GuidanceComplianceRegulatoryInformation/Guidance

4 Hormone Receptor Status and Breast Cancer Treatment

Early in the morning, Claire, a woman in her 40s, starts running the water for her shower. As the steam rises in the bathtub, she feels her breast sway as she pulls away from turning the knob. Something is different. She feels a small tug, or an imbalance in her breast. It is barely perceivable. As she stands in the shower and runs water over her head, she raises her hands over the top of her head to be sure the water distributes across all of her hair. As she does so she feels the slight weighty pull in her breast again. Curious, she touches her breast. It feels tender. She is not sure, but with slight pressure from her hand, she thinks she feels a lump. Could this be cancer? As she showers, her imagination runs ahead a bit. What would treatment be like? Would she require surgery? Radiation? Chemo? She thinks of a friend or two she knows who have had breast cancer. She thinks of her children, and shudders. She decides to put it out of her mind for later consideration. She has a lot to do today; she will make an appointment.

This scene is played out hundreds of thousands of times a year in the US and around the world. Women know that the first sign of breast cancer is usually a lump, found by women or their partners, or their doctors during regular manual breast exams. While breast self-exams (BSEs) are often promoted, two randomized clinical trials showed no difference in survival between them and those who were not (Thomas *et al.*, 2002; Semiglazov *et al.*, 2003). In both studies, the number of biopsies of benign lumps was nearly doubled by BSEs. In women under 45 years of age in the US, 71% of breast cancer cases are found by the patient; 9% by routine clinical exams, and 20% by routine mammography (Coates *et al.*, 2001).

Breast cancer used to be, like many cancers still are, a near death sentence for most patients. Survival rates in the US began to improve slightly in the 1980s, and then jumped dramatically in the 1990s due to increased, regular use of mammograms. Today, a woman in the US diagnosed with breast cancer has an 89.2% chance of five-year survival (SEER, 2014). Early detection, improvements in surgeries and refinement in the use of chemotherapies are, in large part, responsible for improved outcomes. But her odds of survival depend on whether she belongs to the 90% of women whose cancers express one of three particular hormone receptors. If she is among the 10% less fortunate women whose breast tumors do not express one of these hormone receptors (triple-negative breast cancer), her treatment options are more limited, and her chances of survival to five years are much lower because endocrine therapy is not an option. There were 232,000 new breast cancer cases, and over 40,000 women in the US died of breast cancer in 2014 (SEER, 2014). By comparison, in Japan, breast cancer incidence and mortality has increased from very low to nearly as high as the US since 1970. This is attributed to two factors: women having fewer children, and a westernized diet (Okazaki, 2013).

The story of how hormone receptor status has improved outcomes for breast cancer patients has all of the hallmarks of a successful translational research program. The first hallmark is improved survivorship. Medical practice can be separated roughly along a dimension of stages of care. For cancer, this dimension usually follows prevention, diagnosis, treatment, some of which are sufficiently advanced along the translational dimension to include reports on disease-free survival, overall survival, and long-term survival.

Red Light, Green Light

Claire drives away from her appointment rather shaken. Her doctor's words ring in her ears. "We'll have to do a biopsy to see if it's benign, or malignant." She tries to rationalize the fear away, with denial. "It's probably benign. I really don't need this right now," she thinks, as tears well up in her eyes. She slams on the brakes — she almost ran a red light. She chokes back the tears, clears her throat, and becomes a bit more resolved. "We'll just have to wait and find out, I guess!" she thinks. The light turns green. She drives on.

The Hallmarks of Translational Success in Cancer Research

In clinical practice, the later stages of care are highly dependent on the earlier stages. Early detection is key to long-term survival and, of course, selection of the most effective treatment is also key to better outcomes. Chemotherapy may be used to shrink a tumor sufficiently to allow safer surgery, for example, to reduce the chance of involvement of blood vessels, or to keep the tumor away from other tissues such as chest muscles, as in breast cancer. My oncologist friends and colleagues, and their patients, are waging a constant battle with time for information on the results of the last treatments.

For any cancer, research on the later stages of care is also highly dependent on success in the earlier stages. A larger number of options for diagnosis, for example, should lead to an understanding of which methods of are more accurate, and which can detect cancer earliest. Further studies would reveal which combinations of methods of diagnosis led to earlier and more accurate detection. These improvements in diagnosis then could by augmented by clinical research studies on which modes of treatment — and options within each mode — are associated with the best outcomes for the patient. Clinical studies often focus on surgery, chemotherapy (many options) and radiation.

When these kinds of studies are successful, then we can start to see studies that focus on the combined modalities and treatments. Studies on identifying biomarkers that can predict which therapies are likely to be successful for specific patients are then possible. Finally, we should see an increase in the number — and percentage of studies — that report increased survivorship.

One of the services provided by the NIH is the National Center for Biotechnology Information (NCBI). This service provides computational resources for researchers and the public. Pubmed is perhaps the most used specific research resource of any kind in the world. It is a searchable, heavily cross-indexed, user-friendly interface on a database that includes research papers, editorials, and position papers from all indexed journals. It is a big deal for a journal to acquire Pubmed listing; it means that it has passed the stringent test of having appropriate, objective peer review. When the journal I envisioned and helped create with Tim and Tom Hill (*Cancer Informatics*) became listed in Pubmed due to the rigorous industry-standard peer-review system we had put into place, I silently celebrated its inclusion among the ranks of other well-accepted research journals. My mom's legacy was intact, and would be long-lasting.

Searching Pubmed is easy; if you can use Google, you can use Pubmed. Pubmed is often used to study trends in publication. I used it to study the number, and percentage, of studies on 10 types of cancer, over the various terms indicative of a study's focus on stages of cancer care: Prevention, Risk, Diagnosis, Treatment, Metastasis, Recurrence, Survival. I found the total number of studies that focused on a particular cancer type by searching Pubmed. For example, for pancreatic cancer, I searched for "pancreatic" + "cancer."

First, the number of studies on each stage of care topic, for each cancer, is roughly humped-shaped over the axis of Stages of Cancer Care (Fig. 4.1). There are few studies on prevention, more on diagnosis, about the same number on treatments, but few on metastasis and fewer on survival (Fig. 4.1).

I was curious about what proportion of all studies in each cancer type focused on each stage of cancer. Then, for each stage of cancer care, I searched for studies focused on each cancer type that contained words reflecting each particular Stage of Care. For example, for studies of metastatic pancreatic cancer, I searched Pubmed for "Pancreatic" + "Cancer" + "Metastasis." This gave me the total number of studies for each

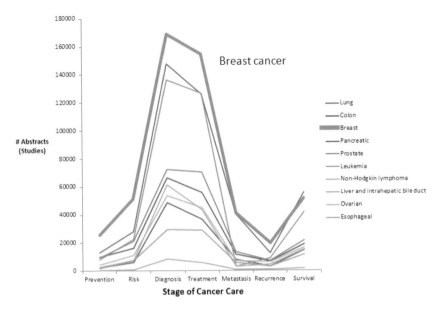

Fig. 4.1 Distribution of published studies in Pubmed (all journals) mentioning cancer types and various stages of cancer care. Note the hump-shaped distribution, reflecting a relative dearth of studies focused on Prevention, Risk, Metastasis, Recurrence and Survival relative to the number of studies focused on Diagnosis and Treatment.

cancer type that focused on each stage in cancer care; these numbers showed a similar humped-shaped pattern reflecting the distribution of effort on each topic results for all studies focused on receptors (not shown).

However, when I calculated the *percentage* of all studies that focused on receptors for a particular Stage of Care for each cancer, what I found was remarkable. Breast cancer is the only cancer that, over the time period I studied, shows a clear hallmark of translational success: It is the only cancer that shows a steady increase in studies from prevention through to survival (Fig. 4.2). I interpret this to reflect, in large part, the high degree of translational success due to the focus on receptors in breast cancer research.

Translational success in breast cancer associated with decades of optimizing treatments based on receptor-status has informed clinical care.

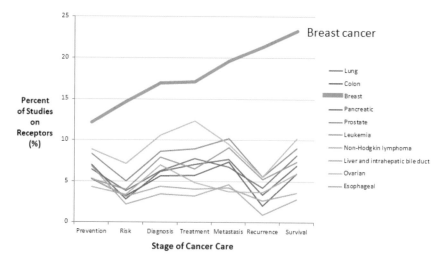

Fig. 4.2   A signature of translational success in breast cancer due to receptor research is reflected in the elegant increase in studies that consider Metastasis, Recurrence and Survival relative to other cancers. The absence of a linear increase in proportion of studies focused on receptors in cancers other than breast cancer reveals critically important new directions for many other cancer types.

Breast cancer rates worldwide have tended to increase. That is, until recently. Lozano *et al.* (2012) studied global trends of 235 causes of death in 2012 and found that breast cancer rates jumped from 640,000 in 1980 to more than 1.6 million in 2010. The most rapid increases in some countries, such as Japan, are attributed to a westernization of diet. In the US, the greater incidence of breast cancer risk is usually attributed to changes in lifestyle factors, specifically westernization of diet (high fat, calorie-dense foods), increased BMI due to increasingly sedentary lifestyle, smoking, and estrogen exposure, early menarche, late child bearing, fewer pregnancies. Detection is increased via mammography screening.

Mortality due to breast cancer in more developed countries is not as high as would be predicted given the higher incidence (Torre *et al.*, 2015), and is declining. This, of course, is a factor in any ultimate measure of translational success. It is widely known that early detection is key to the improvement of outcomes, however this knowledge has not yet translated to the world's poor — rural women in India, for example, suffer very high mortality compared to their urban counterparts due to a lack of access to screening programs. The same pattern is repeated in Brazil, where poor, uneducated women have much higher mortality due to breast cancer (Albrecht *et al.*, 2013).

There are countries with patterns different from global trends, including Japan, Australia, some countries in Africa, and some of the former Eastern Bloc countries (Bray *et al.*, 2004; Jemal *et al.*, 2010; Torre *et al.*, 2015).

There is increasing interest in the study of hormone status in other cancers in hope of repeating the translational success in breast cancer. Each of the communities focused on research problems in all types of cancers would do well to increase the focus of that research on prevention, risk prediction, outcomes-related studies in metastasis, recurrence, and survival.

Hormone-Receptor Mediated Chemotherapy

Claire's biopsy of her mass will be thoroughly scanned by a pathologist to determine if it is malignant (potentially life-threatening) or benign. It will also be tested for certain proteins. Breast tissue is amazing — at puberty, it undergoes a second stage of growth in response to hormones. During pregnancy, another set of hormones activate milk glands. Many women know that their breasts change in firmness as a matter of routine as hormones change over the course of their menstrual cycles. Many are also aware that breast density changes over their lifetime. About half of women in a recent survey reported knowing that breast density can have an impact on cancer detection (Rhodes *et al.*, 2015). So it is no surprise that breast tumors may also be highly responsive to hormones.

One of the greatest advances in molecular medicine has been the use of hormone status in breast cancer to help choose appropriate therapies. The proteins the oncologist is interested are hormone receptors — proteins in the cellular membrane that latch onto hormones, including estrogen, progesterone. We refer to these proteins as ER (estrogen receptor) and PR (progesterone receptor). Drugs used to treat ER and PR expressing cells include tamoxifen. Aromatase inhibitors are also used to starve the tumors of the estrogen that signals them to grow.

In 1979, a third protein, human epidermal growth factor 2 (Her-2 Neu), was found to be an indicator for another type of drug. Dr. Dennis Slamon found the anti-Her-2 Neu targeting drug Herceptin (trastuzumab) targeted cells expressing Her-2 Neu, and that Her-2 Neu+ breast cancers can be expected to respond to Herceptin.

The history of how hormone receptor targeting became *en vogue* in breast cancer is fascinating. In 1875, in Scotland, a young future Sir George Thomas Beatson, M.D. made several astute observations and inferential leaps. Farmers and shepherds at the time knew that when cows and sheep had their ovaries removed (oophorectomy) after giving birth, they would continue to produce milk even after their calves or kids would wean. Beatson had done experiments on the degeneration of fat in the lactating breasts of rabbits. He realized that the presence of ovaries in lactating mammals influences the growth and activity of breast tissues. The brilliant deductions Beatson made from his key observations led him to perform three oophorectomies on women with late-stage breast cancer; one patient's breast cancer went into remission (cured), the other two showed dramatic improvement. Shortly thereafter, others took up the practice with a larger number of patients, and endocrine therapy was born (Stockwell, 1983). He was one of the Sherlock Holmes of cancer research of his time.

Fast forward to 1967. A medical researcher named Dr. Elwood Jensen working at the University of Chicago in the Ben May Laboratory for Cancer Research developed a means to measure the estrogen receptor protein in breast cancer tissues. Jensen was originally a chemist who had previously worked with poison gas during World War II. He discovered the true biological nature of estrogen receptors — turning over (incorrect) common knowledge about their function and activity in the human body. Jensen reported that a climb on the north face of the Matterhorn inspired him to try alternative approaches. When stuck on a particular molecular problem (say, localization of a hormone), he would think outside the box a little — and begin asking about the localization of that hormone in patients who, for other medical reasons, had the right organ removed to allow him to deduce, via observation, the correct mechanisms of action. The history of the extensive structure activity relationship research leading to the discovery of localization of hormones to specific tissues is outlined beautifully in MacGregor and Jordan (1998).

Then, seven years later, a medical doctor named Dr. William McGuire from Medical School at San Antonio in Texas developed a new method to make quantitative measures of ER. At the time, numerous doctors had observed that about a third of women with late-stage (metastatic) breast cancer would go into remission if they had their ovaries, adrenal glands, or pituitary glands removed. With the new, more robust type of data, McGuire made two key additional observations. McGuire (1973) correctly hypothesized that the presence of ER in breast cancer tissue may indicate the likelihood of response to some form of endocrine (i.e., hormone) therapy. McGuire wrote:

> *Precise quantitation of EBP in all human primary tumors may prove to be an excellent prognosticator of endocrine therapy in metastatic breast cancer.*

He concluded with:

> *In summary, specific quantitative assays for EBP in human breast cancer are now available. Data from such assays correlated with future clinical responses should lead to a better understanding of endocrine-induced breast cancer regression as well as a more rational approach to therapy.*

These findings indicated foresight into the fields of targeted therapeutics and personalized medicine.

Here, McGuire also set the bar fairly for the full utility of ER "status." He knew that the concentration of ER exhibited a wide variation in breast cancer tissues at various stages (early, primary vs. late, metastatic). So, he insisted the technology used to measure be both accurate and precise (i.e., quantitative, not qualitative).

Accuracy is the ability of a measurement to be on-target in an unbiased manner. Precision is the ability of a measurement to be easily repeated, with little error. Measurements made these days tend to relatively sloppy — semi-quantitative at best.

We have settled for nearly 20 years for proxy measurements, like gene expression values made in unknown dimensions from scans of fluorescence intensity. Measurements that are both accurate (unbiased), and

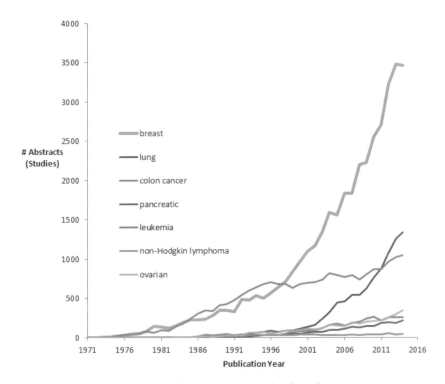

Fig. 4.3 Increasing trend in number of receptor studies focus by cancer type in various cancer types in the National Center for Biotechnology Information's Pubmed resource (1970–2014). Percent of all cancer type values show similar trends.

precise (low error), and that are properly calibrated and quantitative, are needed.

Dr. William McGuire and many others went on to work out the HER2-neu how another protein could inform doctors on the optimal treatment for breast cancer. In 1987, McGuire, then at the University of Texas Health Science Center, and Dr. Dennis Slamon at the University of California Los Angeles (UCLA), working with Dr. Axel Ullrich at a company called Genentech, noticed that breast cancer patients who had high rates of relapse and low rates of survival also had high levels of the HER2 protein (Slamon *et al.*, 1987). Then, at the National Cancer Institute (NCI), Dr. Pier Paulo di Fiore and Dr. Stuart Aaronson discovered that HER2 causes normal cells to become similar to aggressive tumor cells (di Fiore *et al.*, 1987). Dr. Larry Norton at the Memorial Sloan Kettering Institute for Cancer Research searched for combinations of chemotherapy that might work especially well on HER2-neu positive cancer cells (e.g., Baselga *et al.*, 1997), while at the same time searching for HER2 antibodies for use in characterizing tumors, eventually finding that they augment some forms of chemotherapy (Slamon *et al.*, 2001). Dr. Richard Pietras at UCLA found that some drugs appeared to be more effective when used in combination with HER2 antibodies, and defined the antibody treatment mechanisms of response to DNA repair (Pietras *et al.*, 1998). Finally, in 2006, after a series of impressive clinical trials (e.g., Slamon *et al.*, 1998), the FDA approved Herceptin, a HER2 antibody, for use in the treatment of HER2-neu+ positive breast cancer. Well-known and closely monitored side effects include heart and lung problems.

About one-third of breast cancers do not express any of these receptors. Knowing that a tumor will not respond to specific treatments based on their receptor status can save a woman time in her treatment regime, and she and her doctors can then consider other therapies that might have more success. This is called targeted therapy, and via individualized medicine, will likely become the primary approach to care in some form for all cancers.

If Claire's biopsy comes back as malignant, the report will include her ER, PR and Her-2 neu status. It will include information on the size of the tumor, and from this and the description of the cells and the extent of the tumor, it will be staged. Stage 1 is small, limited to a local area within the breast. Stage 2 is more diffuse, but localized. Stage 3 indicates involvement of tissue outside the breast (such as nearby lymph nodes), and Stage 4 is distant metastasis (such as lung, liver, or brain).

From the ER, PR and Her-2 Neu status, the oncologist can begin choosing an appropriate route to chemotherapy. He or she will discuss surgery and radiation options with her, depending on the degree of infiltration, muscle tissue involvement, and other factors. She may even consider a radical mastectomy. Some women with triple-negative breast cancer (ER-, PR- and Her-2 Neu-) may opt for this because it is a type that is very likely to recur with additional *de novo* tumors, especially if she carries a BRCA1 or BRCA2 variant associated with breast cancer.

The legacy of these early researchers is long-lasting and widespread, and continues to grow. Refinements on techniques for the measurement of ER are still ongoing (Wolff and Dowsett, 2011). This chapter is being written in March 2015; a quick scan of Pubmed for research on targeted therapies in breast cancer alone results in 305 hits in Pubmed. A detailed look at those studies reveals a sampling of the numerous targets being studied across the world (Table 4.1). Hormone receptors are being studied in different kinds of cancers as well.

A great deal of the translational success in breast cancer detectable by the publication trends is due to the use of molecularly mediated and targeted chemotherapies. Other advances that have contributed to translational success have included advances in detection, such as improved sensitivity and specificity of mammography, the use of ultrasound for diagnosis, improvements in surgical techniques, and advances in radiation. A better understanding of the role of nutrition and vitamins to modulate the toxicity of chemotherapy has also helped. An aggressive campaign for research by the Susan G. Komen Foundation has driven much of this research forward.

Table 4.1   Select Targeted Therapies in Breast Cancer

Target(s)	Mechanism	Reference	
INOS	inhibition	Granados-Principal et al.	*Breast Cancer Res* (2015) **17(1):** 527
CDK11, CK2	RNA interference	Kren	*Breast Cancer Res* (2015) Dec; **17(1):** 524
Various	nanoparticles	Islamian	*Asian Pac J Cancer Prev* (2015) **16(5):** 1683–6
Various	microtubule stabilization	Pabla and Sparreboom	*Clin Cancer Res* (2015) March 15; **21(6):** 1237–9
PI3K/mTOR	inhibition	Nagaraj, Ma	*Breast Cancer Res Treat* (2015) March 12
CDK4/6	inhibition	Nagaraj, Ma	*Breast Cancer Res Treat* (2015) March 12
HER2	receptor blocking	Dawood, Sirohi	*Future Oncol* (2015) March; **11(6):** 923–31
AurA	mediation of anti-mitotic effects	Tentler	*Mol Cancer Ther* (2015) pii: molcanther.0538.2014
Various	microtubule inhibitor	Burns	*Mol Pharm* (2015) March 13
Various receptors	agonists/antagonists	Rodrigues-Ferreira	*Front Pharmacol* (2015) **6:** 24
NPR-1	RNA interference NPR-1	Han et al.	*Mol Med Rep* (2015) March 3

People sometimes make claims such as: *"Doctors don't want a cure, they want treatment, because never-ending treatment means more money for them!"* This type of speculation is often made out of abject ignorance of the many success stories in which biomedical research has brought findings from basic studies forward into improvements in clinical practice. "We cure cancer all the time," an oncologist friend once told me. The speculation on the part of the public belies the complexity of cancer as a disease; each primary tumor in each patient is a unique biological event. It also shows that the public is not sufficiently informed of the hard-won successes that do occur. The worst that can be said for cancer researchers working to identify ways to improve clinical care, I think, is that they suffer from weak public relations campaigns to the general public. The discoveries that shape the clinical options available today took a century to develop. The NIH and the NCI have not done a good job informing the American public of the successes due to sustained effort. This has been a mix of individual and collaborative efforts, and such efforts are ongoing. Refinements that fine-tune the customization of breast cancer treatment options are forthcoming, at a faster rate than ever before.

Funding for receptor-mediated treatment research across all cancer types should be prioritized, and greenlighted, especially if the mechanisms of cancer drugs may be blocked by the lack of expression of specific receptors.

Given the difficulties of translating the subtle nuances of high-end clinical trials, and the specific molecular mechanisms of and effects profiles of modern medicine, the public relations campaign has to become more aggressive, with a balancing act of education, information, and not leading anyone to the conclusion that funding rates for research can now drop because we have had these successes. Our society has made, over the past 30 years, massive investments. Much more funding is needed to sustain this effort, to allow the promise of knowledge gained by hard work and long hours to translate into improved outcomes for patients. The people deserve to know how NIH and NCI funding has made a difference in their lives. I am advocating for a return to funding increases; a 20 percent increase in the NIH budget every year for the next five years — focused on the doing of science, not the building of buildings — will work wonders for translation of that knowledge into further improvements across all types of cancer. But this success will only be likely if we heed the advice of Dr. William McGuire: Accuracy, precision, and calibration all matter, so if we're going to measure it, we should make it quantitative. If all researchers could combine such high standards with the perspicuity of Sir George Thomas Beatson, with focused follow-up research by others over the span of decades, we would likely see more tailored and targeted (precision) treatment advances in all types of cancers.

References

Albrecht CAM, *et al*. (2013) Breast cancer mortality among patients attending a cancer hospital, Vitoria, ES. *Rev Bras Epidemiol* **16:** 582–91. [http://dx.doi.org/10.1590/S1415-790X2013000300003]

Baselga J, *et al*. (1997) HER2 overexpression and paclitaxel sensitivity in breast cancer: therapeutic implications. *Oncology (Williston Park)* **11(3 Suppl 2):** 43–48.

Beatson GT. (1896) On the treatment of inoperable cases of carcinoma of the mamma: suggestions for a new method of treatment, with illustrative cases. *Lancet* **148:** 162–65.

Bray F, McCarron P, Parkin DM. (2004) The changing global patterns of female breast cancer incidence and mortality. *Breast Cancer Res* **6(6):** 229–39.

Coates RJ, *et al*. (2001) Patterns and predictors of the breast cancer detection methods in women under 45 years of age (United States). *Cancer Causes Control* **12(5):** 431–42.

di Fiore PP, *et al*. (1987) erbB-2 is a potent oncogene when overexpressed in NIH/3T3 cells. *Science* **237(4811):** 178–82.

Jemal A, *et al*. (2010) Global patterns of cancer incidence and mortality rates and trends. *Cancer Epidemiol Biomarkers Prev* **19(8):** 1893–907. [doi: 10.1158/1055-9965.EPI-10-0437]

Jensen EV, *et al.* (1967) Estrogen-receptor interactions in target tissues. *Arch Anat Microsc Morphol Exp* **56:** 547–69.

Jensen E. (2012) A conversation with Elwood Jensen. Interview by David D. Moore. *Annu Rev Physiol* **74:** 1–11. [doi: 10.1146/annurev-physiol-020911-153327]

Lozano R, *et al.* (2012) Global and regional mortality from 235 causes of death for 20 age groups in 1990 and 2010: a systematic analysis for the Global Burden of Disease Study. *Lancet* **380(9859):** 2095–128. [doi: 10.1016/S0140-6736(12)61728-0]

MacGregor JI, Jordan VC. (1998) Basic guide to the mechanisms of antiestrogen action. *Pharmacol Rev* **50(2):** 151–96.

McGuire WL. (1973) Estrogen receptors in human breast cancer. *J Clin Invest* **52:** 73–77.

Okazaki A. (2013) Survey: Breast cancer death rate drops for the 1st time in 2012. *The Asahi Shimbun.* [http://ajw.asahi.com/article/behind_news/social_affairs/AJ201309130080]

Pietras RJ, *et al.* (1994) Antibody to HER-2/neu receptor blocks DNA repair after cisplatin in human breast and ovarian cancer cells. *Oncogene* **9(7):** 1829–38.

Rhodes DJ, *et al.* (2015) Awareness of breast density and its impact on breast cancer detection and risk. *J Clin Oncol* pii: JCO.2014.57.0325.

Semiglazov VF, *et al.* (2003) (in Russian) [Results of a prospective randomized investigation [Russia (St.Petersburg)/WHO] to evaluate the significance of self-examination for the early detection of breast cancer]. *Vopr Onkol* **49(4):** 434–41.

Slamon DJ, *et al.* (1987) Human breast cancer: correlation of relapse and survival with amplification of the HER-2/neu oncogene. *Science* **235(4785):** 177–82.

Slamon D, *et al.* (1998) Addition of Herceptin (humanized anti-HER2 antibody) to first line chemotherapy for HER2 overexpressing metastatic breast cancer markedly increases anticancer activity: a randomized, multinational controlled Phase III trial. *Proc of ASCO* #377, 17:98A.

Slamon DJ, *et al.* (2001) Use of chemotherapy plus a monoclonal antibody against HER2 for metastatic breast cancer that overexpresses HER2. *N Engl J Med* **344(11):** 783–92.

Stockwell S. (1983) Classics in Oncology: George Thomas Beatson, M.D. (1848–1933). *CA: A Cancer Journal for Clinicians* **33(2):** 105–107.

Thomas DB, *et al*. (2002) Randomized trial of breast self-examination in Shanghai: final results. *J Natl Cancer Inst* **94(19):** 1445–57.

Torre LA, *et al*. (2015) Global cancer statistics, 2012. *CA Cancer J Clin*, 2015 March, **65(2):** 87–108. [doi: 10.3322/caac.21262]

Wolff AC, Dowsett M. (2011) Estrogen receptor: a never ending story? *J Clin Oncol* **29(22):** 2955–58.

More Information about Sir Beatson and the Beatson Cancer Institute:

The Beatson Cancer Institute in Glasgow, Scotland was in part founded by Sir George Beatson. From the Institute's website:

> *The foundations for the Beatson Institute were laid at the end of the 19th century when, in 1890, a new cancer hospital was opened in Glasgow. Sir George Thomas Beatson — a surgeon of considerable talent — soon became head of the institution and in 1912 established a research department.*
>
> *In 1967 — under the directorship of Dr John Paul — the department became the Beatson Institute for Cancer Research and moved to its present location at the Garscube Estate in 1976. Prof John Wyke became Director in 1987 and worked to develop links between the Beatson Institute and the University of Glasgow — in particular with the departments of Medical and Radiation Oncology. Prof Karen Vousden was appointed as Director at the end of 2002.*

http://www.beatson.gla.ac.uk/about/history.html (Accessed 3/2015)

MacMahon CE, Cahill JL. (1976) The evolution of the concept of the use of surgical castration in the palliation of breast cancer in pre-menopausal females. *Ann Surg* **184:** 713–16.

Sir Beatson's contributions are described in greater detail by MacMahon and Cahill (1976) and by Stockwell (1983).

5 Fecal Microbiota Transplantation

Imagine undergoing surgery, say, for a hip replacement. Your surgeon will, as matter of routine, prescribe antibiotics to protect you from any incidental infection that may have occurred during surgery. The doses are usually very strong to insure efficacy. After a week of taking the medication, you develop severe diarrhea, uncontrollable vomiting, and high fever. You try over-the-counter medication, and initially it seems to help. But then nothing seems to stop it, and you start vomiting as well. You lose tens of pounds in the first week. You don't want to eat. You have trouble sleeping. You can't concentrate. You can't go to work, and your sick time is being used up, and you are now at risk of losing your job. As time passes, you feel weaker and weaker. No one knows why you're sick, and weeks pass before you receive any sign of a diagnosis.

Patients taking antibiotics to prevent or treat infection can sometimes develop a serious, long-term, life-threatening condition called *C. difficile* infection (CDI), or *Clostridium difficile* colitis. *Clostridium difficile* is spore-forming bacterium that can produce toxins. The colitis caused by pathogenic (disease-causing) *C. difficile* can occur when the large intestine loses its natural community of bacteria species. The intestines can, especially in hospital settings, become inflamed due to overpopulation by one or more strains of *C. difficile* that are resistant to antibiotics.

The symptoms of CDI are profuse diarrhea, uncontrollable vomiting and high fever. It is difficult to get an accurate diagnosis because these symptoms are also consistent with food allergies, diabetes, Crohn's disease, irritable bowel syndrome, ulcerative colitis, food poisoning, and any of a myriad of forms of non-*C. difficile* gastroenteritis (a.k.a. "stomach flu").

Besides threatening their lives, the toll these diseases can take on people can be absolutely disruptive. There are over 340,000 cases of CDI in the US each year, and the annual death toll is around 14,000. These infections are very difficult to treat; patients lose massive amounts of weight and can die from associated causes. The repeated and varied attempts at classical treatments (antibiotics) cost in excess of $1 billion a year. Patients often have rounds and bouts of treatment and recurrence and, as the disease takes over their lives, they cannot function as their normal selves at home or at work. The condition is quite distressing as formerly extremely robust and healthy patients can literally waste away. These types of disease take a serious, long-lasting psychological toll (McCombie, 2015).

CDI is not new. Case studies in the 1950s were not uncommon, and in 1958, researchers in Colorado attempted a unique form of therapy for CDI. They transplanted feces from a healthy person into the colon of four patients with hard-to-treat gastrointestinal infections. Remarkably, the patients all recovered.

Fecal microbiota transplantation (FMT) involves collection of stool from a tested donor, and preparation of an infusion. The transplantation is done either by colonoscopy, endoscopy, sigmoidoscopy, enema, or capsule. The goal of the treatment is to restore populations of healthy bacteria. Strong courses of antibiotics can wipe out the normal healthy biome in the gut. *C. difficile* is reduced as well, but returns more efficiently from spores. The species can overpopulate, leading to serious malfunctioning of the normal bacterial processing of waste in the gut and, most commonly, to intense, prolonged diarrhea. *C. difficile* infection causes about 500,000 cases of gastroenteritis and 14,000 deaths per year in the US (US Centers for Disease Control and Prevention data).

FMT has been used for hundreds of years. Li Shizhen, a Chinese scientist and pharmacologist (1518–1593), used preparations of fecal solutions and fermentations to treat gastrointestinal diseases. In 2003, a study of nine years of experience with FMT at one institution (Aas *et al.*, 2003) revealed that of the 18 patients treated, 15 were cured, one experienced treatment failure, and two died of unrelated illnesses. More recent studies demonstrated the safety and efficacy of FMT for treatment of *C. difficile* (89% cure rate; Kelly *et al.*, 2014).

FMT appears highly effective in treating both chronic constipation and Irritable Bowel Syndrome (IBS). In a study of 55 patients with IBS and IBD treated with FMT, cure was reported in (36%, decreased symptoms in 16%, and no response reported in 47% patients; Borody *et al.*, 1989). In another study, of 45 patients with chronic constipation treated with colonoscopic FMT and subsequent fecal enema infusions, 89% reported relief. Normal bowel movements, without laxative use, persisted in 60% 19 months afterwards (Andrews *et al.*, 1995).

This sensible, low-cost, highly effective (typically >90% cure rate) treatment that provides rapid cure (hours to days) is not yet approved by health insurance companies, in spite of a study published in the *New England Journal of Medicine* (Brandt *et al.*, 2011) in which FMT was given to a treatment group, while the control group was treated with the antibiotic vancomycin or vancomycin with bowel lavage. Diarrhea associated with CDI resolved without relapse after 10 weeks in 15 out of the 16 patients in the treatment group (94% cure). There were only mild side effects. In the control group, cure rates were only 31% for vancomycin and 23% under vancomycin plus bowel lavage. Due to the risk to patients in the control group, the trial was stopped and the control group members were given FMT — 15 of 18 patients who relapsed and subsequently underwent transfusion were also cured (83%). A follow-up study of bacterial species diversity in the feces of patients who had undergone the transfusion showed increased diversity, a sign of a healthy gut.

A cost-effectiveness study (Varier *et al.*, 2015) has demonstrated that not only is FMT more effective than vancomycin tapering, it is also more cost-saving. The US FDA has approved the use of FMT for treatment of *C. difficile* infections that have not responded to standard treatment; there are ongoing double-blind randomized clinical trials at Montefiore Hospital. FMT has shown promise as an effective treatment for dysbiosis (incorrect "bugs" in the intestine) due to cancer treatment (Blackburn *et al.*, 2015) and liver transplant (Wang *et al.*, 2015). FMT is recognized around the world as a success for *C. difficile* infection and is being further studied, and is also recognized for utility in treating a variety of functional gastrointestinal disorders, including irritable bowel syndrome, inflammatory bowel diseases, insulin resistance, multiple sclerosis, and idiopathic thrombocytopenic purpura (Pinn *et al.*, 2015; Matsuoka *et al.*, 2014 (Japan); Smits *et al.*, 2013 and Singh *et al.*, 2014 (Netherlands); Borody *et al.*, 2014 (Australia)). It is being studied in Italy with promising results for ulcerative colitis (Scaldaferri *et al.*, 2015). In China, it has been seen to be effective for pseudomembranous enteritis (Wang *et al.*, 2015) and severe sepsis and diarrhea after vagotomy (removal of all or part of the vagus nerve, which serves the abdominal area; Li *et al.*, 2015).

Initially, the regulatory and legal barriers to FMT adoption in the US were seen as "insurmountable" (Louie, 2008). The cultural resistance that might be expected to exist has primarily been in the area of medical staff, not patients; by the time FMT is considered, patients are willing to try just about anything. Happily, the science behind FMT is robust. In 2013, the FDA reversed its decision to require an "Investigational" New Drug (IND) Application (IND) for the use of FMT to treat *C. difficile* infections (FDA, 2013). Treating physicians should obtain informed consent from the patient for the use of FMT as a treatment, including a statement that the use of FMT products to treat *C. difficile* is investigational, and a review of its potential risks and side effects. The most definitive review of the benefits of FMT is provided by Bakken *et al.* (2011). Some physicians supervise self-administered FMT; do-it-yourself is not recommended, although estimates are that thousands of people have treated themselves without medical supervision.

Possible side effects of FMT include acquiring an infection from the donor. Doctors screen both donors and stool for evidence of infectious agents, naturally, and have the option of selecting a "safe" donor: a spouse, or relative, whose clinical background is well-known to the patient. They also can use the patient's own fecal matter that has been collected prior to exposure to the clinical treatment that might wipe out their intestinal biome.

"Ecobiotics": Lab-Grown Ingestible Live Microbiota in a Pill

Thomas Louie, M.D., a professor of Microbiology and Infectious Diseases at the University of Calgary, spent hours harvesting normal bacterial species for a study in which 31 out of 32 patients who took 24 to 34 of the capsules orally over a 15-minute period were cured of *C. difficile* related gastroenteritis. One patient had a recurrence due to antibiotic treatment for an unrelated infection. Youngster *et al.* (2014) showed the feasibility of using frozen, capsulized FMT taken orally: 18 out of 20 patients were cured.

This approach, which has been called "Ecobiotics" instead of "Probiotics," restores the normal healthy flora to the bacterial ecosystem. Johnson & Johnson Pharmaceuticals is developing a pill form called SER-109. In a Phase I/II study of SER-109, the treatment showed 100% cure rate in the high dose arm of the trial and >90% cure rate in the lower dose arm.

Individualized Medicine and FMT

The movement toward individualized medicine is likely to have a good example in the future use of tailored FMT-like treatments. In the near future, by assaying a patient's microbial gut microbiome, not only will pathogenic species be identified, and removed with species-specific antibiotics, any missing species typically found in a healthy human gut may be replaced with made-to-order FMT pellets or pills. Within five to 10 years, the science of ecobiotics will likely be exact, with precision treatments for specific ailments. Some forms of moodiness and depression have been linked to dysbiosis, and prebiotics appear to reduce cortisol, a signature of stress in humans (Schmidt *et al.*, 2015). The clinical pharmacology community may do well to participate in this area. While repeated treatments might be expected to ensure the microbiome change is successful, by and large it seems likely that single effective and safe high-dose tailored treatments will become commonplace. Herein also lie real opportunities for ecological modelers (community ecology) to study the dynamics of species interactions in the human gut.

A list of providers of FMT is available at the Fecal Transplant Foundation website at the URL listed under References, below, and a list of clinical trials involving FMT for various conditions are available at ClinicalTrials.gov

2015 FMT Trials at ClinicalTrials.gov

https://clinicaltrials.gov/ct2/results?term=fecal+transplant&Search =Search

2015 List of FMT Providers

http://thefecaltransplantfoundation.org/providers-trials/

Hopefully, the FDA will see fit to use FMT as a first case of a "blanket compassionate use" treatment without the need for extensive paperwork.

References

Aas J, Gessert CE, Bakken JS. (2003) Recurrent *Clostridium difficile* colitis: case series involving 18 patients treated with donor stool administered via a nasogastric tube. *Clin Infect Dis* **36**: 580–85.

Andrews P, *et al.* (1995) Bacteriotherapy for chronic constipation — long term follow-up. *Gastroenterology* **108**: A563.

Bakken JS, *et al.* (2011) Treating *Clostridium difficile* infection with fecal microbiota transplantation. *Clin Gastroenterol Hepatol* **9(12)**: 1044–49. [doi: 10.1016/j.cgh.2011.08.014]

Blackburn L, *et al.* (2015) Fecal microbiota transplantation in patients with cancer undergoing treatment. *Clin J Oncol Nurs* **19(1)**: 111–14. [doi: 10.1188/15.CJON.111-114]

Borody TJ, *et al.* (1989) Bowel flora alteration: a potential cure of inflammatory bowel disease and irritable bowel syndrome? *Med J Aust* **150**: 604.

Borody TJ, Brandt LJ, Paramsothy S. (2014) Therapeutic faecal microbiota transplantation: current status and future developments. *Curr Opin Gastroenterol* **30(1):** 97–105. [doi: 10.1097/MOG.0000000000000027]

Brandt L, Reddy S. (2011) Fecal microbiota transplantation for recurrent *Clostridium difficile* infection. *J Clin Gastroenterol* **45(Suppl):** S159–S167.

FDA. (2013) Guidance for Industry: enforcement policy regarding investigational new drug requirements for use of fecal microbiota for transplantation to treat *Clostridium difficile* infection not responsive to standard therapies. www.fda.gov/BiologicsBloodVaccines/GuidanceComplianceRegulatory Information/Guidances/Vaccines/ucm361379.htm

Kelly CR, *et al.* (2014) Fecal microbiota transplant for treatment of *Clostridium difficile* infection in immunocompromised patients. *Am J Gastroenterol* **109(7):** 1065–71. [doi: 10.1038/ajg.2014.133]

Li Q, *et al.* (2015) Successful treatment of severe sepsis and diarrhea after vagotomy utilizing fecal microbiota transplantation: a case report. *Crit Care* **19(1):** 738. [doi: 10.1186/s13054-015-0738-7]

Louie T, Adams PC. (2008) Nature's therapy for recurrent *Clostridium difficile* diarrhea. *Can J Gastroenterol* **22(5):** 455–56.

Matsuoka K, *et al.* (2014) Fecal microbiota transplantation for gastrointestinal diseases. *Keio J Med* **63(4):** 69–74. [doi: 10.2302/kjm.2014-0006-RE]

McCombie AM. (2015) Coping strategies and psychological outcomes of patients with inflammatory bowel disease in the first 6 months after diagnosis. *Inflamm Bowel Dis*, June 19, 2015. [Epub ahead of print]

Pardi DS, *et al.* (2014) Ser-109, An oral, Microbiome-based therapeutic, is efficacious for the treatment of recurrent *C. difficile* and eliminates Enterobacteriacea and Vancomycin-resistant enterococci colonizing the gut. www.icaaconline.com/php/icaac2014abstracts/data/papers/2014/B-1875a. htm

Pinn DM, Aroniadis OC, Brandt LJ. (2015) Is fecal microbiota transplantation (FMT) an effective treatment for patients with functional gastrointestinal disorders (FGID)? *Neurogastroenterol Motil* **27(1):** 19–29. [doi: 10.1111/ nmo.12479]

Scaldaferri F, *et al.* (2015) P398. An Open-label, pilot study to assess feasibility and safety of fecal microbiota transplantation in patients with mild-moderate ulcerative colitis: preliminary results. *J Crohns Colitis* **9 Suppl 1:** S278. [doi: 10.1093/ecco-jcc/jju027.517]

Schmidt K, *et al.* (2015) Prebiotic intake reduces the waking cortisol response and alters emotional bias in healthy volunteers. *Psychopharmacology (Berl)* **232(10):** 1793–801. [doi: 10.1007/s00213-014-3810-0]

Singh R, *et al.* (2014) The potential beneficial role of faecal microbiota transplantation in diseases other than *Clostridium difficile* infection. *Clin Microbiol Infect* **20(11):** 1119–25. [doi: 10.1111/1469-0691.12799]

Smits LP, *et al.* (2013) Therapeutic potential of fecal microbiota transplantation. *Gastroenterology* **145(5):** 946–53. [doi: 10.1053/j.gastro.2013.08.058]

Varier RU, *et al.* (2015) Cost-effectiveness analysis of fecal microbiota transplantation for recurrent *Clostridium difficile* infection. *Infect Control Hosp Epidemiol* **36(4):** 438–44. [doi: 10.1017/ice.2014.80]

Wang J, Xiao Y, Lin K, *et al.* (2015) Pediatric severe pseudomembranous enteritis treated with fecal microbiota transplantation in a 13-month-old infant. *Biomed Rep* **3(2):** 173–75.

Youngster I, *et al.* (2014) Oral, capsulized, frozen fecal microbiota transplantation for relapsing *Clostridium difficile* infection. *JAMA* **312(17):** 1772–78. [doi: 10.1001/jama.2014.13875]

6 Overdiagnosis of ADHD: It's Their Mind, Not Yours

Your child is very active, happy, full of energy and excited about going to school. He/she (typically he) has been in a few tussles with a sibling, or a neighbor. Perhaps they challenge your authority. They may act up in school, and you have one or more sessions with a school counselor. You find them difficult to manage, and so while the news from the school is a disappointment, it is not a surprise, either. You worry. You meet with the teachers. They discuss the behavioral problems as "disruptive to other students' classroom experience." You cry. It's eating you up inside. You buy books on parenting. You lose sleep. Nothing seems to help. You want to help. You try to blame the teacher. You try to blame yourself. You try every tool in your parenting toolbox — you love your child, but nothing you try seems to help. So you seek some counseling. Or, on the advice of a counselor or teaching, or a parent with a child within similar behavior, you seek a diagnosis.

Your child is diagnosed with attention deficit hyperactivity disorder (ADHD). A physician offers a treatment, such as a prescription for Ritalin, or Adderall. Initially, the stimulant seems to calm the ADHD. Your child seems more attentive to the teacher, is to be able to focus better at school, and can sit down after school and complete their homework. They're doing better on their tests. Their grades improve. You are amazed at how simple the treatment is, and you might even berate yourself a little for not trying it sooner. But, overall, you feel great. You've made the right call, you can see the improvement. The improvement in class attentiveness is so dramatic, you feel that there might not be any more need for counseling. Your child feels better, too.

Over time though, you notice that your child becomes increasingly agitated, and restless, especially at night. The drug given to your child is, after all, a stimulant. So your counselor or doctor prescribes a sleep aid. Most likely, according to a study in 2010 by researchers at Brown Medical School in Providence, RI (Owens, 2010), they tend to prescribe alpha agonists (medications like clonidine).

If you accept the sleep aid for your child, you may not realize it, but your child is now on a pharmaceutical roller coaster: an "upper" to stay "normal," a "downer" to sleep. Initially the sleep aid seems to help. But the sleep is chemically induced sleep, not the deep, rapid eye movement (REM) sleep that is so important for a healthy mind. In fact, some sleep aids can shut down low-wave sleep patterns for months. Your child begins to suffer additional symptoms.

Without the proper amount of REM sleep, they may exhibit personality inconsistencies. They may suffer emotional detachment, become depressed. They are diagnosed with a "mood disorder." They may begin to hallucinate, develop suicidal ideation, or exhibit violent behavior. One in five children treated with these two combinations of drugs become aggressive or violent. Some become homicidal.

Your child may even be diagnosed with bipolar w/psychotic features. You're devastated, and you are told that it's imperative to get your child "help." The solution?

Most likely, *another* prescription for these symptoms (perhaps Zyproxa, or Rixpridol or drugs for depression).

According to the Owens study, children with mood disorders are most often treated with antipsychotics (e.g., Abilify), anticonvulsants (e.g., Tegretol or Neurontin), and short-acting hypnotics (e.g., Ambien). They are now on drugs to stay awake, drugs to fall asleep, and drugs to tolerate the side effects of these drugs.

In a very disturbing finding, Olfson and colleagues at Columbia University, in New York City, found that many youths diagnosed with bipolar disorder had taken one of these drugs a year before their diagnosis of bipolar disorder:

During the year before the new diagnosis of bipolar disorder, youths were commonly diagnosed as having depressive disorder (46.5%) or disruptive behavior disorder (36.7%) and had often filled a prescription for an antidepressant (48.5%), stimulant (33.0%), mood stabilizer (31.8%), or antipsychotic (29.1%).

Humans have been parenting children for as long as humans have existed on the planet. Some kids are highly spirited. Most kids struggle from time to time with school. Some kids can't sleep. Some kids may, in fact, have ADHD, and some kids are even bipolar. There is no doubt that these can be serious conditions. But there is also no doubt that these are also very serious drugs. Medication of children for behavioral issues was unheard of until the latter half of the 21st century.

The effects profile of a drug is the list of effects on the human mind and body, including side effects. The effects profile of the drugs most commonly prescribed for ADHD are identical to those of amphetamines (a.k.a. "speed"). Known side effects include delayed onset of sleep, mood swings and irritability. This treatment for ADHD robs your child of their sleep. ADHD patients tend to either have involuntary sleep disorders (such as restless leg syndrome), or apparently voluntary sleep disorders, such as REM behavioral disorder (willfully staying up too late, for example, playing video games or watching TV in their bedrooms).

What is ADHD?

ADHD is considered a developmental disorder with age-inappropriate behaviors, such as the inability to exhibit self-control, exhibiting disruptive behaviors, making quick decisions, restlessness, distractibility, and an inability to stay on task toward a specific goal, i.e., to focus. It is considered by some to be a permanent disorder, readily treatable with drugs.

The bulk of children do not have ADHD and, in a perfect world, accurate ADHD diagnosis would pick out those children who would benefit from some type of treatment from those students who do not qualify under established diagnostic criteria in the *DSM-V* and *ICD-10*.

When parents hear from teachers that their student can do better in school when given a treatment that will help them stay focused and achieve their goals, the temptation must be high. Every parent wants to help their children. Most parents can relate to an inability to capture and keep their children's attention, and get them to do what you tell them to do. How can they know whether the normal distractibility of their child — after all, they are not adults — is a developmental disorder worthy of clinical intervention?

Why is REM so Important?

Studies of REM interruption have shown that it can result in irritability. Extended periods of no sleep can result in a loss of a sense of being in touch with reality, and in psychosis. Sleep deprivation is so powerful it used as a tool in interrogation and "brainwashing." Children diagnosed with ADHD need REM sleep for learning and, more importantly, for proper brain development. Pre-adolescence and adolescence are the period of time in which the human mind learns methods for coping with the stresses of life. The hormones that cause puberty have a powerful effect on the human brain: The neocortex disassembles, and the re-assembly process takes time.

The science behind brain function and sleep support the notion that disrupted REM sleep can have profoundly negative influences. Studies have shown that when our brains are well rested due to proper REM sleep, we are better able to synthesize new knowledge with old (Karni, 1994). A lack of a good night's sleep, even if voluntary, is associated with poorer academic performance (Lee *et al.*, 2015). It appears that efficient (not long) sleep improves academic performance (Gruber *et al.*, 2014). We undergo cycles of brain wave patterns throughout the night. It is thought that these repetitive cycles are the brain reinforcing input it experienced during the day to create long-term memory.

The consequences of sleep deprivation on cognitive function have been very well studied (e.g., Durmur, 2005). These studies report a slew of broad cognitive performance deficits the result from sleep deprivation (Table 6.1).

The listed side effects of prescription sleeping pills such as Lunesta, Sonata, Ambien, Rozerem and Halcion may include daytime drowsiness, "impairment the next day," mental slowing or problems with attention or memory, and unusual dreams.

Restless leg syndrome (RLS) is found in a large percentage of ADHD patients (Durmur *et al.*, 2005; Gagliano *et al.*, 2011; Silvestri *et al.*, 2009; Chervin *et al.*, 2002). It is possible that sleep disorder leads to inattentiveness; thus, ensuring a good night's sleep and avoiding stimulants may be essential for treatment of ADHD (Chervin *et al.*, 2002). Teasing apart cause and effect can be tricky; that's why studies often

Table 6.1. Summary of Broad Cognitive Performance Effects of Sleep Deprivation

- Involuntary microsleeps occur
- Attention-intensive performance is unstable with increased errors of omission and commission
- Cognitive slowing occurs in subject-paced tasks, while time pressure increases cognitive errors
- Response time slows
- Both short-term recall and working memory performances decline
- Reduced learning (acquisition) of cognitive tasks
- Performance requiring divergent thinking deteriorates
- Response suppression errors increase in tasks primarily subserved by prefrontal cortex
- Response perseveration on ineffective solutions is more likely
- Increased compensatory effort is required to remain behaviorally effective
- Tasks may be begun well, but performance deteriorates as task duration increases
- There is growing neglect of activities judged to be nonessential (loss of situational awareness)

report "associations" and tend not to define one factor as a cause and the other as an effect.

However, RLS is known to be caused by diphenhydramine (Benadryl). So when increased incidence of RLS in ADHD patients is induced by a sleep aid, the known high rate of RLS in ADHD patients might be made worse, contributing further to sleep loss. We will revisit the potential links among the use of sleep aids, the reduction in REM sleep and the increased incidence of RLS in ADHD patients.

Effects of Amphetimine-Like Stimulants: Bad Sleep, More Drugs, More Side Effects

The stimulants typically used to "treat" ADHD are classified by the FDA in the same category as addictive drugs like amphetamines and cocaine. These drugs are known to cause a buildup of dopamine, and can lead to drug-induced psychosis or schizophrenia.

Dopamine is a key player for a good night's sleep. It is produced in the pineal gland — the seat of the body's internal clock. At night, it interacts with its receptors and stops the effects of norepinephrine, leading to release of melatonin. A more complete picture of how dopamine interactions with other proteins to prepare the brain for sleep, and how they interact to serve as a signal for the brain to wake up, is now available (Sergio González *et al.*, 2012).

Ritalin, Adderall and similar drugs act to increase dopamine, and they do lead to increased focused attention over the short-term. For patients with a *bona fide* genetic profile that predicts low dopamine production, increasing dopamine can work wonders for their academic performance in the short term.

However, playing with dopamine levels is tricky. In Parkinson's disease, cellular degeneration occurs in an area of the brain that produces dopamine (the substantia nigra). It is well known that in patients with Parkinson's treated with too much L-dopa, a precursor of dopamine, we can see schizophrenia-like psychosis (McKenna, 1997; Hasett *et al.*, 2005).

Side effects of drugs targeting dopamine production (L-dopa, Pramipexole and Ropinirole) include insomnia, hallucinations, and augmentation (worsening of the condition over time). They are no longer considered the first line of treatment for sleep disorders. The sedative hypnotic drug alternatives (Zaleplon, Zoplidem and Clonazepam) come with a risk of dependence and depression, and respiratory suppression. These drugs do not treat restlessness; they merely help your child sleep through the symptoms of nighttime restlessness. Alpha2 agonist drugs such as Catapres (Clonidine) bypass the dopamine system altogether and focus on impairing the sensation of nighttime restlessness itself.

ADHD is Overdiagnosed

In his book *Anatomy of an Epidemic*, Robert Whittaker points out that the rates at which Americans who would qualify under disability rules for psychiatric disabilities from 1900 to present are roughly as follows:

1900   1/1000
1950   1/500
2000   1/50

Is it even possibly correct that one in 50 Americans need some form of therapy or medication to correct a mental illness? This is tough question that is answered, in part, by a sobering statistic: 50% of seniors in nursing homes around the country are on some type of psychotropic drug. Can 50% of our elders really be so out of their minds that they need to be doped? A study in 2010 reported that within three months of admission, 71% of nursing home patients in Florida were being given at least one form of psychoactive medication, even if they had not previously been on those meds. Only 12% were on behavioral therapy. Remarkably, 15% were on *four or more such drugs* within three months of admission (Molinari *et al.*, 2010). Other statistics are chilling: The Centers for Medicare and Medicaid Services reported in 2010 that 39.4% of residents with no diagnosis of psychosis received antipsychotic drugs nationwide. Incredibly, 39.4% of people in nursing homes with no diagnosis of phychosis, and 15.9% of people with no cognitive impairment or behavior problems receive antipsychotic drugs (CMS, 2010). A smaller, but still significant percentage of residents not at high risk (15.6%) received antipsychotic drugs (CMS, 2010).

Currently, the percentage of residents in nursing home facilities on such medications that are given specifically antipsychotic drugs ranges from around 9.6% in Hawaii to over 25.3% in Texas (national median around 19%; NPR; Centers for Medicare and Medicaid Services; data for June 2014).

In 2005, the FDA issued a "Black Box" warning that atypical antipsychotics were never approved for use in the cases of dementia-related psychosis, and that the practice of their use in nursing homes should be stopped. These drugs are sometimes called "chemical restraints," leaving residents in a stupor, stripping them of any sign of their personality and of their dignity.

The inappropriate use of drugs imposes a heavy financial burden on Medicare and increases the likelihood of death of people in nursing homes due to falls, heart failure, stroke and infection. The FDA conducted a meta-analysis (FDA, 2009) and found that the use of atypical antipsychotics were associated with higher mortality in patients with behavioral disturbances in nursing homes. Around the same time, Liperoti *et al.* (2009) found that the use of classical antipsychotics was associated with higher mortality than even that associated with atypical antipsychotics.

"Why is Everyone so Lifeless around Here?"

These studies and statistics can tell only part of the story. Scenic Shores is a little facility (33 beds) in Two Harbors, Minnesota. In 2006, the facility hired a new nurse named Eva. In her first days at the facility, she observed how odd it was that she did not hear a single sound from any of the residents. Puzzled, she turned to her co-workers, and she asked simple questions: "Why is everyone so lifeless around here?" They are sedated, she was told. "Why is everyone sedated?"

The answer to the first question was that none of the patients were able to be responsive to their environment, or to those around them, because each one of them was on medicines that prevented them from interacting with others. The answer to the second question surprised her, and most of the staff. When she and the others at the facility began to look into the cases, they realized that few of the patients had a diagnosis accompanying their prescription that could support the treatment as clinically appropriate. Patients with no indication of psychosis were on antipsychotics; people with very little indication of behavioral issues were on hypnotics.

Eva and the others on the Scenic Shores staff approached the management with their observations. It was clear to all that, for both ethical and legal reasons, something had to change.

Through collaborative effort, mutual support and teamwork, the observations and concerns eventually led, in 2008, to a $3.1 million dollar 15-site pilot program funded by the Minnesota Department of Public Health. The goal of the pilot program was simple: to reduce the incidence of medication without supportive diagnosis.

In nursing homes around the country, many of our elderly are chronically medicated for symptoms presented months or years before the present, without regular case review. Thus, the relevance of their "treatment" is questionable, and their chronic unresponsiveness is a severe impediment to updating any real updates to clinical psychological care. In short, they are in both chemical and clinical limbo. At the beginning of the pilot program, the baseline percentage of residents in all 15 facilities that were medicated without clinical cause was 44%. Through mechanisms such as self-report score cards (with third-party validation), the program had a modest goal of a 20% reduction in inappropriate medication. By the end of the first quarter, the percentage dropped by 80%. By the end of the first year, the program had succeeded in reducing the rate by 90%.

Some of the most commonly asked questions about the program reveal the entrenchment of the incorrect and dangerous idea that nursing home residents require medication. "Surely you don't mean taken off medicine, you just changed the diagnosis, right?"

This is type of question most often fielded by Maria Reyes, a former nurse at one of the pilot sites for the Awakenings™ Program, and now it's Director.

I had the pleasure of chatting with Maria about the program's history, origins, and operations, and the science behind the studies. The answer to the skeptics' question, she says, is "No." Most patients who are taken off meds are not automatically put on new medicines. Most of the time, there is no new diagnosis. The focus is on reversing the adverse effects of unnecessary psychotropic drugs on the quality of life of the residents.

Again, statistics tell only part of the story. Sites where most of the residents were catatonic became filled with people smiling, talking, and interacting with the staff and with each other. Maria said yes, there were some behavioral episodes. When I asked how they were handled, I was not prepared for the very basic, but important reminder of the lessons on the sanctity of human life and respect for the dignity of the human spirit.

We learned that we — meaning the staff, and the management — were responsible for each and every behavioral episode in each patient.

I wondered how this could be so.

Every behavioral episode — outburst, anger, sulking, crying — was due to some specific, identifiable, unmet human need. As caregivers, it was our responsibility to meet those needs. We challenged ourselves to identify, and meet them. When the needs were fulfilled, the episodes stopped.

The elegant simplicity and obvious correctness of these thoughts made me pause and wonder what unmet human needs the children of our nation have that cause them to become over-medicated. Here was an organization will to take responsibility — and to do their jobs.

Maria said that the program succeeded in the pilot phases in most part because of the positive attitude adopted by all involved. They sensed that they could have a positive impact on many people's lives. If they were taking away the drugs, she said, they needed to provide good processes and alternative techniques to allow the staff to meet the human needs of the residents. In this sense, the program began fulfilling the provider needs of the staff, making them much more relevant to the well-being of the residents.

Maria sees the changes that were needed as the major cultural shifts they were. I asked her what the most important things were that helped the staff accept the pilot program. "Leadership, support from the top," she said. "We needed to adopt a judicious way of thinking. In the end, we decided to make physicians advocates of the residents."

Nurses, she said, were asked to question diagnoses and treatments. They were trained to ask questions of the doctors, such as "Why is this patient on these medicines?", and to question the diagnosis. They would ask: "Is a dose reduction possible?" If a patient had been on the same medicines for many years, they would ask: "Do we know if this diagnosis is still accurate, and that these medicines are still relevant?"

Alternatives to Sedative Geriatric Care

The program operates by transforming the environment and schedule of the patients to promote activity. The program includes social events, music therapy, art, light therapy, massage therapy, aromatherapy, and foot massages with lavender oil. "It sounds like a place I'd like to spend the weekend," I joked to Maria.

And that's exactly the point. These are care services for *people*, who are not automatically *patients*. "Many of the solutions that will help people," Maria said, "have been known to work for years".

"So these options are considered techniques," I asked. "What's the difference between a technique and a treatment?"

"A technique is a procedure that is used during the course of a treatment," she replied. "It's important, because you can get a technique wrong and do more harm than good. For example, if you walk into a room and a resident is crying, you can give them a hug and reassure them, all appropriate."

"Do you mind if I ask you a tough question?" I asked.

"Sure, I'm ready!" came the reply.

"Well," I started, "I have a sort of a crystal ball, and I can see, in the not-too-distant future, some of the people working for the drug companies complaining that it's not fair, the practitioners can offer these therapies while they have to spend millions on clinical trials every year. Won't they demand evidence from randomized placebo-controlled clinical trials? Won't they demand a warning letter from the FDA because these programs will cut into their profits?"

She was indeed ready.

We have a number of clinical studies focused on these non-pharmacological practices. First, researchers at Notre Dame are validating our reported findings. Second, a long-term prospective clinical trial is being conducted by the University of Minnesota. They will quantify outcomes according to specific measures — not general ones like answers to questions such as "do you consider anyone here to be your friend?"

"Do you mean, like the number of activities participated in per day, number of self-care steps taken per day, or number of conversations per day?"

"Yes, those would all be good measures of outcome," she replied enthusiastically.

One of the most touching aspects of the program is that the staff place familiar but surprising items — treasures — in drawers in the back of the room, so residents — many of whom are experiencing dementia — can satisfy the common, agitated urge to look for "something." Quite often, when they "discover" a trinket, a toy, a recipe book or a small stuffed animal, their reaction is one of "aha, this is what I have been seeking!" and they are calm and satisfied.

This is one of those rare cases in which observational science may be sufficient. There is no control group; it would unethical to give any of these patients psychotropic drugs without a prescription, and knowing that there is no diagnosis to support the administration of these drugs takes ethical and moral precedent over the strictures of clinical research. The comparison to baseline analyses — comparing the outcomes in the before-and-after setting is the only type of analysis that could be done. Comparison of levels of activities to any other nursing home in the Ecumen system should compel individuals involved in providing care to the ethical discontinuation of any drug not supported by a diagnosis. The differences, however, are obvious.

Keeping the majority of nursing home patients on antipsychotic and hypnotic drugs may soon be a thing of the past. Under these drugs, residents are extremely unresponsive to stimuli — they don't do things, they don't talk, they don't explore their surroundings. This program has transformed the lives of the participants. I am not sure how to measure that kind of beauty, but the contrast to inappropriately sedated elderly people is impressive.

In addition to talking, interacting, and doing small but important things for themselves, they even start taking care of themselves. The program is a stunning success, with 97% reduction in the use of drugs to manage residents. These drugs are not used to *treat* patients; they are used to control them. Certainly due to the FDA's warning that antipsychotic drugs are not to be prescribed as treatment for people with dementia, nursing homes cannot return to the past in which drugs are used so easily just to keep residents calm.

In the US, the CMS is exploring similar approaches for a national program, including the use of Individualized Music Therapy — providing residents with access to music they preferred before their entry into the nursing home. Music has the ability to transform quiet, unresponsive patients into smiling, laughing and singing individuals. I have witnessed this transformation personally — I occasionally play music at nursing homes around the Pittsburgh region. One evening, a few days before

Christmas, my friend and sometime music partner Richard Kobertz played an evening of Christmas music at Orion Nursing Home, and to match interest with the crowd, we played a few John Denver songs, and some originals. One resident in particular seemed to be enjoying herself especially. During a break, the staff came to us in tears, stating that she had not smiled, or laughed, or even moved in the two-year period prior to our performance. I was moved to tears myself.

What are we doing to our seniors by denying them a life of social interactions so they are more easily "managed?" We are denying them an existence. Even criminals in prison are given recreational time, exercise and social activities.

The Awakenings Program appears to be a viable alternative to sedative geriatric care. In 2012, CMS announced a partnership to improve dementia care in nursing homes, including time outdoors and planning individualized activities with a goal of reducing inappropriate use of drugs in the care of the elderly nationwide. During her descriptions of the alternative programs, Maria used the words "techniques" and "non-pharmaceutical practices."

This is the language and culture that must translate over into education.

Maria was fiercely proactive in her position, positive, and filled with hope. She shared with me the similarities of the resistance on the part of the staff for the adoption of non-pharmaceutical practices in elderly care and the resistance she experienced in just talking with teachers about what might be done to help her son's apparent ADHD without prescription.

I was told they didn't have the staff, the class sizes were too big. And I understand. Schools today are very different then when I was in school. They have so many things to deal with that we didn't, with school shootings, and the effects of social media. It's not like a school anymore — there are more security and control issues, it's very different than when I was in school.

What are we doing to our childrens' brains and minds by making them more attentive in school with drugs? I'm a scientist, and my goal in setting out to write this book was to identify medically successful translational successes in biomedical research in the context of profit-driven research. As I researched ADHD, it rapidly became apparent to me that this would be a tall order. Where in the ADHD research is the silver lining? The public cannot feel good about diagnosis rates of ADHD, and the effects of psychotropic drugs on our children. What did the clinical trial research say?

In reviewing the history of the controversy of the question of ADHD overdiagnosis in the US, I found that retaining my objectivity was doubly difficult. I am the father of two sometimes spirited adolescents. As a product of an abusive home, however, I have found the spirited youth for my boys to be both challenging, and fulfilling. Keeping up with them is sometimes hard, but I'm only their dad, so I try to keep up.

Maria's son was originally diagnosed with ADHD; she told me that he "outgrew" it, and that while he was on it, Ritalin did little for his attention, as far as she could tell. The first response in many crises, she says, seems to be to seek the answer in a pill. So I asked her what she thought it would take to bring this culture of care to the problem of ADHD overdiagnosis.

> First, you need 100% buy-in from the top. You need a change in the way of thinking. While there is more work up front, I tell my staff that I'm not asking to do extra. I let them know that I'm asking them to do things differently. And the cost savings to payers is huge. In the first pilot program, we saved payers — families, insurance companies, and Medicaid/Medicare — $250,000 to $380,000 per month.

That's right. *Per month.*

Those were just the cost savings from the cost of the actual prescriptions. Add to that the fact that patients on these drugs have high accident rates (falls), comorbidity due to stroke, pneumonia, diabetes, and other side effects, and the cost is much higher. Maria described how using psychotropic medicines actually leads to a lot more work — the residents are not "there" to help you help themselves.

"It's all about planning the seeds of change," Maria said.

It is clear that making the caregivers the advocates of the residents as residents first, and as patients second (contingent upon a fully accurate diagnosis) was critical in the operation. Who are the advocates for the students as students first, patients last (checking and insuring an accurate diagnosis)? The school nurse? The teachers? The clinicians? The parents? I believe the answer has to be all of the above.

I went into this review of the literature hopeful that I could find some good news. After digesting the facts, the trends, the controversies, and the studies, the best phrase that I can think of to describe the early years of the controversy is "street fight." We'll come back to that later.

There are numerous instances in which people working on behalf of drug companies claim to know that ADHD is not overdiagnosed in the US. It's easy to say that the ADHD drug market is a multi-million dollar market worldwide. That in and of itself cannot be used to condemn the practice of treating ADHD with drugs. However, for the proponents of medication, the rates of ADHD in America are not too high. National estimates stand at between 10% and 14%, depending on the source; in some places, 20% of boys have been diagnosed with ADHD.

Over the last decade, however, the number of cases of childhood ADHD in the US has increased 40%. It has increased over 50% in the last 25 years.

When those numbers are compared to the global estimates of rates of ADHD of 5% (Polanczyk *et al.*, 2007), something seems terribly wrong. While we can't dismiss an increased awareness of mental issues, which could explain increased rates of detection, these rates in the US fly in the face of reason. A study in 2010 estimated that as many as one million children in the US are misdiagnosed with ADHD (Elder *et al.*, 2010).

Given the seriousness of the effects of the drugs for treating ADHD, we must take a closer look at the research that has been done.

Are Females Really Underdiagnosed?

Proponents of the medication route often cite the lower rates of diagnoses in females as evidence of a "problem" of underdiagnosis of females in the US. However, this interpretation requires first that we accept that the rate of diagnosis in males is correct, a dubious conclusion at best.

Citing rates, however, is mere argumentation and can lead only to stalemate, because no one knows the true percentage of children with ADHD. Critics of the reports of surveys showing increased rates of diagnosis have, in the past, made the counter-claim that expressions of concern of overdiagnosis may prevent children with ADHD from getting the treatment they need by scaring parents away from the drugs.

From a purely logical, scientific point of view, that position does not make sense, and it begs the question of overdiagnosis. The role of scientists should be to determine, for any medical diagnostic, the true positive rate (sensitivity), the false positive rate (specificity), and other performance evaluation characteristics. For severe cases of ADHD, psychotropic drugs may indeed help. But given the serious nature of adverse events (undesirable development or worsening of a medical condition) associated with these drugs, widespread concern of overdiagnosis and overtreatment, numbers like 10–14% ADHD with 85% psychotropic drug treatment seem too high.

Perhaps an analogy away from ADHD would help with the seriousness of this wrongful medication. Some institutions have been charged with overdiagnosing women for pap smears. Pap smears are follow-up tests for cervical cancer. A potentially positive cervical exam leads to a secondary test (the smear) that is used as evidence for, or against, cervical cancer. Any institution that has too high a false positive rate given the cervical exam could be charged with being a "pap smear mill."

But the analogy does not go far enough. Overdiagnosis is one thing. Over treatment of a population is another thing altogether. In the case of cervical cancer, patients will certainly have had a confirming biopsy. Some might have had their uterus removed. Pathologists examine every cell in slices of the cervical tissue to full characterize the nature and extent of the cancer.

Now imagine for a moment if this confirmatory step were omitted. If cancer were treated like ADHD, suspicion of cancer would lead chemotherapy. There would be no confirmatory test; the diagnosis could be based on initial observations, and the patient would be given life-altering and life-threatening drugs without, evidently, any concern whatsoever as to whether her diagnosis is correct. Imagine chemotherapy without confirmation. That's what diagnosing 14% of children (or more, locally) and treating 85% of children diagnosed with ADHD with psychostimulants is like: It's not overmedication. It's *wrongful* medication.

Lee and *Lacasse Castigate* the New York Times as *Complicit via Shallow Reporting*

In a stunning indictment of modern journalism, two experts in cognitive sciences, Lee and Lacasse, take the *New York Times* to task for coming late to the party on reporting ADHD overdiagnosis — by 15 years. Their article (Lee and Lacasse, 2015) hits hard:

> *The pharmaceutical companies are not alone when it comes to promoting the medical model. "The New-York-Times" has a long history of giving preferential treatment to the idea that ADHD is a fundamental flaw in a person's biology. Only recently can one sense skepticism of this idea within the pages of the "Times". Over the past several years*

they have started to publish more guest commentaries critical of the ADHD label, and even their own newsroom staff is starting to take a broader view of ADHD. Alan Schwarz, a Times reporter, has recently written a series of provocative articles on ADHD. His articles have covered overdiagnosis, the adverse effects of psychiatric medication, and the marketing of ADHD. Mr. Schwarz's articles have attracted substantial attention and he has appeared on media programs such as "Democracy-Now" to publicize his work.

As academics who have published critiques of the ADHD enterprise over the past 15 years, we have watched the Times' coverage with great interest. It is heartening that they are finally taking a broader view of the issues. However, the fact that the Times has finally begun to report on ADHD with some skepticism, echoing what critics have been saying for decades — calls attention to the belated nature of their current reporting. Even with their new found skepticism, instead of acknowledging the extensive community of ADHD critics, the Times still turns to the original proponents of ADHD for commentary.

They include references to the *Times'* continued use of so-called Key Opinion Leaders even after the consensus of overdiagnosis was sealed, including one who had been found to have participated in a ghost-written study on Paxil that eventually led a US Department of Justice to impose a US$3 billion dollar fine on GlaxoSmithKline (GSK). GSK was found to have conducted research fraud and to have used illegal advertising in which they misstated facts and made false claims about Paxil's efficacy for children. Lee and Lacasse made note that the *Times* made use of Dr. Harold Koplewicz as a mental health expert six years after the GSK finding.

What brought about this type of retrospective analysis? Lee and Lacasse were reacting, in part, to an article published in the *Times* in December 2013, "The Selling of Attention Deficit Disorder," in which Schwarz reports the entire terrible fiasco leading to an epidemic of false diagnosis and overmedication.

What Causes ADHD?

Those who have argued against the evidence for overdiagnosis also attempt to minimize the effects of the environment. For them, ADHD is a neurogenetic disorder, and those with the disorder are destined to continuously be disabled in their ability to focus. For them, one cannot outgrow ADHD. There have been at least 16 studies that have shown a child's environment can influence the degree of ADHD (Nigg *et al.*, 2010). It is worth noting that there are at least 16 genes that have variants that are associated with ADHD (Nigg *et al.*, 2010). This alone suggests that individualized treatment — treating the actual source of the symptoms, guided by molecular genotyping — should be taken up in the future. However, Nigg *et al.* also summarize environmental factors supported by the 16 studies: They list four prenatal, four perinatal, and 11 post-natal environmental effect candidates for ADHD:

- *Prenatal: Tobacco use, alcohol use, pollution, maternal stress.*
- *Perinatal: Perinatal complications, low birth weight, hypoxic ischemia, parenchymal lesion.*
- *Post-natal: Lead exposure, manganese exposure, mercury exposure, diet, parenting, family/marital conflict, adversity, maltreatment, and TV/video.*

Social factors matter in the appearance and the severity of ADHD. Genetic X Environment interaction (G x E) involve interaction of genes and environmental factors, derived from variation impacting bona fide ADHD patients. Such factors would likely include parenting style, parenting behavior (modeling), teaching styles, and genetics. The rational position to adopt in the absence of evidence is not to dismiss environmental factors; instead it is to state ignorance, and call for the research to be done.

That said, there is evidence that for *bona fide* ADHD patients, genetic factors do appear to play a role. Having a genetic factor, however, does not make it a deterministic trait; it can be modified by other genes, and the environment. There is wide variation geographically in the rates of ADHD diagnosis, and heterogeneity in its expression among patients.

Given the complex nature of this disorder, for a proper diagnosis of ADHD, the behavior must be

- Persistent (lasting more than six months),
- Pervasive (not restricted to a single setting, such as school)
- Impairing (affecting school performance and/or ability to learn life skills), and importantly
- Not attributable to other conditions or factors.

On the face of it, it is hard to accept that 14% of any nation's population of children have a mental disorder sufficiently serious to warrant psychotropic drugs. If there is systemic overdiagnosis of ADHD, what could be driving it?

Are Teachers Partly to Blame for Overdiagnosis?

The short-term positive effects of stimulants on academic performance are not in question (e.g., Molina *et al.*, 2009); their combined utility on patients with *bona fide* ADHD, in combination with behavioral modification and therapy, is well known (e.g., Kolko *et al.*, 1999). There is some question as to the long-term differences between those medicated and those given only therapy. The side effects of stimulants are well-characterized as well; they include delayed growth, which would likely influence any adolescence's self-esteem. The higher incidence of RLS in ADHD patients, loss of REM sleep and use of sleep aids in ADHD patients deserves close scrutiny, especially because the upswing in ADHD overdiagnosis is likely artificial (cultural), not biological.

However, a study of the approval process of drugs like Adderall and Ritalin conducted at Boston's Children's Hospital (Bourgeois *et al.*, 2014) found that the FDA has been extremely lax on the standards used for the approval of drugs for ADHD. Many trials had far too short of a duration to assess any long-term negative (adverse) effects. Also, many were too small to provide sufficient power (ability to detect) adverse effects. Quoting directly from their study:

> *A total of 32 clinical trials were conducted for the approval of 20 ADHD drugs. The median number of participants studied per drug was 75... Eleven drugs (55%) were approved after 100 participants were studied and 14 (70%) after 300 participants. The median trial length prior to approval was 4 weeks (IQR 2, 9), with 5 (38%) drugs approved after participants were studied 4 weeks and 10 (77%) after 6 months. Six drugs were approved with requests for specific additional post-marketing trials, of which 2 were performed.*

These findings are remarkable, given the FDA's long-standing preference and requirement of large studies with sufficient focus on adverse events. Bourgeois (*et al.*, 2014) also reported a stunning fact:

> *Biphetamine was previously approved as an anorectic in adults, but the original approval package does not include safety assessments in children and ADHD was added as an indication in product labels starting in 1979 <u>without supporting clinical trials</u>. Adderall was originally approved in 1960 as an anorectic under the trade name Obetrol before being marketed without FDA approval as Adderall for the treatment of ADHD. Approval was subsequently obtained **<u>without clinical trials assessing its safety in children or efficacy in ADHD</u>**.*

Subsequent trials, they report, fell far below the standards for market approval. Essentially, these drugs are at Phase II of the typical drug approval process. If therapists and parents knew of the lax standards by which ADHD drugs were approved by the FDA, they would never prescribe these drugs because we do not really yet know the long-term effects.

That means that these drugs are prescribed off-label to treat a condition for which they were never approved. While that it not illegal, it is illegal for drug companies to advertise the use of these drugs to treat conditions for which there is no Phase III evidence.

To avoid serious consequences of withdrawal, concerned parents should never remove their child from these types of drugs without close supervision of a therapist.

Factors Contributing to Overdiagnosis in the US

One of the hypotheses for the cause of overdiagnosis of ADHD comes from the observation of mechanisms of funding in school- and state-wide performance levels on standardized tests and the ADHD rates (Hinshaw *et al.*, 2009). Disturbingly, they found that ADHD tends to be more frequently found in students in schools that operate under the threat of funding cuts due to low overall standardized test performance. This was a study in which the authors cite the correlative finding as a "smoking gun." No factor other than the pressure from standardized testing correlated with ADHD diagnosis rates. The authors of that study have written a book *The ADHD Explosion* (Hinshaw *et al.*, 2014) that reviews the trends of overdiagnosis in much greater detail.

The push for higher performance in school and the need for a good night's sleep may be satisfied by something as simple as a later start time for school. Meltzer *et al.*, (2010) found that students who started school later and who did not have technology in their bedrooms had better sleep hygiene habits.

There is also a pattern within schools: Teachers tend to refer younger students for consideration for ADHD diagnosis with higher frequency, further revealing teacher perception bias (Elder, 2010). This is the same finding of LeFever *et al.* (1999): Among the elementary students in Virginia Beach elementary school, children who were young for their grade were 23 times more likely to be medicated for ADHD. A remarkable 63% of "young for grade" students were being medicated for ADHD at the time.

Anxious Parents Give More than Genes: Compound Gene/Environment Interactions as Risk Factors?

But the "blame" for overdiagnosis and overtreatment, if there is any to be had, cannot rest on the shoulders of educators alone. The diagnosis of ADHD is also higher in families with anxious and stressed mothers (Glover, 2011). Here things get tricky, in light of the findings of genetic links to the risk of ADHD.

If ever there was a phenotype that was plastic, the mind is the place to look. Phenotypic plasticity is the conditional expression of a genotype in the context of an environment. The presence of a stressed parent may be correlated with increased ADHD diagnosis. It has also been noted that stressed parents may be more prone to accepting the recommendation of a solution for behavioral problems in the form of a pill. That is not to say they have not tried other routes, but it is to say that both parents and doctors have tended to perceive the option of giving children pills as being relatively easy.

There is another reason why parents of spirited children may be less able to cope with the anxieties of parenting, thus contributing to the likelihood of the phenotypic expression of an ADHD genotype. The nature of the genetic association itself making teasing apart causal factors challenging; however, a child with a genetic profile correlated with ADHD is more likely to have one or more parents with a similar genetic profile; therefore, is the occurrence of ADHD in the child due to the mind functions of the child (i.e., a genetic disease burden), or is it the product of an ADHD parent's poor parenting style? The overall genetic risk contribution is 20%, not nearly 80% as some drug proponents would have us believe. Children learn boundaries when consequences for undesirable behavior are clear, consistent, and delivered in a timely manner after the undesired behavior. It may also be a response on the part of the parent to the suggestion that a drug can "fix" what's "wrong" with their child — followed by a relative inability to see cause and correlation for the lack of sleep due to the stimulant, the up/down/withdrawal cycles that occur due to stimulant/depressants cycles, and the final bipolarity that may be likely due to a failure of proper brain development due to improper rest. Bipolar disorder may be comorbid with ADHD treatments, as opposed to ADHD.

Some authors (e.g., Warner, 2012) are worried that discussion of the impact that parents might have on their children could lead to a return to an era of stigmatization of parents who are held accountable for their inability to parent effectively. My analysis of the issues with overdiagnosis does not include those parents that Judith Warner, in her book *We've Got Issues* (Riverhead), cites as having held out as long as possible before medicating their children. The risk of stigmatization may be real, but can we really expect to come to understand complex mental issues like ADHD if any one of a child's major environmental influences is off the table?

Parental behavior has never been considered a taboo subject for objective, empirical research. It is an oft-studied factor in other areas such as alcohol use (Sørensen *et al.* 2011), tobacco use (Scherrer *et al.*, 2012), sexual risks (Elkington *et al.*, 2011; Murry *et al.*, 2013), smoking and antisocial behaviors (Pagani *et al.* 2013), smoking and inner ear infection (Hammarén-Malmi *et al.*, 2005; Murphy, 2006, and many recent studies), smoking and leukemia (Chang *et al.*, 2009), modes of expression of anger (Feldman *et al.*, 2011), adolescent self-esteem (McClure *et al.*, 2010), eating disorders (Horesh *et al.*, 2015; Tseng *et al.*, 2014) and suicide (Torjesen *et al.*, 2015). The knowledge that a parent's behavior can influence such behaviors adds significantly to the tools in the toolbox for reducing the incidence of bad outcomes.

First Alternatives to Drugs

Are some parents more prone than others to seek a diagnosis in the first place, and are some more ready to accept a drug treatment for something as complex as a developing child's mind? This must be made into, and considered, a scientific, not a cultural question. Taking individual parents out of it, the scale of the rates of misdiagnosis and over-medica-tion of children make these issues a matter of public health. If parents are never offered alternatives by the teachers, counselors, or therapists, what other options do they have?

Pharma's Illogical Responses

It is important to realize that the issue in ADHD is one of overdiagnosis. While many diseases may be mis-diagnosed, this is not an acceptable excuse for willfully ignoring the resulting overmedication. The concern of overdiagnosis cannot be answered with arguments such as "but the medication works, and ADHD patients benefit." Such argumentation does not address the point of the question: the potential harm done via wrongful medication when the diagnosis is incorrect.

Further, the question of parental contribution is met with charges that someone is trying to "blame" the parents. I don't know of anyone who is serious about research in ADHD who thinks of parental contri-bution to a child's environment as "blame." The question is not one of blame; it is one of increased understanding of environmental factors. The "diagnose and drug" advocates want us to believe there is noth-ing that can be done with or for a child in their environment that can help with ADHD. They would like us to believe ADHD is 80%–100% genetic, and that there are no environmental influences at all. According to their talking points, nothing a parent does can help alleviate their child's suffering from ADHD.

One "Key Opinion Leader" recently sarcastically told a group of parents that if he hears one more time that meditation can help with ADHD, he was "going to puke." While the statement elicited laugh-ter from the parents, this was not a professional, serious objective and logical assessment of the realities of what is known and what is not yet known of the interactions between genes and the environment on some-thing as complex as the human mind. It's not science. It's showmanship, evocative of emotion, and pure advertisement. Scientists do not need to resort to such raw, emotive statements to elicit understanding. The position that ADHD is a fixed condition, unalterable by any change in child's environment, could be taken by some to relieve parents of any responsibility whatsoever for helping their children cope.

Some parents believe that a good test of attentiveness for any child is whether they can sit still and play video games for hours on end. The field has attributed the attentiveness that a child can display on video games to "addiction." But where is the objective scientific evidence that the type of attentiveness a child can display at video games is not the same type of attentiveness needed to learn? A study by Bioulac *et al.* (2014) compared the focus ability of ADHD-diagnosed children with a non-ADHD control group of children at two tasks: playing three commercial video games and a "continuous performance test" called the CPT II. Compared to commercial video games, the CPT II is extremely dull, monotonous, and repetitive. The user is simply asked to press the space bar or click a button if any symbol other than "X" appears on the screen. Without, I hope, appearing to sound as if I am romanticizing ADHD, do we really want to "normalize" our children so they are better able to perform dull, monotonous, meaningless tasks like the CPT-II? Or do we want prepare our children for a dynamic world with multiple information inputs and demands on complex problem solving?

Another study (Haghbin *et al.*, 2013) examined the relationships among self-control, video game addiction and academic achievement comparing normal and ADHD-diagnosed students. They failed to find a strong direct causal association between video game addiction and academic performance in either group, though they did note that a correlative effect likely exists in that children who spend excessive time playing video games have less time availabe to engage in academic work. A more recent study (Brunborg *et al.*, 2014) observed that when "addiction" is distinguished from "extensive use," a clear association is found between addiction and academic performance, but not overall time spent, but those authors, also, balked at the use of the word "cause." The field consensus is that demonstration of cause vs. correlation will be very difficult in this population to tease apart — a high degree of collinearity exists among the variables, and the timing of events in life is important (e.g., ADHD patients, who already demonstrate lower academic performance, may turn to video game use as a result of their perceived low performance, desire for control over the time, etc.).

A company in Boston, Akili Interactive Labs, is turning the prevailing view that video game "addiction" in ADHD patients is bad on its head. They have created a video game that gets harder — challenges the player more the better they get. Its purpose is to activate multiple types of higher-order cognitive processes and problem solving, which can give the very active mind the satisfaction at problem solving such a mind can crave. The game currently provides a score that reveals the mind's "multitasking deficit." An ADHD mind will exhibit an inability — in the context of the game — to pay attention to multiple types of information. It is being studied in clinical trials for diagnosis of cognitive function deficits in both Alzheimer's disease and ADHD. While the game is not prescriptive, however, speculation is that it could be made into a biofeedback tool that might help train the brain to be better able to multitask. If children can stay attentive given sufficient stimulating problems to solve, it would seem warranted to conclude that under the right stimuli, their brain can, in fact, focus appropriately without medication. The entire repertoire of children's behaviors should be considered by physicians, counselors, and parents, not just during times when a teacher wishes that they could sit still and focus.

Are Key Opinion Leaders de Facto Advertisements for Off-Label Use?

In July 2013, GlaxoSmithKline was fined $3 billion for promoting antidepressants and other drugs for unapproved uses; a month later, Johnson & Johnson agreed to a $181 million consumer fraud settlement with

36 states and the District of Columbia over its off-label marketing of Risperdal, an antipsychotic drug.

The Key Opinion Leader in question leaves the distinct impression of a walking billboard for amphetamine use for off-label treatment of ADHD. The longitudinal studies that have been done, in fact, do not support the efficacy of long-term amphetamine use, and they indicate and support serious adverse effects. Most clinicians are familiar with the first year report of the MTA study, but few seem to be aware of the more important follow-up sixth and eighth year reports. The most important study, and the one that all practicing clinicians should read and digest in its entirety, was published in 2009 in the *Journal of the American Academy of Child and Adolescent Psychiatry* (Brooke *et al.*, 2009). In these reports, the initial benefits of amphetamine were observed to decline over time, drawing into question the efficacy of psychotropic drugs for the treatment of ADHD.

The study used randomly selected students similar to those enrolled in the treatment group. The expectation was that the MTA protocol for community-supervised administration of medications would help alleviate, in the long-term, the symptoms of ADHD. The study failed to find this outcome. Instead, they reported:

- Increased psychiatric hospitalizations
- Lower GPA
- Increased delinquency
- Increase in arrests
- Increased grade retentions

In fact, the medicated group scores were worse than control on 91% of the variables tested. The authors concluded:

> *Our findings suggest that community treatments can improve ADHD symptoms and associated impairment, but even when preceded by intensive medication management and/or behavioral therapy for*

14 months, continuing community interventions are unable on average
to "normalize" children with ADHD.

The science done in the study was haphazard; the study became an observation study mid-course, with families being allowed to adhere to the treatments based on their choice, not based on their enrollment. Rather than accept their own results at face value, the authors tended to cite a lack of evidence of support for "community administered medication" as opposed to the lack of efficacy of the medication. Further, they cite a *potential* (i.e., unmeasured, untested for) source of bias called selection bias as a likely factor responsible for the result. In essence, without any additional data, they concluded that somehow the students in the treatment group self-selected toward the variables in question in their decision to continue or discontinue medication. However, if the patients in the study tended to discontinue the use of medication, they cite poor adherence to medication across the board in ADHD patients, and thus the finding of inefficacy and poor outcomes are highly relevant for the clinical population. There does appear to be a minority of ADHD-diagnosed students who did well, but this would be post-hoc subset analysis, which is generally eschewed by the FDA.

In their new book *Psychiatry Under the Influence: Institutional Corruption, Social Injury, and Prescriptions for Reform*, Whittaker and Cosgrove (2015) further dissect the inconsistencies in the reporting of the results in the Abstract (summary) of the study compared to the results reported in the full paper.

Key Opinion Leaders who push amphetamines also (1) down-play overdiagnosis, (2) do not also share the key findings of the long-term MTA study, and thus are very likely to be presenting sponsored endorsements, a.k.a. advertisements. While off-label use by doctors is legal, providing misleading written statements on the safety and efficacy of drugs to doctors and consumers off label is illegal.

Verbal speech is another matter. The courts in the US have sided with drug companies in their efforts to retain first amendment freedom of speech rights of paid personnel (salespersons) for discussing off-label uses. In 2005, a salesperson named Mr. Caronia for Orphan Medical (now acquired by Jazz Pharmaceutical) was recorded by a doctor, who was also a government informant, of promoting a drug called Xyrem as a treatment for insomnia, fibromyalgia and other conditions. The drug was only approved for use in the treatment of narcolepsy (sudden sleep syndrome). Mr. Caronia was convicted by a jury in 2008, and appealed his conviction claiming freedom of speech violations.

The Food, Drug and Cosmetic Act (1938, and amended) gave the FDA the authority to regulate drugs. Misbranding drugs and selling a drug specifically to treat conditions not listed on the label is illegal. While doctors may prescribe a drug for any use, Mr. Caronia was tried, and convicted, on the grounds of showing intent for the sale of Xyrem for off-label use. The Second Circuit overturned the conviction, citing among other things that free speech violations were evidence (basically stating that discussing (verbally) off-label use does not show intent, that only actual mis-labeling a drug is required to prove intent to break the law).

"The government clearly prosecuted Caronia for his words — for his speech," the majority wrote, adding that "the government cannot prosecute pharmaceutical manufacturers and their representatives under the FDCA for speech promoting the lawful, off-label use of an FDA-approved drug."

The Matter of Wrongful Treatment in ADHD

It's legal to play fast and loose with verbal statements, and it is of course legal to offer incorrect and misleading interpretations of data from clinical studies that go against commercial interest. We live in an open society, and therefore we are subject to the gains and pains of debates and discussions — including the risk of being lied to. However, while off-label use of amphetamines may be legal, and discussions of off-label use may be protected by the First Amendment, unwarranted treatment of a patient without a condition is not legal, even if a clinical writes a script (see Chapter 1). If most of our discussions focus on the aspects of incomplete diagnoses leading to inappropriate treatments, we will likely see reform, and more children will be protected from harm.

Overtreatment, wrongful treatment, and legal issues aside, the main point of this chapter is ADHD overdiagnosis because it leads to wrongful treatment. Science that could also be done to help answers questions on the problem of overdiagnosis has not been done. No one, for example, has asked about the factors in schools that might make a teacher more or less likely to suggest a diagnosis of ADHD to parents. Beyond the fact that teachers should never diagnose a student because they are not professional clinicians, there are interest questions. Do teachers of different subjects (Science, Math, Reading, English, History, Art, Physical Education) all suggest counseling or clinical help for children that they suspect may have ADHD at the same rates, or are there differences? If there are differences, what can they attributed to? Are there significant differences between the referral rates of teachers who teach morning and afternoon? Does teacher gender play a role? What can be done to the curriculum to mitigate the effects of the structure of the curriculum on the true positive ADHD students in the classroom? Should students be given physical activity first thing in the morning? Is there an interaction between specific subjects and the time of day that they are taught for optimal overall education? These are *scientific,* not *cultural* (i.e., blame game) questions, and are not beyond the conveyance of objective scientific inquiry.

Parents and teachers alike should be made aware that there are additional first options that they may wish to try — with persistence — before turning to drugs. When I was a child, my teacher would, most days, pull the curtains and have the entire class put their heads on the desk for five or 10 minutes. The effect on the classroom was remarkable. Humans have gland that is responsive to light (the pineal gland), and reducing the light for even a brief period of time can have a calming effect. Meditation is a powerful technique that can be used to be more mindful and achieve more control over one's thought processes.

A number of studies have found that mindful meditation can reduce self-reported symptoms of ADHD, including clinician ratings of ADHD and executive function symptoms (Zylowska *et al.*, 2008; Mitchell *et al.*, 2013). This science flies in the face of the "diagnose and drug" part of the ADHD community. Two randomized clinical trials support yoga as effective in helping ADHD patients (Haffner *et al.*, 2006; Jensen *et al.*, 2004). Again, a counterpoint study exists that should be cited by anyone presenting information to parents of ADHD children. A 15-week course in Tai-chi exercises has been shown to improve attentiveness, but not impulsivity, in ADHD in young adults (Converse *et al.*, 2014). Anyone who ignores these studies and presents visceral disgust at the idea of such techniques as a counter-argument in lieu of rational discourse should be seen as motivated to willfully dismiss possibilities, especially if they have financial conflicts of interest.

Frank (i.e., true) ADHD does have a heritable component — but not as high as often reported (heritability — as high as 70%). What portion is genetic and what portion is adoption of behavioral norms within families is not sufficiently studied. A study of genetic variants concluded that only up to 9% of all ADHD patients are likely to benefit from stimulants (Arcos-Burgos *et al.*, 2010a) via a specific molecular mechanism involving the latrophilin 3 gene (LPHN3). Most cases of ADHD do not have the same variant, and thus it is a heterogenous condition with likely a multitude of possible metabolic pathways to the same symptoms. At least 10 different genes have been found to have variants associated with ADHD risk (Arcos-Burgos *et al.*, 2010b). Thus, even a correct diagnosis of "ADHD" could lead to an ineffective or counterproductive treatment — the wrong drug aimed at the wrong patient.

Mental health treatment and research on treatments should certainly include consideration of parenting style, parent self-assessment of anxiety and stress, and in-home and in-school environmental factors. If the findings indicate increase risk due to anxious and stressed parents, the illness is better understood and, even better, it may prevented in some cases via modification of those factors. Once a *bona fide* diagnosis of ADHD is made, including the exclusionary criteria (which parents should expect to be informed of), the need for careful, gene-guided therapies for personalized ADHD seems to be a promising future for the rare cases of actual ADHD.

Evidence that ADHD is Grossly Overdiagnosed

In one study of 92 children referred to an ADHD clinic with a diagnosis of ADHD, 41% were found to not fit the accepted criteria for ADHD after more comprehensive evaluations (Cotuono, 1993). In another study, 62% of suspected ADHD referrals were not confirmed as ADHD (Desgranges *et al.*, 1995). Different diagnostic criteria have been found to lead to inconsistent estimates of the rates of ADHD (Wolraich *et al.*, 1996). ADHD diagnosis rates vary significantly. One study found a comparatively low rate of ADHD diagnosis in Utah, which is understandable as the state ranked 44th nationally for Ritalin consumption at the time (LeFever *et al.*, 2003).

Good News on ADHD Overdiagnosis? Now We Know

While studies suggest a tendency for overdiagnosis in the clinic, to really understand whether ADHD is overdiagnosed or misdiagnosed, one would have to study the accuracy of the practitioner population when presented with sets of clinical features representing patients with and without ADHD, given standard diagnostic criteria. That's just what a group of researchers (Bruchmüller *et al.*) did in 2012. They hypothesized that therapists might diagnosis ADHD patients on inclusion criteria while ignoring exclusion criteria. So they sent four "vignettes" (descriptions of patients) to 1,000 therapists — four case descriptions to 1,000 child psychologists, psychiatrists, and social workers — and requested a diagnosis. Incredibly, 16.7% of therapists diagnosed ADHD in the two case studies that did not fulfill the full criteria for ADHD. Moreover, if the gender was indicated as male for these "patients," the therapists were twice as likely to diagnose ADHD for the case than for otherwise identical female vignettes. Exclusion criteria were downweighted in the assessments. Chilakamarri *et al.* (2011) also found a gross overdiagnosis of ADHD in a mixed group of patients of ADHD, bipolar disorder, and major depressive disorder children and adolescents.

These lines of evidence should have been sufficient cause for rapid dissemination of a call to change clinical practice. Some psychiatrists, however, will suggest treatment for ADHD without so much as an attempt at a formal diagnosis. Ironically, while writing this chapter, I received news from my sister that her 16-year-old son was being considered for treatment for ADHD — without a formal diagnosis.

A study just out in 2015 promises to change ADHD diagnosis for the better. In 2015, Snyder and colleagues (Snyder *et al.*, 2015), all working at geographically diverse locations, studied rates of "ruling out" by a multidisciplinary team tasked with case reviews after referrals. What they found was astonishing: 34% of cases originally "diagnosed" with ADHD did not hold up to scrutiny by the multidisciplinary team. Then, these researchers tested the use of EEG (electroencephalography) on the same patients to determine if they could rule out false positive ADHD patients, just as the multidisciplinary team did.

Importantly, they found that the use of electroencephalography on suspected cases of ADHD was nearly as good as ruling out likely false positive diagnosis (97% concordance with experts, with EEG increasing accuracy over clinical referral alone to 88%). This study should be replicated prospectively at numerous sites to insure generalizability. Their study design was a thing of beauty — a design to beat all designs. It was a prospective, *triple-blinded*, 13-site, clinical cohort study. That means that the patients were added to the study before any diagnosis was made, that a third independent party maintained a seal of records like EEG so the initial diagnosis was not informed by that technique.

For me, this settles the issue: ADHD overdiagnosis is real, by as much as 34% (~1/3). Estimates of national rates of ADHD in the US should all be revised downward by at least 1/3. During the time of the build-up of the epidemic of false positives of ADHD in the US, the exclusionary criteria were all but ignored by many clinicians. Before accepting recommendations of a diagnosis of ADHD, parents should demand a consideration of Exclusionary Criteria, including:

- Several symptoms present before the age of 12 years;
- Several symptoms present in two or more settings, (e.g., at home, school or work; with friends or relatives);
- Clear evidence that the symptoms present interfere with, or reduce the quality of, social, school, or work activities;
- Symptoms do not appear only during the course of schizophrenia or any other psychotic disorder. That is, the symptoms should not be better explained by another mental disorder (e.g., Anxiety Disorder, Dissociative Disorder, Mood Disorder, Personality Disorder).

Studies indicate that overdiagnosis is due to the failure of therapists to pay attention to these exclusionary criteria. The following lines of evidence all point to what should be considered to be a translational success of monumental importance for our society: ADHD is grossly overdiagnosed.

- *the massive increase in rates of diagnosis of ADHD (53% increase over the last decade, US Centers for Disease Control and Prevention data, 2013);*
- *the "incidence" of ADHD in the US vastly exceeds that of global estimates;*
- *high rates of misdiagnosis have been confirmed in multiple studies;*
- *when clinicians pay sufficient attention to the criteria for proper diagnosis of ADHD, as many as 1/3 of "cases" are then ruled out.*

The risks of the medicated route to treatment have been made especially well-known thanks in large part to two books, *Medication Madness* by Dr. Peter Breggin (St. Peter's Press) and *Brain-Disabling*

Treatments in Psychiatry (Springer). Another worthwhile read is Marilyn Wedge's book *A Disease Called Childhood: Why ADHD Became an American Epidemic* (Avery, Penguin).

The question of overdiagnosis of ADHD requires knowledge of the question of the expected percentage of students who, in modern schooling practices, with children sitting still in large numbers, might *normally be expected to exhibit these symptoms*, including repeated incidents of boredom, pre-adolescent and adolescent political intrigue, and inattentiveness over the span of six months. Certainly that number cannot be expected to be zero. In other words, it is reasonable to expect, from parents and teachers, some degree of false positive identification. This would lead to the "medicalization" of behaviors that fall within the normal range of most people at some point in their lives. Note especially that both DSM-V and ICD-10 exclusionary criteria emphasize that symptoms of ADHD begin in childhood (DSM-IV was before the age of 6, updated to DSM-V before age 12; ICD-10, 2015).The increase from age 6 to 12 means that a dramatically higher population-wide incidence of misdiagnosis, as much as 37%, is likely to occur.

Concern for Overdiagnosis Disparaged in Favor of Scripts

Some see the public's misunderstanding of the uncertainty of the diagnosis of the disease as a "barrier" to the treatment of children who need stimulants (Bussing, 1998; Bussing, 2001), and provide a counterpoint that claims that because some children with ADHD are missed, that it is "underdiagnosed." This is not a logical response to overdiagnosis. In fact, logically, it does not even address the issue. I cannot imagine an oncologist treating a patient with chemotherapy unless they are certain of the diagnosis of cancer.

This form of counter-argumentation conflates the question: The answer to the question of overdiagnosis cannot be that treatment of *bona fide* ADHD cases will be missed (first, do no harm?). The *miss rate* is a characteristic of the true clinical subpopulation (all children who really have ADHD), whereas the false positive rate (*overdiagnosis*) is a characteristic of the entire population (say, of all children in the US). The miss rates, when expressed as a percentage, seem high (e.g., in one survey "only 47% of ADHD children are receiving treatment"). It should be remembered that not all frank (verified) cases of ADHD require medication. However, this is a much smaller number of children than the number of children who would erroneously receive medication due to a high false diagnosis rate in the entire population.

ADHD may be a symptom, not a condition: The condition may be in many cases a lack of good, restful sleep. I see the need for balance as a call for more detailed research, improved methods for diagnosis. Checklists should be followed closely as an aid for improvements in the accuracy of diagnosis, and not the subjective or "gestalt" opinion of the therapist.

Are We Witnessing a "Pharmacaust?"

References to Hitler, and to the WWII Holocaust of Jews and others at the hands of the Nazi regime, seem to come too easy to people in public discourse of late. However, many have noted that the use of psychotropic drugs by individuals seems to be associated with dramatic changes that threaten lives. The comparison is made with a deep respect for both the suffering and deaths of the individuals lost during genocide, and their loved ones, and for the suffering and loss of those whose lives have forever been altered due to misdiagnosis and inappropriate treatment, and for their loved ones, too. The scale of misdiagnosis of ADHD also vastly outnumbers any incidence of outright, unthinkable genocide, and thus the comparison to the Holocaust is not made casually.

When a child is diagnosed with a mental illness, they now have a life-long condition of mental illness, with (on average) 25 fewer years in life expectancy, with an increased risk of suicide up to age 25. If the psychotropic drugs have caused bipolar disorder, their future medical, psychological and personal fates are forever changed. What about the life-long effects on a person thinking they require psychotropic drugs to be "normal?" Only 5% of children diagnosed with ADHD — now, keep the overdiagnosis rates in mind — make it through college. The diagnosis alone is not likely to be causal. The question is whether the comorbidity and mortality rates are due to the disease, or to the effects of the drugs on their developing minds?

Correll *et al.* (2011) reported that the number of clinical trials on ADHD in the recent past has increased to a remarkable extent. These trials are finding many adverse outcomes of psychotropic treatments for ADHD for children and adolescents compared to adults. They are also finding that therapy alone works as well as, or better than, the medications for some students. A number of people have noted the high frequency of psychotropic drug use by people involved in mass killings; individual case studies of suicide, suicide ideation, and homicide ideation report first-time instances after exposure to some ADHD drugs. There is likely to be a correlative link here: People who have conducted mass shootings are unwell, and therefore likely to be taking some form of psychotropic meds. Some think the connection is causal; others believe the correlation is that mentally unwell people are likely to be receiving psychiatric care. A causal connection between the side effects of the drugs and behavior leading to harm to the patient and to others is known: Suicidal and homicidal ideation are often listed among the possible side effects (Gibbons *et al.*, 2012; see Terrell, 2013 for a more thorough treatment).

A study conducted in 2015 (Crockett *et al.*, 2015) found a way to determine whether psychotropic drugs affect the moral judgement of people under its influence, specifically in a way related to aggression. The study, which was the first of its kind, used a unique exchange rate for determining the effects of certain drugs on the economic cost of increasing a dose of moderately painful shock to themselves, and to other people — basically, how much a person would lose in pay to avoid harming themselves or harming others.

Study participants receiving the placebo were willing to forfeit, on average, 55 cents per shock to avoid harming themselves, and 69 cents to avoid harming others. This shows that harm aversion was greater for others than for the self.

The two drugs tested were citalopram (a serotonin enhancer used to treat depression and obsessive compulsive disorder) and levodopa (used to treat Parkinson's disease). Both drugs are neuromodulators that influence social behavior. Citalopram enhances serotonin neurotransmission by blocking its reuptake and prolonging its actions in the synapse. Levodopa is converted into dopamine after crossing the blood-brain barrier.

The effect of citalopram was to nearly double the subjective cost per shock, both for self and others. Subjects on citalopram chose to deliver, on average, 30 fewer shocks to themselves and 35 fewer shocks to others over the course of the experiment, relative to subjects on placebo. Levodopa caused patients to be just as likely to shock others as themselves. The study authors concluded that levodopa can cause a loss of hyperaltruism.

Another study found the rates of violence during the first psychotic episode — prior to treatment — were much higher than the rates seen during and after treatment (Nielssen O and Large, 2010). Thus, while those propagating the idea that psychotropic meds are behind school shootings can cite convincing-looking lists of cases, that style of presentation of data does not include violent events in which the perpetrator was not yet being treated and those in which they had been treated but stopped. Thus, rates cannot be calculated from such lists alone, and care must be taken to not jump to conclusions and participate in fear-mongering.

Given the known side effect risks and the absence of sufficient large, long-term prospective studies for drugs used to treat ADHD (Bourgeois *et al.*, 2014) each of the drugs deserves closer scrutiny with additional research on safety, and therefore extreme care should be used in deriving a diagnosis of ADHD in the first place.

What Good Does Reporting Conflicts of Interest Do if the Views of those with Deep Financial Conflict Are Not Scrutinized?

In science and medicine, when someone publishes a research paper or an opinion article on a given topic, it is standard practice to expect that they will disclose potential conflicts of interest (more benign-sounding "competing interest," or even less suggestive "disclosures"). It is generally now accepted, even by vocal defenders of Ritalin, that ADHD is overdiagnosed (Hallowell, 2012).

Concerns over conflicts of interest appear to dissipate when the disclosures are made, and the norm is to procure a "Conflict of Interest Management Plan." However, such plans do not remove profit motives from the participants in the conversation, and their positions should be seriously down-weighted in light of the existence of such conflicts. Those who use their position within a medical system to secure contracts for companies they own, or in which they otherwise hold a financial interest, have a serious bias, and it is dubious that they can manage their own financial interests against the patient's true best interest. There are no substantive differences between the outcomes of two identical disclosure statements when the underlying motives differ. Such, disclosure, therefore, is often a mere formality, and violations are rarely prosecuted or otherwise corrected.

"Kill the Messenger": Early Warning Doctor Vindicated

The opinion of medical doctors who have weighed in on the debate on overdiagnosis rates who have conflicts of interest, therefore, should carry very little weight. However, this has not always been the case. In the mid-1990s, a Dr. Russell Barkley, PhD, participated in a highly questionable series of events that contributed to the dismissal of a Dr. Gretchen LeFever Watson (who now goes by the name of Dr. Gretchen Watson) of Eastern Virginia Medical School (EVMS). In her research, she had discovered a dramatic increase in the rates of diagnosis of ADHD in her region. She recounts this in sordid, painful detail in an article in 2014

(*J Contemp Psychother* **44**: 43–52). However, after Dr. Barkley visited the EVMS campus, Dr. LeFever Watson's supervisor then abruptly canceled all of her cases, told her peers she no longer worked at EVMS, and then, without administrative approval (i.e., without due process), demanded her resignation.

These were very unseemly and suspicious circumstances. As LeFever *et al.* (2014) recount:

> *It is unclear how many people knew then (or realize now) the significance of the fact that a sizeable proportion of Barkley's taxable income came from the pharmaceutical industry. Barkley's own website once showed, for example, that approximately 8% of his taxable income came from Eli Lilly alone. Eli Lilly manufactures Strattera, a commonly prescribed medication for ADHD. Other income categories that were explicitly tied to the pharmaceutical industry accounted for approximately 19% of his income... Like other ADHD opinion leaders, Barkley also has had extensive support from Children and Adults with Attention-Deficit/Hyperactivity Disorders (CHADD) — a prominent advocacy group that is supported with funds from the manufacturers of ADHD medications.*

Dr. Barkley clearly had a serious conflict of interest. Dr. Watson's findings had led to an effective community intervention program, which was all but dismantled due to her unwarranted dismissal from the EVMS. Dr. Barkley, by the way, is the same Key Opinion Leader who tried to use the threat of vomiting to try to convince parents that ADHD is 100% genetic. In the absence of scientific evidence, I suppose any evocative statement will suffice.

Added concerns mounted when an anonymous person levied allegations of data fabrication. An investigation ensued. In sum, after a thorough scouring of her study files and data, a typo in an Appendix of one publication was found. It was determined that this typo had no impact on the study results or conclusions. Nothing was ever found that supported the anonymous allegations against Dr. Watson, but serious damage had been done to her academic career.

The logic of arguing against the fact of overdiagnosis does not hold up to reasonable scrutiny with logic. Those who argue against the reality of overdiagnosis switch to emotive appeals to ensure that ADHD patients can get the treatments they presume they need. This position begs two important questions: Is the treatment of the few true positive (i.e., frank ADHD patients), who are likely 3–5% of the population, nominally, worth the inappropriate, off-label treatment of many more (the >10% of the population of children who are misdiagnosed)? In no other field of medicine would this type of wrongful medication be tolerated.

The Translational Success Story in ADHD as of 2015

Perhaps the greatest translational success that can be recognized is that findings of overdiagnosis in the research of Dr. Watson and colleagues has now been validated, and she is now completely vindicated. Frances (2010) reviews the phenomenon of overdiagnosis of mental illnesses overall, including ADHD; Kirk evaluated DSM criteria and found an *expected* overdiagnosis of 37% false positives, with only 4% expected false negatives.

Dr. Watson's credibility should be seen by the community as higher than Dr. Barkley's, and higher than those practitioners who too easily provide scripts for psychotropics off-label with questionable diagnosis. It is now nearly universally accepted that ADHD is overdiagnosed in the US. Even an ardent defender of Ritalin (Hallowell, 2012) acknowledges overdiagnosis (i.e., "pseudo-ADHD"), even as he argues for continued treatments with stimulants. Dr. Watson should be (and is) invited to speak at conferences, to editorial boards, and should be considered a viable candidate for a leadership position in the reform of ADHD diagnosis and treatment.

The state of the science of treatment of ADHD is that we are now perhaps on a pathway to success. New sophisticated methods for confirmatory diagnosis are being developed to help reduce misdiagnosis (Anderson *et al.*, 2014; Bohland *et al.*, 2012; Brown *et al.*, 2012; Dey *et al.*, Johnston *et al.*, 2014; O'Mahony *et al.*, 2014; Peng *et al.*, 2013; Sidhu *et al.*, 2012; Synder *et al.*, 2015; Tenev *et al.*, 2014). That literature should be well-studied by any clinicians who claim to seek the humane care of their clients.

Modifying Risk Factors First

At best, then, being in a school in which standardized testing results determine funding, having an anxious parent, and having a particular genetic profile can be seen as "risk factors." Risk factors are not only for use in predictive diagnosis — identifying patients likely to have a specific disease. Modifying risk factors can also reduce the occurrence of disease (such as the effect of quitting smoking on lung cancer, or of losing weight on heart disease). Obviously, removing children from homes of stressed parents is not an option; however, if parents are stressed or anxious, the teacher/counselor might suggest family counseling for their own stresses, or parenting support groups, before jumping to a diagnosis of ADHD for children. Also, uncoupling funding from standardized testing would relieve teachers of the stress for their students to perform. Again, if a lack of sleep is a risk factor, sleep habits might be a more appropriate clinical starting point.

Rather than stimulate children during the daytime, it may be preferable to conduct a sleep study on potential ADHD patients first. Other diagnoses may be become apparent, and if directly treated (without stimulant), may prove much more effective. Owens *et al.* (2010) reported that 30% of therapists prescribed melatonin for ADHD, a more natural remedy for sleep pathologies.

Need for National Reform on ADHD Diagnosis and Wrongful Treatment

The US Centers for Disease Control and Prevention have reported that ADHD is, in fact, overdiagnosed. This translational success is due in large part to the activities of pioneers and thought leaders such as

Dr. LeFever Watson. Our society owes her a debt of gratitude for her efforts. The *New York Times* was severely criticized by Lacasse and Leo (2015) for dragging their feet in letting go of the idea that ADHD is not overdiagnosed, and for relying on KOLs after they had been discredited.

After I wrote this chapter, I had the pleasure of speaking with Dr. Watson about her experience and the current state of the practice, and we shared war stories. She is veteran strengthened by fire and composed by experience. Her passion for the truth is undaunted.

Dr. LeFever Watson shared with me her personal experiences of the wrongful dismissal, and the effects of the successful bid by Dr. Barkley and whomever he was working on behalf of to discredit and bury her work. Their attempt at delaying the current widespread acceptance of ADHD overdiagnosis of fact, however, is a failure. While it put money in the pockets of those profiting from the wrongful medication of our children, it has not stopped other scientists from going forward and validating the original findings. Dr. LeFever Watson herself never ceased, or even paused in her mission to help others. Her dedication and perseverance is a sign of personal greatness. She is the type of clinician I would want my sons to interact with, if necessary.

More so, she is the type of person I would want to see leading a national reform in education of new psychiatric physicians. Her immediate response to the personal crisis in her life due to the wrongful dismissal was, naturally, to help others. In spite of the fact that her former colleagues avoided her company in public, she felt compelled to continue to promote awareness of the problem of overdiagnosis. She knew her data was correct. I asked her what kept her going.

People would ask me: Why are you still smiling? Why are you still standing? Why are you still fighting? Given how strongly they came after me, it reaffirmed not only that I was on to something, but I was on to something terribly important. I already knew that my research must be correct, but that there was more at stake than I had initially realized.

She also knew that, because she had conducted objective research, time would eventually bear her findings out. While compiling the growing evidence of overdiagnosis from other researchers around the country year after year, study by study, she took a job at Regent University, where she quickly rose in the ranks to a leadership position in her department. She was the first faculty member to win a federally funded grant: $1.25 million dollars to work on teacher preparation for career switchers. That proposal, she says, was then "given" by a dean to another, male, faculty member. She continued work in the area of patient safety, and she watched the field of clinical psychiatry slowly but surely decay toward clinical pharmacology. She was invited to speak at conferences on ADHD overdiagnosis. Her colleagues at one conference insisted that she publish her story. With trepidation, but due to dismay at the take-over by the pharmaceutical industry of her former profession and science, and with respect for her former university (EVMS), she finally relented, and the original co-authors joined her in publishing her story (Watson *et al.*, 2014). I not only recommend the paper to every reader but to every entry-level graduate student in any science or clinical training program.

Dr. Watson and her colleagues were at least 15 years ahead of their time. Her opinion on clinical matters, especially in care of ADHD, now carries great weight with her colleagues. Her primary concerns are to revamp the training and education of the next generation of practitioners. She has observed that (1) new clinical psychologists are being taught without the benefits of real evidence-based medical research, including the research that indicates ADHD overdiagnosis; (2) they are being offered relatively new degrees ("PsyD degrees") that provide clinical training, but do not require adequate exposure or training in research or statistical analysis to substantiate the scientist-practitioner model that clinical psychology espouses; (3) the faculty in the most prestigious degree-awarding institutions who are in charge of the curriculum commonly have financial ties with the pharmaceutical industry; (4) the curriculum de-emphasizes studies like the MTA studies showing overdiagnosis and adverse effects of amphetamines. She fears that each of these factors will continue to weaken the entire profession.

The public cannot feel good about the lax approval of ADHD drugs, nor about the fact of ADHD overdiagnosis and its overtreatment. However, they can feel good that we now know, as a result of multiple lines of evidence including a triple-blinded prospective randomized trial, that ADHD is overdiagnosed by as much as one-third in the US. Dr. Watson's earlier work has been completely vindicated. She was eventually cleared of all allegations of scientific misconducted (Lenzer, 2005; 2008).

This means that we can, and we must — for both ethical and legal reasons — do something about it in terms of standards of care (require exclusionary criteria, require EEG scans) and reform in training. This is a matter of public health.

The public can also feel good that after the egregious *ad hoc* dismissal of early reports of overdiagnosis of ADHD, the question is settled. ADHD is overdiagnosed — there is no longer any question about it. Cavalier diagnosis and writing scripts without overt demonstration of consideration of exclusionary criteria is dangerous practice, and could be made grounds for sanctions. Alternatively, a national program, perhaps modeled after the Awakenings™ nursing home program, could be implemented whereby the diagnosing physicians interact with advocates of the student body within each school with the aim of ensuring the proper diagnosis of any suspected ADHD cases. Perhaps the school psychiatrists, counselors, and nurses could be asked to do what they do differently, and given the authority and resources to do it. Ideally, while the implementation would be different, the operational model of the nursing home staff focused on the question of overmedication of nursing home residents could provide a model. According to Maria Reyes:

> *If you want change, it can be done. You just have to stick to your goals, stay with your positions. It can be done. You have to want it.*

The field is moving toward molecular diagnosis, and parents will be able to expect that their clinician will provide them with a specific, molecular subtype of any diagnosis, with a corresponding recommendation for treatment. The advocates would have to keep up with these advances. The public should currently expect that their doctors/therapists be aware that a diagnosis of ADHD requires evidence of multiple symptoms of disruptive inattentiveness that persists for six or more months in at least two settings (home and school), before the age of seven.

Parents can also expect therapists and clinicians to be more than sufficiently attentive to Criterion E. Clinicians should not diagnose ADHD subjectively: ALL of the criteria should be fulfilled, or they risk misdiagnosis and missing proper diagnosis of potentially treatable other conditions. Parents should refuse to accept a diagnosis of any kind from a teacher, and they should resist treatment with stimulants until their child is given a sleep study to determine if he or she is getting proper rest. When in doubt, parents should consider whether they would allow an oncologist to give their child a chemotherapeutic agent without a complete diagnosis.

Advances in Treatment of ADHD

Other advances in the treatment of ADHD exist as well. Some subtypes can be treated effectively with dietary supplements. A study in Germany (Widenhorn-Müller *et al.*, 2014) found that Omega-3 fatty acid supplements improved working memory function. This is important because working memory is the placeholder for motivation and intention. The study, however, showed no net positive effect on measures of attention. However, they may have missed an important finding for a subtype of ADHD. A Swedish study (Johnson *et al.*, 2009) found that, astonishingly, a full 26% of ADHD patients respond well to Omega-3 fatty acids added to the diet within three months. After six months, 47% responded. The initial response was a 25% reduction of ADHD symptoms, and a drop of CGI (Clinical Global Impression) scores to the *near-normal range*. After six months, 47% of all showed such improvement. The patients who showed the best response were ADHD inattentive subtype with comorbid neurodevelopmental disorders. While these results tend to be minimized by paid pro-drug advocates, given the additional benefits of Omega-3 fatty acids on cardiovascular health, the importance of these finding cannot be understated. In addition to Omega-3 fatty acids, zinc supplements and neuro-feedback may be useful (Searight *et al.*, 2012). Yes, these approaches take more effort than a pill. But they are harmless if ADHD is misdiagnosed.

As unnatural as it may seem, parents should separate their own ego from that of their child's. Their children, after all, are the ones who have to take the drugs and live with the potential life-altering side effects.

A Message to Parents

I understand concern for our children; I have two adolescents of my own. Here are some things that parents can consider doing for their children:

(1) First, take a deep breath, and understand that parenting can be challenging, but growing up can be challenging, too, for any child. Someone parented you. Now it's your turn.

(2) Parents can request a sleep study prior to an attempted diagnosis of ADHD. If your child isn't getting good, restful sleep, they just may not be able to focus the next day.

(3) Parents should never accept a diagnosis of any illness of psychological condition from their child's teacher. The high false-positive rate means that teachers who "know ADHD when they see it" are learning what ADHD is from a mix of students with frank ADHD and false positives.

(4) Parents must advocate for a correct diagnosis. They should ask to see a checklist of symptoms in their child under accepted criteria and make sure that each and every condition for diagnosis of ADHD is fulfilled. They can hold the doctors accountable to properly execute the diagnosis of ADHD in the first place, *and ask them to focus on the exclusionary criteria as well as the inclusion criteria.* Therapists and doctors are supposed to weigh all diagnostic criteria in

both the *DSM-V* and the *ICD-10* categories for ADHD equally, *as a requirement for diagnosis*. Doctors should not weigh the criteria according to their subjective understanding about the disorder, but they do (Bruchmüller & Meyer, 2009; Kim & Ahn, 2002; Meyer & Meyer, 2009; Schmidt *et al*, 2005).

(5) Parents of preschool children should never accept a diagnosis of ADHD; their children are too young for accurate diagnosis, and many suspected cases resolve in a year or two.

(6) If your child is diagnosed with ADHD, they still need a good night's sleep. Behavioral modification therapies should be tried first, and melatonin. Try to avoid the "upper/downer" roller coaster at all costs. But you can also ask for a genetic profile analysis in search of possible mechanisms. It might help your doctor form a personalized route to treatment.

(7) Psychotropic drugs should never be used in combination unless there have been randomize clinical trials demonstrating their safe combined use (Guevara *et al.*, 2002). No such trial has successfully demonstrated the long-term efficacy and safety of these medications for ADHD.

(8) Omega 3/6 fatty acids may help, and cannot hurt, your child's cognitive functions, especially if you stick with the additive for at least six months, combined with external aids for working memory (lists, time pieces). Concrete reminders of the tasks at hand will prove useful.

Parents who are averse to any drugs can help their children get good sleep, too. Before accepting a prescription for poor sleep, parents should discuss with their child the links between good sleep and daytime attentiveness. Then, depending on the child's age, they should remove all electronic media from a child's bedroom (laptops, cell phones, television) one hour before bedtime for three months' time — and stick to it. For adolescents, it will be important to incentivize them and teach them the link between a little downtime before sleep, a good night's sleep, and their academic performance. Studies have reported that a low dose of over-the-counter melatonin given half an hour before bedtime can help. Once they begin a good sleep pattern, the body's normal melatonin production may take over. Note that melatonin has been shown in many studies to help ADHD patients sleep better, but it has no effect on the inattentiveness symptoms for *bona fide* ADHD patients.

A Message to Educators and Pharma

The issue of academic performance should first and foremost be seen as academic, not medical, and legislators, parents and teachers alike should never overtly or otherwise put the onus of low standardized test scores on the neurobiology of developing adolescent minds. Those minds are our future and should be protected from harm from drugs of all kinds.

The lax use of diagnostic criteria often leads to the abuse of ADHD drugs by students in high school and in college. Students feel that their academic performance may be improved and may sample Adderall or Ritalin obtained from a peer. They can seek "referrals" — names of counselors, for example — that they think might be willing to prescribe these powerful drugs. In some cases, such abuse can lead to the types of psychoses, violence and suicide mentioned at the beginning of the chapter. Parents should be alert to these trends and talk with their children at a young age about this issue.

The hard-won translational knowledge should cause parents to be extremely cautious about accepting these powerful prescriptions for their children. Similarly, teachers should not be in the position to suggest diagnoses, and therapists should be extremely conservative in diagnosis of ADHD without first conducting a sleep study. That is not to say that some severe cases of *bona fide* ADHD will not be helped by prescription drugs. It is also not to say that ADHD does not exist. The effects can be debilitating if the condition is untreated. However, and this cannot be stressed strongly enough:

These are Strong Drugs

The effects of these drugs can be debilitating on those who do not need them, i.e., those who are misdiagnosed. I am reaching out here to the ADHD community that identifies themselves with the condition: There are good reasons to understand that the causes of ADHD may affect sleep first. When we look at what's *behind* ADHD and not merely focus on the treatment of the symptoms, many patients with a preliminary diagnosis will benefit.

It is also a caution to parents, who are initially told that the stimulants are given just to "help their child focus," and yet they often end up unwittingly committing their child to an expensive future of never-ending scripts and copays — often without assurance of the accuracy of the diagnosis.

It is also to caution teachers, therapists and parents from unleashing the entire pharmacopeia of psychotropic drugs on something as precious as a developing human brain. Our society's approach to this problem stands in stark contrast to the problem of overmedicating seniors in nursing homes. Why, as a society, are we willing to admit the need for change, and then explore changes in the care of our elderly to prevent overmedication, while we are willing to turn a blind eye to the inappropriate medication of children who are misdiagnosed with ADHD? Just like we have for protecting our elderly from wrongful medication in nursing homes, we need a national task force (perhaps international) focused on the goal of reducing the misdiagnosis of ADHD in our schoolchildren to protect them from wrongful medication, and on providing effective means of meeting the unmet educational needs of our students.

It's their mind, not yours.

Further Reading

LeFever GB, Arcona AP, Antonuccio DO. (2003) Evidence of over diagnosis and overuse of medication. *SRMHP* **2:1** http://www.srmhp.org/0201/adhd.html

Dr. Watson's (and colleagues') original study demonstrated overdiagnosis.

Molina BSG, *et al.* (2009) The MTA at 8 years: Prospective follow-up of children treated for combined type ADHD in the multisite study. *Journal of the American Academy of Child and Adolescent Psychiatry* **48(5)**: 484–500. [doi: 10.1097/CHI.0b013e31819c23d0]

The long-term MTA study in which results summarized in the abstract do not match those described in the paper.

Terrell R. (2013) Psychiatric Meds: Prescription for Murder? *New American,* March 06. www.thenewamerican.com/usnews/crime/item/14655-prescription-for-murder

A rather sensationalist, but thought-provoking article.

Watson GL, Arcona AP, Antonuccio DO, Healy D. (2014) Shooting the messenger: the case of ADHD. *J Contemp Psychother* **44:** 43–52. http://link.springer.com/article/10.1007%2Fs10879-013-9244-x

Dr. Watson's (and colleagues') representation of events surrounding the end of her career as a practicing clinician and academic researcher.

References

Anderson A, *et al.* (2014) Non-negative matrix factorization of multimodal MRI, fMRI and phenotypic data reveals differential changes in default mode subnetworks in ADHD. *Neuroimage* **102 Pt 1:** 207–19. [doi: 10.1016/j.neuroimage.2013.12.015]

American Psychiatric Association. (2013) *Diagnostic and Statistical Manual of Mental Disorders, 5th edition.* Arlington, VA.

Arcos-Burgos M, *et al.* (2010a) A common variant of the latrophilin 3 gene, LPHN3, confers susceptibility to ADHD and predicts effectiveness of stimulant medication. *Mol Psychiatry* **15(11):** 1053–66. [doi: 10.1038/mp.2010.6]

Arcos-Burgos M, Muenke M. (2010b) Toward a better understanding of ADHD: LPHN3 gene variants and the susceptibility to develop ADHD. *Attention Deficit and Hyperactivity Disorders* **2(3):** 139–47. [doi:10.1007/s12402-010-0030-2]

Balasubramaniam M, Telles S, Doraiswamy PM. (2012) Yoga on our minds: a systematic review of yoga for neuropsychiatric disorders. *Front Psychiatry* **3:** 117. [doi: 10.3389/fpsyt.2012.00117]

Bohland JW, et al. (2012) Network, anatomical, and non-imaging measures for the prediction of ADHD diagnosis in individual subjects. *Front Syst Neurosci* **6:** 78. [doi: 10.3389/fnsys.2012.00078]

Bourgeois FT, Kim JM, Mandl KD. (2014) Premarket safety and efficacy studies for ADHD medications in children. *PLoS ONE* **9(7):** e102249. [doi:10.1371/journal.pone.0102249]

Brown MR, et al. (2012) ADHD-200 Global Competition: diagnosing ADHD using personal characteristic data can outperform resting state fMRI measurements. *Front Syst Neurosci* **6:** 69. [doi: 10.3389/fnsys. 2012.00069]

Bruchmüller K, Margraf J, Schneider S. (2012) Is ADHD diagnosed in accord with diagnostic criteria? Over diagnosis and influence of client gender on diagnosis. *J Consult Clin Psychol* **80(1):** 128–38. [doi: 10.1037/a0026582]

Brunborg GS, Mentzoni RA, Frøyland LR. (2014) Is video gaming, or video game addiction, associated with depression, academic achievement, heavy episodic drinking, or conduct problems? *J Behav Addict* **3(1):** 27–32. [doi: 10.1556/JBA.3.2014.002]

Bussing R. (2001) Barriers to help-seeking and treatment for ADHD. Program and abstracts of the American Psychiatric Association 53rd Institute on Psychiatric Services; October 10–14, 2001; Orlando, Florida. Lecture 13.

Bussing R, et al. (1998) Children in special education programs: attention deficit hyperactivity disorder, use of services, and unmet needs. *Am J Public Health* **88:** 880–86.

Chang JS. (2009) Parental smoking and childhood leukemia. *Methods Mol Biol* **472:** 103–37. [doi: 10.1007/978-1-60327-492-0_5]

Chervin RD, et al. (2002) Associations between symptoms of inattention, hyperactivity, restless legs, and periodic leg movements. *Sleep* **25(2):** 213–18.

Chilakamarri JK, Filkowski MM, Ghaemi SN. (2011) Misdiagnosis of bipolar disorder in children and adolescents: a comparison with ADHD and major depressive disorder. *Ann Clin Psychiatry* **23(1):** 25–29.

CMS, MDS Quality Measure/Indicator Report, Psychotropic Drug Use, July/ September 2010, Measure 10_1_HI.

Converse AK, et al. (2014) Tai chi training reduces self-report of inattention in healthy young adults. *Front Hum Neurosci* **27;8:** 13. [doi: 10.3389/ fnhum.2014.00013]

Correll CU, Kratochvil CJ, March JS. (2011) Developments in pediatric psychopharmacology: focus on stimulants, antidepressants, and antipsychotics. *J Clin Psychiatry* **72(5):** 655–70. [doi: 10.4088/JCP.11r07064]

Crockett MJ, *et al.* (2015) Dissociable effects of serotonin and dopamine on the valuation of harm in moral decision making. *Curr Biol* pii: S0960-9822(15)00595-3. [doi: 10.1016/j.cub.2015.05.021]

Dey S, Rao AR, Shah M. (2014) Attributed graph distance measure for automatic detection of attention deficit hyperactive disordered subjects. *Front Neural Circuits* **8:** 64. [doi: 10.3389/fncir.2014.00064]

Elkington KS, Bauermeister JA, Zimmerman MA. (2011) Do parents and peers matter? A prospective socio-ecological examination of substance use and sexual risk among African American youth. *J Adolesc* **34(5):** 1035–47. [doi: 10.1016/j.adolescence.2010.11.004]

Elder TE, *et al.* (2010) The importance of relative standards in ADHD diagnoses: Evidence based on exact birth dates. *Journal of Health Economics.* [doi: 10.1016/j.jhealeco.2010.06.003]

FDA Public Health Advisory. (2009) Deaths with antipsychotics in elderly patients with behavioral disturbances. http://www.fda.gov/Drugs/DrugSafety/PublicHealthAdvisories/ucm053171.htm

Feldman R, Dollberg D, Nadam R. (2011) The expression and regulation of anger in toddlers: relations to maternal behavior and mental representations. *Infant Behav Dev* **34(2):** 310–20. [doi: 10.1016/j.infbeh.2011.02.001]

Frances A. (2010) Psychiatric fads and overdiagnosis. *Psychology Today* blog: DSM5 in distress. [http://www.webcitation.org/6D5Fqr2Ot]

Frances A. (2013) *Saving Normal: An Insider's Revolt against Out-of-Control Psychiatric Diagnosis, DSM-5, Big Pharma, and the Medicalization of Ordinary Life.* New York, Harper Collins.

Gagliano A, *et al.* (2011) Restless Leg Syndrome in ADHD children: levetiracetam as a reasonable therapeutic option. *Brain Dev* **33(6):** 480–86. [doi: 10.1016/j.braindev.2010.09.008]

Gibbons RD, *et al.* (2012) Suicidal thoughts and behavior with antidepressant treatment: reanalysis of the randomized placebo-controlled studies of fluoxetine and venlafaxine. *Arch Gen Psychiatry* **69(6):** 580–87. [doi: 10.1001/archgenpsychiatry.2011.2048]

Glover V. (2011) Annual Research Review: Prenatal stress and the origins of psychopathology: an evolutionary perspective. *J Child Psychol Psychiatry* **52(4):** 356–67. [doi: 10.1111/j.1469-7610.2011.02371.x]

González S, *et al.* (2012) Circadian-related heteromerization of adrenergic and dopamine D4 receptors modulates melatonin synthesis and release in the pineal gland. *PLoS Biology* **10(6):** e1001347. [doi: 10.1371/journal. pbio.1001347]

Gruber R, *et al.* (2014) Sleep efficiency (but not sleep duration) of healthy school-age children is associated with grades in math and languages. *Sleep Med* **15(12):** 1517–25. [doi: 10.1016/j.sleep.2014.08.009]

Guevara J, *et al.* (2002) Psychotropic medication use in a population of children who have attention-deficit/hyperactivity disorder. *Pediatrics* **109:** 733–39.

Haffner J, *et al.* (2006) [The effectiveness of body-oriented methods of therapy in the treatment of attention-deficit hyperactivity disorder (ADHD): results of a controlled pilot study]. *Z Kinder Jugendpsychiatr Psychother* **34:** 37–47. [doi: 10.1024/1422-4917.34.1.37]

Haghbin M, *et al.* (2013) A brief report on the relationship between self-control, video game addiction and academic achievement in normal and ADHD students. *J Behav Addict* **2(4):** 239–43. [doi: 10.1556/JBA. 2.2013.4.7]

Hallowell E. (2012) Dr. Hallowell's Response to NY Times Piece "Ritalin Gone Wrong." www.drhallowell.com/blog/dr-hallowells-response-to-ny-times-piece-ritalin-gone-wrong/

Hammarén-Malmi S, Tarkkanen J, Mattila PS. (2005) Analysis of risk factors for childhood persistent middle ear effusion. *Acta Otolaryngol* **125(10):** 1051–54.

Hassett AM, Ames D, Chiu E. (2005) *Psychosis in the Elderly.* Taylor and Francis, Boca Raton.

Hinshaw SP, Scheffler RM. (2014) *The ADHD Explosion: Myths, Medications, Money, and Today's Push for Performance.* New York: Oxford University Press.

Horesh N, *et al.* (2015) Father-daughter relationship and the severity of eating disorders. *Eur Psychiatry* **30(1):** 114–20. [doi: 10.1016/j.eurpsy. 2014.04.004]

ICD-10-CM Diagnosis Code F90.9. 2015. http://www.icd10data.com/ICD10CM/Codes/F01-F99/F90-F98/F90-/F90.9

Jensen PS, Kenny DT. (2004) The effects of yoga on the attention and behavior of boys with attention-deficit/hyperactivity disorder (ADHD). *J Atten Disord* 7: 205–16. [doi: 10.1177/108705470400700403]

Johnson M, *et al.* (2009) Omega-3/omega-6 fatty acids for attention deficit hyperactivity disorder: a randomized placebo-controlled trial in children and adolescents. *J Atten Disord* 12(5): 394–401. [doi: 10.1177/1087054708316261]

Johnston BA, *et al.* (2014) Brainstem abnormalities in attention deficit hyperactivity disorder support high accuracy individual diagnostic classification. *Hum Brain Mapp* 35(10): 5179–89. [doi: 10.1002/hbm.22542]

Karni A, *et al.* (1994) Dependence on REM sleep of overnight improvement of a perceptual skill. *Science* 265(5172): 679–82.

Kirk SA. (2004) Are children's DSM diagnoses accurate? *Brief Treatment and Crisis Intervention* 4(3): 255–70.

Kolko DJ, Bukstein OG, Barron J. (1999) Methylphenidate and behavior modification in children with ADHD and comorbid ODD or CD: main and incremental effects across settings. *J Am Acad Child Adolesc Psychiatry* 38(5): 578–86.

Lacasse JR, Leo J. (2015) The New York Times and the ADHD Epidemic. *Social Science and Modern Society* 52: 3–8. [doi 10.1007/s12115-014-9851-5]

Lee YJ, *et al.* (2015) Academic performance among adolescents with behaviorally induced insufficient sleep syndrome. *J Clin Sleep Med* 11(1): 61–8. [doi: 10.5664/jcsm.4368]

LeFever GB, Arcona AP. (2003) Evidence of overdiagnosis and overuse of medication. *SRMHP* 2: 1 [www.srmhp.org/0201/adhd.html]

Lenzer J. (2005) Research cleared of misconduct. *BMJ* 331: 865 [http://dx.doi.org/10.1136/bmj.331.7521.865]

Lenzer J. (2008) Truly independent research? *BMJ* 337: a1332. [doi: 10.1136/bmj.a1332]

Liperoti R, *et al.* (2009) All-cause mortality associated with atypical and conventional antipsychotics among nursing home residents with dementia: a retrospective cohort study. *J Clin Psychiatry* 70(10): 1340–47. [doi: 10.4088/JCP.08m04597yel]

McClure AC, *et al.* (2010) Characteristics associated with low self-esteem among US adolescents. *Acad Pediatr* **10(4):** 238–44.e2. doi: 10.1016/j. acap.2010.03.007.

McKenna PH. (1997) *Schizoprenia and Related Syndromes.* Psychology Press, New York.

Meltzer LJ, Shaheed K, Ambler D. (2014) Start later, sleep later: school start times and adolescent sleep in homeschool versus public/private school students. *Behav Sleep Med* **14:** 1–15.

Mitchell JT, *et al.* (2013) A pilot trial of mindfulness meditation training for ADHD in adulthood: impact on core symptoms, executive functioning, and emotion dysregulation. *J Atten Disord*, Dec 4: 1–24. [doi: 10.1177/ 1087054713513328]

Molina BSG, *et al.* (2009) The MTA at 8 years: prospective follow-up of children treated for combined type ADHD in the multisite study. *J Am Acad Child Psy* **48(5):** 484–500. [doi: 10.1097/CHI.0b013e31819c23d0]

Molinari V, *et al.* (2010) Provision of psychopharmacological services in nursing homes. *J Gerontol B Psychol Sci Soc Sci* **65B(1):** 57–60. [doi: 10.1093/ geronb/gbp080]

Murphy TF. (2006) Otitis media, bacterial colonization, and the smoking parent. *Clin Infect Dis* **42(7):** 904–6.

Murry VM, *et al.* (2013) Contributions of family environment and parenting processes to sexual risk and substance use of rural African American males: a 4-year longitudinal analysis. *Am J Orthopsychiatry* **83(2 Pt 3):** 299–309. [doi: 10.1111/ajop.12035]

Nielssen O, Large M. (2010) Rates of homicide during the first episode of psychosis and after treatment: a systematic review and meta-analysis. *Schizophr Bull* **36(4):** 702–12. [doi: 10.1093/schbul/sbn144]

Nigg J, Nikolas M, Burt SA. (2010) Measured gene-by-environment interaction in relation to attention-deficit/hyperactivity disorder. *J Am Acad Child Psy* **49(9):** 863–73. [doi: 10.1016/j.jaac.2010.01.025]

Olfson M, *et al.* (2009) Mental health treatment received by youths in the year before and after a new diagnosis of bipolar disorder. *Psychiatr Serv* **60(8):** 1098–106. [doi: 10.1176/appi.ps.60.8.1098]

O'Mahony N, *et al.* (2014) Objective diagnosis of ADHD using IMUs. *Med Eng Phys* **36(7):** 922–26. [doi:10.1016/j.medengphy.2014.02.023]

Owens JA, *et al.* (2010) Use of pharmacotherapy for insomnia in child psychiatry practice: a national survey. *Sleep Med* **11(7):** 692–700. [doi: 10.1016/j. sleep.2009.11.015]

Pagani LS, Fitzpatrick C. (2013) Prospective associations between early long-term household tobacco smoke exposure and antisocial behaviour in later childhood. *J Epidemiol Community Health* **67(7):** 552–57. [doi: 10.1136/jech-2012-202191]

Partridge B, Lucke J, Hall W. (2014) Over-diagnosed and over-treated: a survey of Australian public attitudes towards the acceptability of drug treatment for depression and ADHD. *BMC Psychiatry* **14:** 74. [doi: 10.1186/1471-244X-14-74]

Peng X, *et al.* (2013) Extreme learning machine-based classification of ADHD using brain structural MRI data. *PLoS One* **8(11):** e79476. [doi: 10.1371/journal.pone.0079476]

Polanczyk G, *et al.* (2007) The world wide prevalence of ADHD: a systematic review and metaregression analysis. *Am J Psychiatry* **164:** 942–48.

Scheffler RM, *et al.* (2009) Positive association between ADHD medication use and academic achievement during elementary school. *Pediatrics* **123:** 1273–79.

Scherrer JF, *et al.* (2012) Parent, sibling and peer influences on smoking initiation, regular smoking and nicotine dependence. Results from a genetically informative design. *Addict Behav* **37(3):** 240–47. [doi: 10.1016/j.addbeh.2011.10.005]

Schwarz A. (2013) The Selling of Attention Deficit Disorder. *The New York Times*, Dec 14, 2013. [www.nytimes.com/2013/12/15/health/the-selling-of-attention-deficit-disorder.html]

Sclar DA, *et al.* (2012) Attention-deficit/hyperactivity disorder among children and adolescents in the United States: trend in diagnosis and use of pharmacotherapy by gender. *Clin Pediatr (Phila)* **51(6):** 584–89. [doi: 10.1177/0009922812439621]

Searight HR, *et al.* (2012) Complementary and alternative therapies for pediatric attention deficit hyperactivity disorder: a descriptive review. *ISRN Psychiatry* **2012:** 804127. [doi: 10.5402/2012/804127]

Sidhu GS, *et al.* (2012) Kernel Principal Component Analysis for dimensionality reduction in fMRI-based diagnosis of ADHD. *Front Syst Neurosci* **6:** 74. [doi: 10.3389/fnsys.2012.00074]

Silvestri R, *et al.* (2009) Sleep disorders in children with Attention-Deficit/ Hyperactivity Disorder (ADHD) recorded overnight by video-polysomnography. *Sleep Med* **10(10):** 1132–38.

Sørensen HJ, *et al.* (2011) The contribution of parental alcohol use disorders and other psychiatric illness to the risk of alcohol use disorders in the offspring. *Alcohol Clin Exp Res* **35(7):** 1315–20. [doi: 10.1111/j.1530-0277. 2011.01467.x]

Sroufe LA. (2012) Ritalin gone wrong. *The New York Times*, Jan 28, 2012.

Snyder SM, *et al.* (2015) Integration of an EEG biomarker with a clinician's ADHD evaluation. *Brain and Behaviors.* [doi: 10.1002/brb3.330]

Tenev A, *et al.* (2014) Machine learning approach for classification of ADHD adults. *Int J Psychophysiol* **93(1):** 162–66. [doi: 10.1016/j.ijpsycho. 2013.01.008]

Torjesen I. (2015) Children whose parents attempted suicide are at raised risk of similar behaviour, study finds. *BMJ* **350:** g7862. [doi: 10.1136/bmj. g7862]

Tseng MC, *et al.* (2014) Co-occurring eating and psychiatric symptoms in Taiwanese college students: effects of gender and parental factors. *J Clin Psychol* **70(3):** 224–37. [doi: 10.1002/jclp.22014]

US Centers for Disease Control and Prevention. (2015) Attention-Deficit/ Hyperactivity Disorder (ADHD). http://www.cdc.gov/ncbddd/adhd/data.html (Last accessed 3/23/2015)

Warner J. (2012) ADHD: Is stigma back in style? *Time Magazine*, Feb 3, 2012. [http://ideas.time.com/2012/02/03/adhd-is-the-stigma-back/]

Widenhorn-Müller K, *et al.* (2014) Effect of supplementation with long-chain ω-3 polyunsaturated fatty acids on behavior and cognition in children with attention deficit/hyperactivity disorder (ADHD): a randomized placebo-controlled intervention trial. *Prostaglandins Leukot Essent Fatty Acids* **91(1–2):** 49–60. [doi: 10.1016/j.plefa.2014.04.004]

Wolraich ML, *et al.* (1996) Comparison of diagnostic criteria for attention-deficit hyperactivity disorder in a county-wide sample. *J Am Acad Child Adolesc Psychiatry* **35(3):** 319–24.

Zylowska L, *et al.* (2007) Mindfulness meditation training in adults and adolescents with ADHD: a feasibility study. *J Atten Disord* **11(6):** 737–46.

Chapter 7

Vaccination Programs: Eradication of Infectious Diseases

The panel of vaccines on the pediatric schedule in the US includes those for a variety of diseases: Poliovirus, Rotavirus, Hepatitis and Hepatitis B1, diphtheria, tetanus, pertussis, *Haemophilus influenzae*, Pneumococca, Meningococcal, measles, mumps, rubella, and *Varicella*. The combined net good of reduced human suffering and lives saved from vaccinations against these diseases over the last decade in the US alone is estimate at 322 million illnesses, 21 million hospitalizations and 732,000 deaths (US Centers for Disease Control and Prevention). Worldwide, vaccines have saved millions of lives directly and many more by reducing the rate of spread of deadly contagious and infectious diseases. According to the World Health Organization, tetanus, measles, and pertussis are still among the top causes of deaths worldwide in children under five years of age (WHO, 2011).

Herd immunity is the protection that individuals enjoy from infection with a communicable disease when a high enough proportion of a population is vaccinated. The proportion needed for a given disease in a given population is called the "target percentage." There is no specific target percentage that applies to all populations for all diseases; the number depends, among other factors, on the population density, the modes of transmission, and the basic reproductive rate (R0) of the infectious agent. In general, infectious agents with higher R0 values also have higher target percentages. Another factor that influences the target percentage is population density.

In a report in October 2014, the US Centers for Disease Control and Prevention reported high variation among states in reaching the target percentage of vaccinations for measles, with percent vaccinated ranging from >99% to as low as 93%. Last year, in California, a measles epidemic is sweeping the country. Numerous diseases, including polio, and measles, had been all but eradicated in the US due to the vaccination program. Measles is more than just a collection of red welts on the skin; it comes with high fever, and can also result in pneumonia and fatal brain swelling. Some of the afflicted can go blind or lose their hearing.

In the Ebola-stricken countries of West Africa, because of the disruption of Ebola to their health infrastructure, measles could claim 16,000 lives beyond the 7,000 which are normally seen (Takahashi *et al.*, 2015). The solution proposed to prevent this outcome is a massive vaccination program. Ebola has destroyed the already fragile health care system in Liberia, Guinea and Sierra Leone. The lingering effects of dogma, superstition and fear of aid workers is likely to afflict these countries for a long time to come.

There is no doubt that vaccinations have been one of the most successful translational research programs in history. The first reported successful use of an inoculum was in China around 1,000 years ago. There is evidence of vaccine use in Turkey and Africa. In 1796, Edward Jenner experimented with the use of cowpox as a vaccine against smallpox. In 1886, Louis Pasteur developed an attenuated vaccine against rabies using rabbits. Its first use successfully saved the life of a young boy who had been bitten by a rabid dog.

There is an increasing number of parents in the US who are decidedly against vaccinating their children against what used to be common childhood diseases: measles, mumps and rubella, for example. In a 2009 survey study (Omer *et al.*, 2009), individuals who declined vaccines listed concerns over autism, over side effects, and over limited additional protection given the rarity of the diseases as factors that contributed to their positions against vaccinating their children. Those who resist vaccinations were also found to tend to be white, affluent, and insured. By adopting this position, some say they put others in the population — the very young (under four months), the immunocompromised (organ transplant recipients), and the elderly — at risk of death by aiding and abetting the virus by providing safe passage of the virus, through their children, to other humans.

The medical doctors who push for untested changes to scheduling, and even advocate taking a "free ride" on herd immunity are, according their critics, directly responsible for the current measles outbreak that started in 2014 in Disneyland in California. Of the initial people traced to the park's outbreak, 85% had either not been vaccinated or had unknown or undocumented vaccination status (US Centers for Disease Control and Prevention, 2015). The strain behind the multi-state outbreak that has infected over 160 people thus far is identical to a strain from the Philippines (US Centers for Disease Control and Prevention, 2015; Zipprich *et al.*, 2015). It is likely, therefore, that a traveler to Disneyland brought the measles to the state from the Philippines, and was transmitting the virus, where unprotected children — and adults — contracted the disease. Some doctors in California had taken the position that in his view, given the low incidence of measles in the US, it was possible to raise an unvaccinated child safely. Accusations have been made against parents for taking a "free ride" whose doctors who do not work to achieve CDC target percentages. That is not to say that the CDC is infallible — I was particularly critical of them in my first book, Ebola: An Evolving Story (World Scientific), for providing misleading and incorrect information to the public, the health care community, and the research community when Ebola hit US shores. Those who prefer to minimize the risk of any perceived or real side effects of vaccines to their children are accused of doing so at the compounded risk of peril to their own children, and to others (those with compromised immune systems). Similar accusations are made against parents who are against vaccinating their teens against HPV infection. At stake is the question of informed consent and the right of individuals to avoid adverse events from vaccines. HPV, or human papillomavirus, is a primary cause cervical cancer (most cervical cancers are caused by HPV), and it is a major cause of other types of cancer. The vaccines that can confer protection against HPV infection, such as Gardasil, which is spread by skin-to-skin contact, usually during sex, are reported to be safe and effective. Vaccines are now multivalent;

Gardasil 9 offers protections against nine strains of HPV. With an earlier version (Gardasil-4), rates of HPV infection were demonstrated to drop in girls aged 14–19, the vaccine-type HPV prevalence (HPV-6, –11, –16, or –18) decreased from 11.5% in 2003–2006 to 5.1% (Markowitz *et al.*, 2013).

There are those who object to vaccinating their child against HPV in part because they fear sending a permissive signal to their children. They tend to feel the same way about educating their teens on the use of condoms. However, parents who are concerned about their children engaging in sex as teens, or experimenting with drugs as teens, should know this: The time to start discussing these topics is not during pre-pubescence. The appropriate time to teach children how to behave safely in their environment is when they are much younger, 5–8 years of age, with frank, non-judgmental, informed discussions about the risks of teen pregnancy, of STDs, of drug addiction — and what they can do to protect themselves. I told my sons that doing drugs damages the brain (my position backed by citations in Pubmed of course!). To drive the point home, I told them that if brain damage was their goal, they could run head-down into a brick wall, and achieve about the same outcome. Scare tactic? No, my sons are now older, and they are not afraid of drugs. They are confident in their knowledge of the effects lists of street drugs because I gave them the facts on the effects of cocaine, marijuana, amphetamines and heroin on the human mind. Their stories are not yet completely written, but I have confidence in them. I told them that one day, they will be offered a joint. Or a pipe. Or a pill. And a beer. Or liquor. By a friend. Most likely, I told them, you will be offered these by one of your current classmates. Or a college friend. And we role-played the act of turning down the offer, with "Thanks, but I'm not into that." And if their friends persist, with peer pressure, I coached them to say that their father would cause great harm to them if I ever found out (they know this is not true). Finally, if their friend or friends continued to persist, I coached them to call me, and whatever I was doing, I would come get them. That they should leave. I have no doubt that they will experience anxiety when these events take place, and I expect them to take a hit — on the popularity scale with their friends.

Parents should understand that peer pressure is very powerful. So the time to give them the protection they need — the information they need to make the right decisions, and the confidence needed to execute in a manner consistent with their parent's wishes — is when they are very young. Parents who speak with their children about sex and STDs from a young age provide a trusting, safe association with the topic so by the time they are teenagers, sex is not a taboo subject; it is not as odd or awkward. The combined message of STD prevalence is a powerful deterrent. Estimates of the number of new infections of HPV range between 5.5 and 6.2 million a year, over the last decade or so. A study in 2012 found 54% of girls aged 13–17 years had received at least one dose of the HPV vaccine series, but only 33% had received all three doses (US Centers for Disease Control and Prevention, 2013). Vaccination of boys nationally was lower, with around 21% of boys receiving at least one dose, but only 6.8% receiving all three (US Centers for Disease Control and Prevention, 2013). No mention is made as to why booster shot attrition is so high.

The success of vaccination programs requires participation by doctors and patients in a proven technique that has saved millions of lives already. Public health officials should call on the population to inform their peers who refuse to vaccinate their children that they are putting the very young, the sick, and the old at risk by declining to participate in what is arguably the greatest medical achievement of all time. Oddly, this is the kind of thing that, for a deadly disease like Ebola, the US Centers for Disease Control and Prevention and other organizations wish to prevent: They want to make survivors of Ebola heroes, regardless of whether that person's behaviors put others at risk. This topic receives extensive treatment in *Ebola: An Evolving Story*.

Of course, the vaccines should be proven safe, and there are major discrepancies in the way vaccines are considered for use in the population that deviate from other drugs and devices. Entire dose schedules are changed without testing, such as the accelerated pediatric program which increased the exposure of children in the US to ethyl mercury from 75 µg in 2003 to 575 µg in 2013 (Kennedy, 2014). In the age of precision medicine, genetic subtype studies conducted by aggregated samples from those with immediate adverse reactions to the HPV vaccines should be conducted. HPV vaccinations, however, may not be the only line of defense. A drug called Isoprinosine is available as a generic medication in Europe. It was demonstrated to be well-tolerated and can clear HPV from the human body: Over 97% of patients treated in a small study showed HPV negative pap smears after two months (Buyanova *et al.*, 2013).

On Autism

In 1998, the English physician Andrew Wakefield suggested that the MMR (measles, mumps and rubella) vaccine invokes a breakthrough infection, harming the intestines of children, causing measles to enter the bloodstream and somehow harming the brain of patients, who then develop meningitis and regressive autism. A news reporter, Brian Deer, broke in 2010 that Wakefield had received large sums of money to conduct the research from lawyers who were planning on a large class-action lawsuit against pharmaceutical companies. Many of the authors on the study were upset by this news and demanded that the paper be retracted. Eventually, it was retracted.

Not many people dig deep enough into this story to understand that certain aspects of the alleged impropriety by Wakefield were conducted to facilitate the study. The blood for some of the autistic patients was taken at Wakefield's son's birthday party; the children were paid for their contributed blood as a reward. Wakefield had in fact received approval from an ethics committee to enroll specific patients into the study, a standard research ethics practice. By selecting autistic children suspected of having MMR vaccination, he was performing a step in study design called "enrichment." This incurs possible selection bias, but he never claimed a randomized study and he called for further study.

An initial look at the vast literature that has resulted will reveal claims that no studies have reproduced the specific findings of Wakefield *et al.*'s study. Briefly, the main points are

- The question of whether persistent measles infection can be detected in autistic patients other than studies in which Wakefield was involved (ISR Committee, 2001).
- Whether exposure of mice to body-weight adjusted post-natal doses of MMR vaccine contributes to a risk of autism-like symptoms or shows ill effects on the developing mouse brain.

Was the Focus on MMR Conflate "Vaccinated" with "MMR Vaccinated"?

It seems likely that the early focus on MMR may have confused "vaccinated children" with MMR vaccinated children. Many other vaccines at the time contained thimerosal, a form of ethyl mercury. Back in 2004, a study showed the specific harm caused by thimerosal in mice is strain-dependent (Hornig *et al.*, 2004). This strongly suggests a genetic component to thimerosal sensitivity. A Chinese study showed that neonatal exposure to 20× the dosages of thimerosal, a mercury-containing preservative used in some vaccines, has profoundly negative effects on the developing mouse brain (Li *et al.*, 2014). Another study demonstrated an increased risk of autism in infants born to mothers with > 6 mercury amalgam dental fillings (compared to those with five or fewer).

Mercury exposure is chronic pre-natal, and episodic post-natal. What if the ability of some to remove mercury from tissues (in short, sequester and remove from cells) is compromised in some patients? Mercury has been shown to exit the cell as part of a complex with reduced glutathione on "endogenous carriers" (Clarkson *et al.*, 2007). Genetic variation can be expected in the genes encoding these protein carriers, and it thus stands to reason (hypothetically) that the mechanism of removal may be defective in some people. If so, a series of what amounts to low-dose exposures for most of us could prove toxic to some.

A study in 2013 showed that a mitochondrial defect can lead to hypersensitivity to thimerosal in humans (Sharpe *et al.*, 2013). The study used B-lymphocytes from autistic people and their kin, and compared the reaction of those cells to cells from members of control families with no autistic family members.

None of these studies replicate or are even perhaps relevant to Wakefield's allegedly flawed and faked study; however, the current move toward individualized medicine includes accepted modification of the purely randomized trial in other contexts. For example, a biomarker-based enrichment study might lead to accrual of children with a mitochondrial defect in one arm, compared to children without the mitochondrial defect. Wakefield's attempt to identify patients likely to reveal a causal link between their autism and MMR vaccines could now, arguably, be called an awkward enrollment criterion that enriches one arm for a likely effect, i.e., to demonstrate the principle, to discover a possible correlation.

These kinds of enrichment studies are valid — as long as their results are not over-interpreted. They are seen as "Discovery" studies subject to validation. Biomarker-informed molecular allocation is being used in clinical trials of the safety and efficacy of cancer treatment studies — why not autism?

Thimerosal and mercury are not used in MMR vaccines in the US; they are, however, still included as an ingredient in vaccines in many other countries, and used in the US in an influenza vaccine that is given only to pregnant women. It is also present in meningitis vaccines. The following research studies seem warranted:

- The weight-adjusted normal dose studies could be repeated with a mouse model of the mitochondrial defect found by Sharpe *et al.* with wild-type mice as controls. If neurological defects associated with autism are found to occur in the mouse model after exposure to thimerosal, the case could be made that some percentage of children are likely to develop autism, and a biomarker assay could be used to prevent risky exposure;

- Indicative of a failed assumption of one model, post-infection, the measles virus is not detectable in autism patients;
- Similarly, mercury is not elevated in the blood of autistic patients (Hertz-Picciotto *et al.*, 2010).

Measles outbreaks can sicken thousands if left unchecked. On the issue of the MMR/autism link, neither camp, however, can safely overgeneralize their position: It is perhaps just as wrong to say that the vaccine "does not" cause autism as to insist that "it does." The two sides seem deadlocked. However, a logic check would reveal that the conclusion that MMR *does not cause* autism is a universal statement falsifiable by a single confirming instance. Large association-type epidemiological studies could bury the effect if there are rare genetic variants that confer a higher risk of autism in face of environmental exposure to mercury, which was present in other vaccines likely to be received by children who had NMR vaccination. What if the correct studies have not yet been done to ask the question:

Does Thimerosal Cause Autism in Some Patients?

The rare adverse events and deaths that occur shortly after HPV vaccination have, for the most part, all been attributed to other factors. However, the question of whether some genetic subtypes may be sensitive to ingredients in vaccines seems natural to post in the age of personalized medicine. The same question applies to HPV: Does HPV have ill effects in *some* patients? Can they be identified with biomarkers or with genome sequencing (with validation)?

There are around 3,900 adverse events per year in the US from vaccinations. However, there are over 10 million vaccinations per year. The overall risk, therefore, is about 0.0004, less than half an event per 1,000 vaccinations. There is no doubt that vaccinations have been a translational success in protecting the population against infectious agents. However, researchers and regulatory bodies should keep in mind that past randomized population-based studies will surely miss effects that are important to a minority of patients, but that minority of patients should not be condemned to any form of disability due to science's weak ability to detect the importance of risk factors relevant for the important and precious few. Research on the molecular causes of adverse events from vaccines may identify biomarkers that will allow doctors and patients to make informed decisions on specific vaccines, further reducing the risk and improving the overall positive impact of vaccination programs. Also, long-term follow-up studies on the safety of HPV vaccination are ongoing; interim analysis (De Vincenzo *et al.*, 2014) show no waning of the efficacy of either of two forms of the vaccine, with strong protection for at least eight years with the quadrivalent vaccine, and at least nine years with the bivalent vaccine, and adverse event rates were similar between the two vaccines (De Vincenzo *et al.*, 2014). The same study reviewed published rates of adverse events in vaccinated and placebo for numerous large studies, none of which found significantly higher rates of adverse events compared to placebo. This, however, does not mean that a subgroup of people do not exist who are ultrasensitive to HP vaccines or their components.

2014 CDC Whistleblower and "Subgroup" Analysis

The US Centers for Disease Control and Prevention Website contains a page that reads as follows:

CDC Statement Regarding 2004 Pediatrics Article, "Age at First Measles-Mumps-Rubella Vaccination in Children With Autism and School-matched Control Subjects: A Population-Based Study in Metropolitan Atlanta"

CDC shares with parents and others great concern about the number of children with autism spectrum disorder.

CDC is committed to continuing to provide essential data on autism, search for factors that put children at risk for autism and look for possible causes. While doing so, we work to develop resources that help identify children with autism as early as possible so they can benefit from intervention services.

CDC's study about age at first Measles-Mumps-Rubella (MMR) vaccination and autism, published in Pediatrics *in 2004, included boys and girls from different ethnic groups, including black children. The manuscript presented the results on two sets of children:*

All children who were initially recruited for the study, and the subset of children who had a Georgia birth certificate.

Access to the information on the birth certificates allowed researchers to assess more complete information on race as well as other important characteristics, including possible risk factors for autism such as the child's birth weight, mother's age, and education. This information was not available for the children without birth certificates; hence CDC study did not present data by race on black, white, or other race children from the whole study sample. It presented the results on black and white/other race children from the group with birth certificates.

The study looked at different age groups: children vaccinated by 18 months, 24 months, and 36 months. The findings revealed that vaccination between 24 and 36 months was slightly more common among children with autism, and that association was strongest among children 3–5 years of age. The authors reported this finding was most likely a result of immunization requirements for preschool special education program attendance in children with autism.

The data CDC collected for this study continue to be available for analysis by others. CDC welcomes analysis by others that can be submitted for peer-review and publication. For more information on how to access this public-use dataset please go to the(sic) this webpage.

Additional studies and a more recent rigorous review by the Institute of Medicine have found that MMR vaccine does not increase the risk of autism.

Vaccines protect the health of children in the United States so well that most parents today have never seen first-hand the devastating consequences of diseases now stopped by vaccines.

However, our 2014 measles count is the highest number since measles was declared eliminated in 2000. We do not want to lose any opportunity to protect all of our children when we have the means to do so.

Why would the CDC publish such a page?

In 2014, one of the authors of the CDC study, Dr. William Thompson, PhD, was recorded by one Dr. Hooker. Dr. Hooker had allegedly spent 10 years since the CDC study petitioning for access to the entire data behind the study.

In the interview, Dr. William Thompson is heard making the following statements:

Oh my God, I cannot believe we did what we did. But we did. It's all there.

The higher-ups wanted to do certain things and I went along with it.

It was the lowest point in my career that I went along with that paper. And I went along with this, and didn't report significant findings.

I have great shame now when I meet families with kids with autism because I've — I've been part of the problem.

The study was an attempt to answer, in a large case vs. control study, whether the risk of autism of children vaccinated at an early age showed in an increased incidence of autism when compared to a control group of children not vaccinated. The study formed the basis of final decisions of the Immunization Safety Review Committee reports published between 2001 and 2014 that led to the current medical consensus that vaccines and their ingredients do not increase the risk of autism.

Dr. Thompson is alleged to have called Dr. Hooker, according to Hooker himself, so he could take Thompson's "confession" as his priest.

After 10 years of trying to get data from a pivotal study that the CDC had conducted, Hooker had finally acquired from the CDC the full data from the original study. In a re-analysis (Hooker, 2014), Hooker performed two types of analysis: the same type as the CDC (conditional logistic regression) and a cohort analysis. In both analyses, a significant association was found in one subgroup of children — African American black males. In Hooker's analysis, African American black babies vaccinated for MMR before the age of 36 months were found to have an increased risk of developing autism by as much as 340%.

According to Thompson, senior scientists at the CDC — his supervisors, and the study authors — forced him to not report the full results of the analysis of the data, and they knew of the result of the increased risk in African American male babies. The fact that this subgroup result was hidden from the public is clear. In slides made available to the public of a presentation made to the Institutes of Medicine of the National Academies of Science, Dr. DeStefano, first author on the CDC paper states, unequivocally:

"No statistically significant associations for any subgroups in this table."

DeStefano's slides were from a presentation to the Institutes of Medicine of the National Academies of Science, available as of June 2015 at the following URL:

https://www.iom.edu/~/media/2F7869D331024709B448D-C3984A216F8.ashx

This matches the results report in the original publication (Stephano *et al.*, 2008):

No significant associations for either of these age cutoffs were found for specific case subgroups, including those with evidence of developmental regression.

It is important to note that the table contained results from subgroup analyses, and it confirms that subgroup analysis — of the type conducted by Hooker — was in fact conducted using the original data prior to the publication.

By not reporting the full set of subset analyses conducted, the CDC scientists failed to alert the scientific and medical communities to the need for further study to confirm the results, and then, if they could be confirmed, to take steps to protect the population that might be affected. They constrained society's options.

Individuals who might try to dismiss Dr. Hooker's re-analysis (Hooker, 2014, retracted) on the ground that doing too many subgroup analyses can lead to false positives must apply the same critique to the original MADDSP MMR/AUTISM study. It is also important to note that the table in question referenced race as a subgroup analysis. The result not was the race/gender subgroup analyses (e.g., white boys, white girls; African American boys, African American girls), which, according to Thompson, had been conducted but were excluded from the MADDSP MMR/AUTISM STUDY publication.

The original study examined rates of autism in vaccinated and unvaccinated children. They had looked at 614 children with ASD and 1,824 children without ASD. Of the 624 children, the following considerations were given re: study design:

The children in the study were born between 1986 and 1993; they were identified through MADDSP with evaluations available up through 1996, and DSM-IV criteria used to classify children. ASD classification was determined by ASD experts. To be included in the study, the patients had to have the following:

- Valid MMR vaccination date from school immunization form.
- DTP vaccination by age 2 from school immunization form.
- Immunization exemption form.

Note that race was never meant to be an inclusion criterion. It was meant to be a covariate, i.e., a variable that might be an important contributor of risk, or a modifier of risk, of autistic regression after early vaccination with MMR.

Comparing children receiving MMR before 36 months to those receiving it after 36 months, DeStefano *et al.* (2004) found that the relative risk of autism was 1.49 (95% confidence interval [CI]: 1.04–2.14) in the early vaccination group. They concluded that the increased risk was due to greater numbers of autistic children receiving timely vaccinations in order to participate in State of Georgia special education services, which is *non-sequitur* and does not rule out causal influence; it just means their vaccinations were earlier.

According to the Thompson's interview with Hooker, and according to the CDC Statement at the beginning of the chapter, the results showing significant overall association of increased risk of autism and MMR vaccination within African American boys were excluded from their own subgroup analysis of African American babies without birth certificates because the birth certificates were used to collected information about variables that may contribute to risk factors, including race, birth weight, age of mother, and the degree of education obtained by the mother. The race "covariate" was intended to be used in the original protocol.

In a statement from his lawyers, Dr. Thompson said (emphasis mine):

FOR IMMEDIATE RELEASE—AUGUST 27, 2014

STATEMENT OF WILLIAM W. THOMPSON, Ph.D., REGARDING THE 2004 ARTICLE EXAMINING THE POSSIBILITY OF A RELATIONSHIP BETWEEN MMR VACCINE AND AUTISM

My name is William Thompson. I am a Senior Scientist with the Centers for Disease Control and Prevention where I have worked since 1998.

I regret my co-authors and I omitted statistically significant information in our 2004 article published in the journal Pediatrics. *The omitted data suggested that African American males who received the MMR vaccine before 36 months were at increased risk for autism. Decisions were made regarding which findings to report after the data was collected, and I believe that the final study protocol **was not followed**.*

I want to be absolutely clear that I believe vaccines have saved and continue to save countless lives. I would never suggest that any parent avoid vaccinating children of any race. Vaccines prevent serious diseases, and the risks associated with their administration are vastly outweighed by their individual and societal benefits.

My concern has been the decision to omit relevant findings in a particular study for a particular sub-group for a particular vaccine. *There have always been recognized risks for vaccination and I believe it is the responsibility of the CDC to properly convey the risks associated with the receipt of those vaccines.*

I have had many discussions with Dr. Brian Hooker over the last 10 months regarding studies the CDC has carried out regarding vaccines and neurodevelopmental outcomes including autism spectrum disorders. I share his belief that CDC decision-making analyses should be transparent. I was not, however, aware that he was recording any of our conversations, nor was I given any choice regarding whether my name would be made public or my voice would be put on the Internet.

I am grateful for the many supportive emails that I have received over the last several days. I will not be answering questions at this time. I am providing information to Congressman William Posey, and of course will continue to cooperate with Congress. I have also offered to assist with reanalysis of the study data of development of further studies. For the time being, however, I am focused on my job and my family.

Reasonable scientists can and do differ in their interpretation of information. I will do everything I can to assist any unbiased and objective scientists outside of the CDC to analyze data collected by the CDC or other public organizations for the purpose of understanding whether vaccines are associated with an increased risk of autism. There are still more questions than answers, and I appreciate that so many families are looking for answers from the scientific community.

My colleagues and supervisors at the CDC have been entirely professional since this matter became public. In fact, I received a performance-based award after this story came out. I have experienced no pressure or retaliation and certainly was not escorted out of the building as some have stated.

After news of Dr. Thomas' revelations, the first author on the CDC study, Dr. Frank DeStefano, was interviewed by CBS News Reporter Sharyl Attkisson. DeStefano, who is now Chief of the Immunization

Safety office, admitted in the September 2014 interview that vaccines may indeed trigger autism in some vulnerable children.

In the meantime, Hooker's publication (Hooker, 2014) was retracted by the journal in which it was published, with the following statement:

The Editor and Publisher regretfully retract the article as there were undeclared competing interests on the part of the author which compromised the peer review process. Furthermore, post-publication peer review raised concerns about the validity of the methods and statistical analysis, therefore the Editors no longer have confidence in the soundness of the findings.

Hooker's publication aside, the CDC individuals have themselves revealed:

(1) That they had found, prior to the 2004 publication of the MADDSP MMR/AUTISM study, using their methods of data analysis, a strong association between early MMR vaccination in African Americans and autism;

(2) That Thompson considered the failure of the publication of the full set of results not only a violation of protocol, but also "lies."

Thompson had revealed to Hooker: *"If forced to testify, I'm not going to lie. I basically have stopped lying."*

Thompson also revealed that he was aware that the vaccine could do damage to at least some part of the population:

There is a vaccine that still uses thimerosal in the US, and it is used in other countries. Thompson to Hooker: *"Do you think a pregnant mother would want to take a vaccine that they know caused tics? Absolutely not!! I would never give my wife a vaccine that I thought caused tics."*

Based on the data that Thompson has seen, he is convinced that *"There is biologic plausibility right now to say thimerosal causes autism-like features."*

Dr. Bernadine Healy, former Director of the US National Institutes of Health, was interviewed in 2008 by then CBS News Correspondent Sharyl Atkisson, and had some insights on the possible negative influences of such activities:

This is the time when we do have the opportunity to understand whether or not there are susceptible children, perhaps genetically, perhaps they have a metabolic issue, mitochondrial disorder, immunological issue that makes them more susceptible to vaccines, plural, or to one particular vaccine, or to one component of vaccines, like mercury. So we now, in these times have to take another look at that hypothesis; not deny it. I think we have the tools today that we didn't have 10 years ago. That we didn't have 20 years ago, to try and tease that out and find out if there is indeed that susceptible group. Why is that important? A susceptible group does not mean that vaccines aren't good. What a susceptible group will tell us is that maybe there is a group of individuals or a group of children that shouldn't have a particular vaccine or shouldn't have vaccines on the same schedule. I do not believe that if we identified a susceptibility group, that if we identified a particular risk factor for vaccines; or if we found out that they should be spread out a little longer, I do not believe that the public would lose faith in vaccines. It is the job of the public health community and of physicians to be out there and to say, "Yes, we can make it safer because we are able to say, this is a subset and we're going to deliver it in a way that we think is safer." I think the government or certain public health officials in the government have been too quick to dismiss the concerns of these families without studying the population that got sick. The public health officials have been too quick to dismiss the hypothesis as irrational, without sufficient studies of causation. I think they have often been too quick to dismiss studies in the animal laboratory, either in mice, in primates, that do show some concerns with regard to certain vaccines and also to the mercury preservative in vaccines. The government has said in a report by the Institute of Medicine, in a report in 2004, it basically said, "Do not pursue susceptibility groups. Don't look for those patients, those children who may be vulnerable." I really take issue with that conclusion. The reason they didn't want to look for those susceptibility groups was because they were afraid that if they found them, however big or small they were, that would scare the public away. First of all, I think the public's smarter than that; I think the public values vaccines, but more importantly I don't think you should ever turn your back on any scientific hypothesis because you're afraid of what it might show. If you read the 2004 report and converse with a few of my colleagues who believe this still to be the case, there is a completely expressed concern that they don't want to pursue a hypothesis because that hypothesis could be damaging to the public health community at large by scaring people. I don't believe the truth ever scares people and if it does have a certain edge to it, then that's the obligation of those who are delivering those facts to do it in a responsible way so you don't terrify the public. One never should shy away from science; one should never shy away from getting causality information in a setting in which you can test it. Populations do not test causality; they test associations. You have to go into the laboratory, and you have to do designed research studies, in animals. What we're seeing is in the bulk of the population vaccines are safe. Vaccines are safe. But there may be the susceptible group. The fact that there is concern that you don't want to know that susceptible group is a real disappointment to me. If you know that susceptible group, you can save those children. If you turn your back on the notion that there's a susceptible group that means that you are...what can I say? (Healy and Atkisson, 2008).

The proper thing for the CDC to have done would have been to reveal their discovery of the association and discuss in their paper the issues that were raised to condemn Dr. Hooker's re-analysis, among them being that subgroup analyses are prone to producing false positives due to multiple hypothesis testing.

These concerns, however, do not indemnify the CDC scientists from their actions in failing to bring the results to light; they, too, performed multiple subgroup analyses, and it is abundantly clear from Dr. Thompson's interviews that he, and the senior personnel on the project, not only knew of the results showing that boys were at a greater risk of receiving an autism diagnosis when they received their first MMR vaccine prior to 36 months of age than black boys receiving their first MMR vaccine at or after 36 months of age: they also knew that they were hiding information that could go against the mainstream momentum of moving toward consensus on the lack of association between vaccination and autism.

Robert F. Kennedy, Jr. reviewed how pointedly unethical the issues became within the CDC, based on audio recordings (Kennedy, 2014):

> *Thompson described in chilling detail to Dr. Hooker, the intense pressure from his CDC bosses after he first broke ranks on vaccine safety. In 2004, he sent a letter to CDC Director, Julie Gerberding alerting her that CDC scientists were breaking research protocols to conceal the links between thimerosal and brain damage in children. Gerberding never responded to Thompson's allegations, but her deputy, Robert Chen, then head of CDC's Immunization Safety Office and Thompson's direct boss, confronted Thompson in an agency parking lot threatening him and screaming, "I would fire you if I could." In 2009, Gerberding matriculated to Merck as Chief of the company's Vaccine Division. Two years prior to the move, she approved Merck's HPV vaccine for pre-adolescent girls — an estimated billion dollar value to the company. Following Thompson's revelations, Merck transferred Gerberding from its Vaccine Division to Executive Vice President for Strategic Communications, Global Public Policy and Population Health.*

The implication here is that Thompson was brushed off, and then put off by the CDC leadership after raising what he thought was a valid scientific concern, and Dr. Julie Gerberding had a serious conflict of interest in this subterfuge because she was planning to move to Merck.

To make matters worse, *Natural News* reported in August 2014 (*Natural News*, 2014, *unverified*) that they had received a copy of an e-mail from Dr. Thompson to colleagues in 2002 who were trying to decide which documents to turn over to the Department of Justice:

From: Thompson, William,

Sent: Friday, October 18, 2002 4:43 AM

To: Wharton, Melinda

Cc: Orenstein, Walt; Lane, Kim (NIP); Malone, Kevin M.; Dozier, Beverly; Chen, Robert (Bob) (NIP); Shay, David; Boyle, Colleen; Bernier, Roger

Dear Melinda:

I am writing you once more regarding the recent Department of Justice (DOJ) request for a broad range of documents associated with MMR, Thimerosal, and Autism. I first spoke with you on September 3rd of 2002 regarding the sensitive results we have been struggling with in the MADDSP MMR/Autism Study. I have tried to bring your attention to some potentially sensitive legal issues surrounding what documents we should provide for this study. We have subsequently been told by both Beverly Dozier and Kevin Malone that we should apply a very broad definition to the documents that we provide to the DOJ.

Therefore, I will provide all documents that I have in my possession including agendas, analysis plans, excel spreadsheets, SAS programs, draft manuscripts, edited manuscripts, and sensitive results that we have been discussing at the National Center for Birth Defects and Developmental Disabilities (NCBDDD) since February 2001 when I started to work on this study at the request of NIP OD. I will also be providing any other documents that I have related to all other MMR, Thimerosal, or autism studies that I have on while at NIP. I will attempt to provide all those documents by COB October 21st. I have not have the time to access whether those documents are sensitive or not. I don't think anyone has broken the law but I was extremely uncomfortable when Dr. Coleen Boyle, a coauthor on our paper, was required to testify before Congressman Dan Burton's Committee in April of 2002 regarding MMR and Autism. I became more concerned regarding legal issues surrounding the MADDSP MMR/Autism Study when individuals from the NCBDDD began to cc Beverly Dozier, an attorney, on e-mails regarding discussions we were having surrounding the provision of appropriate documents to satisfy the DOJ request. I became further concerned when I attended a meeting at the NCBDDD on October 16th at 1:00 PM to discuss the provision of documents and found out that Beverly was a NCBDDD lawyer, not a DOJ lawyer, who was proving legal advice to Dr. Coleen Boyle regarding what documents to provide. Therefore, I will be hiring my own personal attorney to make sure that I am also providing all of the appropriate documents for this study. It is extremely unfortunate that we need to be concerned about whether our own legal rights are covered when participating in a study such as this. My level of concern has also caused me to seriously consider removing myself as an author on the draft manuscript.

Sincerely,

Bill Thompson

-----Original Message-----

From: Malone, Kevin M.

Sent: Thursday, October 17, 2002 9:32 AM

To: Chen, Robert (Bob) (NIP); Thompson, William; Shay, David; Wharton, Melinda

Subject: RE: DOJ Request

I believe that Beverly Dozier and I have the same interpretation of what needs to be provided now and this is to be very broad in identifying relevant documents for DOJ review.

Thompson also made the financial motive clear to Hooker. In a Town Hall meeting in June 2015, Hooker described it thusly:

> *Dr. Thompson also described a culture of fraud in the CDC, an institution with a built-in conflict of interest regarding vaccine update versus vaccine safety. The CDC buys over $4 billion of vaccines each year from the pharmaceutical industry to distribute to the states' public health departments. Vaccine uptake in the US must be high for the CDC to get reimbursed for that purchase. Thus, vaccine safety scientists are under tremendous pressure not to find associations between vaccines and neurological adverse events, among others. He has been specifically told "point blank" from his superiors in multiple instances to not report such findings and to find ways using fraudulent statistical methods to obviate the results and falsely give vaccines a clean bill of health. Dr. Thompson stepped forward due to the agony of over 10 years of lying and covering up the real truth regarding vaccine injury.*

A former pharmaceutical scientist, Dr. H. Ratajczak, performed an extensive literature review (Ratajczak *et al.*, 2011) of all studies published on possible causes of autism and concluded that the hypersensitivity hypothesis — that some individuals may have a genetic basis of hypersensitivity — is a worthwhile theory, and that increases are likely due to early MMR vaccine and an increase in the number of vaccinations in a short period of time. Here is her full abstract:

Autism, a member of the pervasive developmental disorders (PDDs), has been increasing dramatically since its description by Leo Kanner in 1943. First estimated to occur in 4 to 5 per 10,000 children, the incidence of autism is now 1 per 110 in the United States, and 1 per 64 in the United Kingdom, with similar incidences throughout the world. Searching information from 1943 to the present in PubMed and Ovid Medline databases, this review summarizes results that correlate the timing of changes in incidence with environmental changes. Autism could result from more than one cause, with different manifestations in different individuals that share common symptoms. Documented causes of autism include genetic mutations and/or deletions, viral infections, and encephalitis following vaccination. Therefore, autism is the result of genetic defects and/or inflammation of the brain. The inflammation could be caused by a defective placenta, immature blood-brain barrier, the immune response of the mother to infection while pregnant, a premature birth, encephalitis in the child after birth, or a toxic environment.

In other words, a subset of people may benefit from genetic testing prior to vaccination for hypersensitivity. This has been confirmed by an association study of Pink disease (Austin *et al.*, 2014).

It is ironic that the rest of the medical world is moving toward personalized medicine, with genetic clinical subtypes, and biomarker-mediated treatments. According to the FDA (US FDA, 2015), 45% of all new drug approvals in 2013 were for biomarker (mostly genetic) identified subsets or targeted therapies, compared to just 5% in the 1990s. Molecular subtypes, especially genetic molecular subtypes, are critically important in modern medicine.

If there are hypersensitive individuals at risk of any particular type of vaccine, or vaccine component, the appropriate test should be developed to minimize the risk to the clinical subpopulation, or an alternative vaccine developed that does not use the risky ingredient(s).

Dr. Hooker's paper, in which he revealed the association, has been retracted by the journal for concerns over the statistical methodology and an alleged undisclosed conflict of interest between the author (Hooker) and one of the peer reviewers. The subtype analysis that Dr. Hooker performed included what he called a "cohort analysis" as well as a repeat of the type of analysis used for other comparisons in the original CDC study. The association may well be due to selection bias of some sort; it is, after all, only one study. Any such concern would apply equally to the original study. But then again, the association may be real. The correct interpretation of the limited value of subgroup analysis cannot be attributed to low power; when statistical significance has been demonstrated, power has been demonstrated.

This fact makes the CDC's decision to exclude the one significant subgroup result all the more disappointing. Each of their analyses, except for the African American boys, show no higher incidence of autism. The presence of one significant subgroup result — one with the smallest sample size — would seem to lend support that the other subgroups results were valid, because if any association did exist, it would be likely to be found in the larger subgroups.

To me, this one CDC study is not especially convincing either way — it is only one study. The fact that it was a CDC study should not afford it greater importance than any other study. However, the possibility of a genetic risk is a possibility worth considering that requires further study.

First, we need to confirm whether early vaccinations in African American males increase the risk of autism. Naturally, this should be done using retrospective (i.e., already available) data sets. No parent if fully informed would consent to subjecting their child to a prospective study where the side effect could be as devastating as autism.

If additional data from future subgroup analyses can replicate the detected increased risk, we then need to discover which (if any genes) have genetic variants ("mutations") that are associated with autism induced by exposure to mercury or other potentially dangerous ingredient. Austin *et al.* (2014) found variants in genes encoding paraoxanase 1

(PON1) and methylenetetrahydrofolate reductase (MTHFR) associated with sensitivity to mercury in Pink disease — so called due to the immediate effects of mercury exposure to the hands and feet of some infants. People who had Pink disease have also been found to have an increased risk of having children with autism (Shandley and Austin, 2011).

The first task in doing such studies on autism would be to take the data demonstrating potential risk of increased development of autism at face value, not to bury it and hope that no one ever finds out. Such association studies would have to consider both genetics, environmental factors, and vaccination history as contributing factors with potential interactions, rather than competing variables.

Is This the Second Smoking Gun?

Dr. Hooker received, under the freedom of information act, an e-mail from Verstraeten, the scientist conducting research to study association of vaccination and autism. The study underwent three rounds of analysis. In frustration, Verstraeten reported via an e-mail dated December 17, 1999 to the CDC that, in spite of his best attempts to adjust the analysis factors, the persistent relationship between thimerosal and autism could not be explained by other factors. The e-mail subject line was "It just won't go away."

In an e-mail dated Friday, July 14, 2000, from Thomas Verstraeten to the CDC, he also wrote:

I do not wish to be the advocate of the anti-vaccine lobby and sound like being convinced that thimerosal is or was harmful, but at least I feel we should use sound scientific argumentation and not let our standards be dictated by our desire to disprove an unpleasant theory.

Verstraeten *et al.* published the final analysis in 2003 in the journal *Pediatrics*. The study, as published, ultimately found no association of vaccination with thimerosal-containing vaccines.

Whereas the original plan was to conduct the second phase as a case-control study, we soon realized this would be too time consuming.

A Danish study (Madsen *et al.*, 2002) found no association between vaccine and autism only after "correcting for" variables such as low income, low education level in the mother, low birthweight, young gestational age — all factors that arguably could also play a role in African American families in Georgia in the US. Thus, rather than a genetic basis, ethyl mercury-induced autism could be more likely in children from low-income families. The study explained these variables away as confounding variables. However, the increased risk in autism may be visible only when the rate data are not adjusted for these factors. In other words, there could be a significant interaction between the mercury and standard of living, and by "adjusting for" these variables, the Danish study may have missed a finding of extreme clinical importance due to the incorrect removal of *relevant* confounders. The fact that the US exports thimerosal-containing vaccines to other countries, including to low-income populations, is distressing.

Verstraeten *et al.* (2003) and Madsen *et al.* (2002) are retrospective epidemiological studies. Such studies are rarely, if ever, used by the FDA to approve the use of a drug on the population. They require prospective, randomized placebo-controlled clinical trials. The full vaccine schedule has not been studied for safety and efficacy — and the human brain undergoes massive amounts of specialized neurological development.

Department of Justice Investigation?

The CDC went off IRB-approved research protocol; as a result, they hid results that might raise concern over toxicity of thimerosal in some patience. No one has yet been held accountable for the potentially negative impact of that action on our understanding of autism, however, a Department of Justice investigation is possible. The putative association should be studied further, and quickly, by independent groups, and the CDC should apply the same degree of scrutiny to translational potential in their own studies as they do studies from other institutions. Sanctions that apply to perpetrators of scientific fraud should be considered for those involved in the cover-up; the study paper should be retracted or appended with the complete set of results.

The financial incentive of reimbursement for vaccine deployment should be disconnected from research. No one involved in the financial end of business in the CDC should be involved, or have any influence, over the research efforts. No one involved in policy-making at the CDC should be involved in the research that determines that policy. And certainly under the new rules of ethics, no one at the CDC should have any financial conflicts of interest in the outcomes of the results of studies they conduct. No one at any institution in a position to influence public health should ever have a personal financial stake in the outcome of their research — including the NIH, NIAID, the FDA, and the CDC (among others). No conflicts of interest should be tolerated, including those that the individual and their closest peers would wish to grant each other by applying the euphemism "managed conflicts of interest."

How the Public Should Perceive These Issues

First and foremost, the public should not eschew vaccinations, nor should they arbitrarily change their child's vaccination schedule. But they should not join the pejoratively labeled "Anti-vaxxers" simply because one study hid a possible — emphasis on possible — association, pointing to one potentially susceptible group. They can request thimerosal-free vaccines, each and every time (except in West Virginia and in California). And they can communicate their concerns to lawmakers requesting studies of all ingredients in vaccines and demand transparency in scientific reporting by government employees.

The public, especially parents, should understand that while "science is complex," this is not an acceptable explanation when this type of thing happens. But they should not fall into the trap of thinking "all vaccines are bad." Sometimes in complex issues, it is not either/or; vaccines can be excellent overall, and can have a magnificently positive affect on the health of our population, and an ingredient can be highly toxic to some percentage of the population. There is no *a priori* reason to believe that both side are wrong — they both may be correct.

Sometimes government officials and scientists underestimate the public's ability to reason, and in their fear, forget that the loss of trust in government institutions is most often the result of failure to divulge the truth, however unpleasant or confusing. We saw the same kind of "Government knows best" condescension during the 2014 Ebola epidemic, where it seemed that Dr. Tom Frieden, Director of the CDC, could not seem to utter the words "We do not know." The same type of thinking is behind a recent study conducted seeking correlation of media stories and web searches regarding the disease. The author of the study interpreted the frequency of web searches for "Ebola" and "Ebola symptoms" and "Do I Have Ebola" as a sign of "panic" in the public in response to media coverage as opposed to a well-educated public attempting to learn more about a potentially important health topic.

The public's interest was warranted — they were provided conflicting messages from various government agencies, and they were interested in — and deserved to be told — the truth. We live in the information age. People are hungry to get answers to their questions. If more scientists became comfortable with saying "We don't know yet, but to find out, we need to do additional studies that include X, Y or Z. We'll get back to you," a large proportion of the public, educated or not, would see that response as reasonable, and acceptable. When scientists hide the truth, and the truth comes out, public trust is lost, and the public begins to realize that these public servants do not seem to think that they work for American public via their tax dollars; that they are an entity unto themselves, largely unreachable by the great unwashed masses. The public begins to wonder — and worry — if there are other things that they are being lied to about.

No one should strive to perpetuate such an image of an institution as austere as the CDC, the FDA, or the NIH, especially high-ranking individuals within those institutions. When they do act this way, and the truth comes out, they should not kill the messenger or blame the media.

They should let justice take its course. Progressive scientists are more than honest — they are forthright; they do not commit sins of omission. As a result, they tend to be seen as more credible and trustworthy.

We need an era of progressive science in which individuals are sincerely interested in knowledge for the sake of knowledge, *and* for the sake of translation.

Wakefield Loses NAACP and Other Minority Support Groups for Overreach

Dr. Wakefield, whose questionable research practices cost him his career, created a dramatic video in which he likened the continued practice of the use of thimerosal vaccines to the terrible tragedy in the study of the progression of syphilis in afflicted black men in the now-infamous Tuskegee, Mississippi experiments conducted between 1932 and 1972. The Nation of Islam, by comparison, has been positively responsive to Wakefield's message and tone.

The CDC communicated to ABC News in a statement that Dr. Hooker's study contained results that were somehow different from those arrived at in their unpublished subgroup analysis:

Centers for Disease Control and Prevention Statement Regarding Brian Hooker's Reanalysis of its 2004 Study

Aug. 27, 2014 There was no cover up. The study did not find any statistically significant associations between age at MMR vaccination and autism. In the CDC paper, similar proportions of case (children with autism) and control children (no autism) had been vaccinated before 18 months or before 24 months. While slightly more children with autism (93.4%) than children without autism (90.6%) were vaccinated between 24 and 36 months, this was most likely a result of immunization requirements for preschool special education program attendance in children with autism. As this topic was so sensitive and complex, the CDC study published in Pediatrics in February 2004 underwent clearance at CDC, the usual process of internal review for scientific accuracy that all CDC papers undergo. In addition, before submission to the journal, the manuscript was reviewed by five experts outside of CDC and an independent CDC statistician (see acknowledgements section of the paper for specific names). Finally, all reputable journals undergo peer-review of all submitted papers before final publication. The 2004 CDC study was designed as a case-control study. This means, children with autism (cases) were specifically identified, and children without autism (controls) were identified to be similar to the children with autism in other respects. When data are collected in a specific way for a specific type of statistical analysis (a case-control study in this instance), using those data in a different type of analysis can produce confusing results. Because the methods in Dr. Hooker's reanalysis were not described in detail, it is hard to speculate why his results differed from CDC's.

Since the 2004 Pediatrics *paper, CDC has conducted additional studies of vaccines and autism. In 2004 the Institute of Medicine reviewed published and unpublished findings from the US and other countries and concluded that there was no association between MMR vaccination and autism. In 2011, another IOM committee reviewed additional research, and once again found that evidence favored rejection of this association.*

The problem with this statement is that Hooker's methods are explained in perfect detail in the retracted publication and, more damning to the CDC's public relations, the results reached by Hooker are nearly identical to those in the CDC's unpublished subgroup analysis. While Hooker left out sample sizes for each subgroup, the original CDC publication included patient sample sizes.

Let's look at the "differences" between Hooker's results and the CDC's results. In Hooker's paper (retracted), the overall analysis of all children showed no increase in risk of developing autism, regardless of age of vaccination. This result is the same as the CDC's overall results.

Hooker's results in the subgroup analysis (African American males) and the original, unpublished analysis of the same subgroup that

Dr. Thompson said made him feel so guilty and ashamed both DO show a significant association for African American children:

MMR < 36 mo

CDC Black Model	OR	Lower 95th %tile CI	Upper 95%tile CI
	2.25	1.25	4.03
Hooker result	2.30	1.25	4.22

OR is "odds ratio," a standard analysis in this type of association study. Hooker's subgroup analysis also shows that this result is due to a significant association in African American boys when analyzed alone. No association was found in African American girls when analyzed alone.

Credit for this comparison to Jake Crosby, Editor of *Autism Investigated*, who wrote in an online article:

This would eviscerate critics' claims that Brian Hooker's findings are invalid because his reanalysis did not employ the same statistical methods as the original CDC study. Within Dr. Hooker's paper itself, it is also stated that his "results were also confirmed using a conditional logistic regression design similar to the DeStefano et al. (CDC) study". Another common criticism of Brian Hooker's paper that it did not account for low birth weight children is easily refuted by another table of results showing a greater than two-fold risk for African-American boys even when low birth weight children are excluded.

Yet Dr. Hooker's paper remains retracted in breach of the guidelines the publisher claims to follow when considering retractions. Even before the retraction, the publisher BioMed Central (BMC) had deleted the paper online in breach of its own policies on article removal. BMC has never offered any explanation concerning these issues in response to emails from Autism Investigated. *Also yet to comment in response to* Autism Investigated's *inquiries about the retraction is the Committee on Publication Ethics (COPE), whose guidelines BMC claims to follow when considering retractions and breached when it retracted Dr. Hooker's study. (Crosby J, 2015).*

Hooker's full paper is still available online via Pubmed Central: http://www.ncbi.nlm.nih.gov/pmc/articles/PMC4128611/

Hooker's only gaff in his analysis was to call his analysis a "cohort" analysis; the CDC called their analysis a "case-control" study. Having conducted hundreds of case control studies myself, there is no substantial difference other than terminology; this can be seen in the nearly identical results. Hooker likely called it "cohort" analysis due to being accurate in representing which option he selected in the software he used.

The minor differences in the OR scores does not explain the CDC's significant finding away, or why they decided to bury their result.

If the ASM data are the correct CDC results — and this has not been confirmed — then it would appear that the CDC has issued a misleading statement to ABC News. Even so, the lead author on the CDC study has already acknowledged in the September 2014 interview that vaccines may indeed trigger autism in some vulnerable children.

In the meantime, we might want to consider the chemists' view on thimerosal (Geier *et al.*, 2015):

> *The culmination of the research that examines the effects of thimerosal in humans indicates that it is a poison at minute levels with a plethora of deleterious consequences, even at the levels currently administered in vaccines.*

Given that thimerosal is in use in an influenza vaccine given only to pregnant women, the rates of autism should be checked in African American boys whose mothers received the vaccine while the boys were *in utero*.

Citing Negative Evidence and Using What We Know

The susceptibility of fetuses to methylmercury toxicity had already been established before the 2004 CDC study. In fact, it had been established since the early 1970s (Snyder, 1971). Mothers who ingest mercury in their diet pass it to their fetus (Murata *et al.*, 2004), and to their infant via breast milk (Grandjean *et al.*, 1995). Maternal consumption during pregnancy of methylmercury-contaminated fish in Japan and of methylmercury-contaminated bread in Iraq caused psychomotor retardation in the offspring. Studies reveal adverse fetal effects at very low maternal hair mercury concentrations (Marsh and Turner, 1995). The brains of children prenatally exposed to organic mercury show dysplasia of cerebral and cerebellar cortexes, neuronal ectopia and several other developmental disturbances (Geelen and Dormans, 1990). There are concomitant psychomotor symptoms in children born to mothers who had what had been considered "safe" mercury levels in maternal hair concentrations (Grandjean and Weihe, 1998). Neurological disorders in children due to mercury exposure have been reported (Counter and Buchanan, 2004; Johnson, 2004).

Put Wakefield aside. Put Hooker aside. Put the CDC aside. It does not take any further study to determine that mercury has been known to Western culture to be a toxin since the industrial age, and that mercury, in any form, should never be injected into anyone's body.

It appears that the US government was well aware of the risk of side effects of vaccines — they set up a fund via a small tax on every vaccine to pay out compensation for damages to fund a "Vaccine Court" (The National Vaccine Injury Compensation fund; see www.hrsa.gov/vaccine-compensation). Some see this as a disincentive for companies involved in vaccine development to ensure safety of vaccines. Also, commercials on vaccines usually leave out side effects — which is disconcerting, as under the DTC rules, side effects must be reported. There appears to be insufficient oversight — or at least perhaps vaccine programs are given a pass on reporting side effects. Vaccines are the only drug mandated by any US government — and the companies that produce them are protected, by law, from lawsuits for damages.

It takes no further study to show that MMR vaccines save lives and reduce sickness in the majority of the population. It is, however, incumbent on the US FDA to ensure that drugs are safe. The US FDA and the US EPA issued a statement in 2004 that mothers should avoid fish contaminated with mercury. When it comes to thimerosal, however, the FDA has been slow to act. Time and again, they have come close to banning it, but end up with committee conclusions such as

> *full consideration be given to removing thimerosal from any biological product to which infants, children, and pregnant women are exposed.*

This text is from the FDA's current website (FDA. 2015); we see them citing a lack of evidence of toxicity as grounds for relative inaction:

> *Under the FDA Modernization Act (FDAMA) of 1997, the FDA conducted a comprehensive review of the use of thimerosal in childhood vaccines. Conducted in 1999, this review found no evidence of harm from the use of thimerosal as a vaccine preservative, other than local hypersensitivity reactions (Ball et al. 2001).*
>
> *As part of the FDAMA review, the FDA evaluated the amount of mercury an infant might receive in the form of ethylmercury from vaccines under the US recommended childhood immunization schedule and compared these levels with existing guidelines for exposure to methylmercury, as there are no existing guidelines for ethylmercury, the metabolite of thimerosal. At the time of this review in 1999, the maximum cumulative exposure to mercury from vaccines in the recommended childhood immunization schedule was within acceptable limits for the methylmercury exposure guidelines set by FDA, ATSDR, and WHO. However, depending on the vaccine formulations used and the weight of the infant, some infants could have been exposed to cumulative levels of mercury during the first six months of life that exceeded EPA recommended guidelines for safe intake of methylmercury.*
>
> *As a precautionary measure, the Public Health Service (including the FDA, National Institutes of Health (NIH), Center for Disease Control and Prevention (CDC) and Health Resources and Services Administration (HRSA) and the American Academy of Pediatrics issued two Joint Statements, urging vaccine manufacturers to reduce or eliminate*

thimerosal in vaccines as soon as possible (CDC 1999) and (CDC 2000). The U.S. Public Health Service agencies have collaborated with various investigators to initiate further studies to better understand any possible health effects from exposure to thimerosal in vaccines.

The website reports that thimerosal has been removed from or reduced to trace amounts in all vaccines routinely recommended for children six years of age and younger, with the exception of one inactivated influenza vaccine. This is not correct.

Additional retrospective studies are needed that include subgroup analysis to either refute or confirm the finding left out by the CDC. If the increased risk of autism in African American males exposed to thimerosal is confirmed, the CDC scientists should be held to the same level of scrutiny as others who have failed to be forthright in reporting the full set of results.

Postscript: An often-cited study (Burbacher *et al.*, 2005) compared the effects of dosing infant monkeys with ethyl mercury to the effects of dosing them with thimerosal and found that while the monkeys cleared thimerosal from the blood more quickly, thimerosal has an easier time getting to the brain than methylmercury and is more persistent. Doses in that study were not directly comparable, however, so while "total amounts" in blood and brain are difficult to compare, the percent deposition in the brain of organic mercury is higher in thimerosal, and the metabolism of the two types of mercury is shown to be different, making comparisons between safe levels of ethyl- and methyl-forms of mercury unreliable.

In July 2015, a *New York Times* columnist Frank Bruni wrote an OpEd article (Bruni, 2015) in which he described his reactions to his interactions with Robert Kennedy, Jr, who had reached out to Bruni to try to share the transcripts of Dr. Thompson's revelations. In a reply to Bruni's article, Kennedy revealed that he and colleagues had studied 180 research studies demonstrating toxicity of thimerosal and potentially linking its use to increased risk of autism. In that reply, Kennedy reported something in variance to the CDC website regarding the inclusion of thimerosal in all pediatric vaccines:

> *Bruni erroneously suggests that mercury has been removed from all pediatric vaccines. In fact there are massive doses of mercury in some meningitis vaccines-now mandated for all schoolchildren in New York — and in flu vaccines given to pregnant women, infants and, annually, to all public school kids. Mercury remains in mandated pediatric HepB, HIB and DTap vaccines at double the concentrations deemed safe by EPA. Pharmaceutical companies have recently added to the ingredients of those vaccines, aluminum adjuvants that act synergistically to dramatically amplify the neurotoxicity of the remaining mercury. Finally, our pharmaceutical companies only reduced mercury levels in pediatric vaccines given to American children. We continue to send the range of pediatric vaccines fully loaded with mercury to hundreds of millions of children in developing nations in Asia, Africa, Latin America and the Mid East, a policy that will haunt our country in many dreadful ways.*
>
> *In defending thimeresol (sic) safety, Bruni alludes to the debunked industry canard that the ethylmercury in vaccines is less persistent in the body and therefore less toxic than the heavily regulated methylmercury in fish. However, the best and most recent science shows that ethylmercury is twice as persistent in the brain… and 50 times as toxic as methylmercury in fish…*

Kennedy has published a book (Kennedy, 2015) reviewing the peer-reviewed published scientific evidence indicating toxicity of thimerosal, and links to brain damage in animals and humans.

Kennedy reviews the scientific literature and analyzes, in surprising depth, the vaccine health trends in the US. He reports the well-known fact that the rate of autism has increased from 1 in 2,500 people in 1970 to 1 in 68 in 2010. His analysis also points out increases in the rate at which people after the age of six develop autism-like symptoms. This analysis includes the finding that the expected dose of ethyl mercury experienced by children before age 10 due to the CDC's schedule increased from 75 micrograms in 2003 to 575 micrograms in 2013. He reviews the studies that show that thimerosal is neither safe, nor as effective as claimed, and how there are no substantial cost savings due to translational of use of packing options in the clinic. He outlines that safe alternatives to thimerosal exist, and includes copies of letters from the CDC declining changes to the preservative used by SmithKline Beecham, and outlines how thimerosal is still included in more vaccines than is reported by the CDC in spite of the FDA's recommendation of a ban of the toxin in 1984.

The financial motives for the CDC to retain thimerosal in vaccines that are shipped overseas to less developed countries are unclear. The percentage of profits by Pharma from vaccines compared to their full portfolio is low (some estimates are less than 2%). Perhaps there is no financial motive other than to make vaccines more profitable by volume via overseas sales — certainly Pharma has not moved on their own accord to discontinue the use of thimerosal. The questions are why not, and will they?

The FDA lists autism as a side effect of a Diptheria, Pertussis and Tetanus vaccine (US FDA, 2005).

References

Adams M. (2014) Natural News EXCLUSIVE: Bombshell email from CDC whistleblower reveals criminality of vaccine cover-up as far back as 2002. *Natural News*, Aug 26, 2014. [http://www.naturalnews.com/046614_CDC_whistleblower_vaccine_cover-up_criminal_investigation.html#]

Austin DW, *et al.* (2014) Genetic variation associated with hypersensitivity to mercury. *Toxicol Int* **21(3):** 236–41. [doi: 10.4103/0971-6580.155327]

Bruni G. (2015) California, Camelot and Vaccines. *The New York Times*, July 4, 2015. www.nytimes.com/2015/07/05/opinion/sunday/frank-bruni-california-camelot-and-vaccines.html

Burbacher TM, *et al.* (2005) Comparison of blood and brain mercury levels in infant monkeys exposed to methylmercury or vaccines containing thimerosal. *Environ Health Perspect* **113(8):** 1015–21.

Buyanova N. (2013) Treatment of patients with cervical diseases combined with HPV infection. *Archiv EuroMedica* **3:** 7–8 [http://www.ewg-board. eu/archiv-euromedica/archiv-euromedica-02-2013/archiv_euromed-ica_02_2013_maket_06_02_2014_07_08.pdf]

CDC. (2015) Measles Outbreak — California, December 2014–February 2015. February 20, 2015.

CDC. (2013) National and state vaccination coverage among adolescents aged 13–17 Years –United States, 2012. *Morbidity and Mortality Weekly Report*, August 30, 2013, **62(34):** 685–93.

Clarkson TW, Vyas JB, Ballatori N. (2007) Mechanisms of mercury disposition in the body. *Am J Ind Med* **50(10):** 757–64.

Counter SA, Buchanan LH. (2004) Mercury exposure in children: a review. *Toxicol Appl Pharmacol* **15:** 209–230.

Crosby J. (2015) Brian Hooker's findings are confirmed by CDC's results. *AutismInvestigated*.www.autisminvestigated.com/brian-hooker-confirmed-by-cdc/

DeStefano F, *et al.* (2004) Age at first measles-mumps-rubella vaccination in children with autism and school-matched control subjects: a popula-tion-based study in metropolitan Atlanta. Pediatrics. 113(2):259–66.

De Vincenzo R, *et al.* (2014) Long-term efficacy and safety of human papilloma-virus vaccination. *Int J Womens Health* **6:** 999–1010. [doi: 10.2147/IJWH. S50365]

Hertz-Picciotto I, *et al.* (2010) Blood mercury concentrations in CHARGE Study children with and without autism. *Environ Health Perspect* **118(1):** 161–66. [doi: 10.1289/ehp.0900736]

FDA. (2005) Diptheria and Tetanus Toxoids and Acellular Pertussis Vaccines Adsorbed Tripedia. http://www.fda.gov/downloads/biologicsbloodvaccines/vaccines/approvedproducts/ucm101580.pdf (Accessed July 16, 2015)

FDA. 2015. Thimerosal in Vaccines. http://www.fda.gov/BiologicsBloodVac-cines/SafetyAvailability/VaccineSafety/UCM096228#act

FDA. (2015) White Paper. FDA and Accelerating the Development of the New Pharmaceutical Therapies. www.fda.gov/AboutFDA/ReportsManu-alsForms/Reports/ucm439082.htm

Geelen JA, Dormans J. (1990) The early effects of methylmercury on develop-ing rat brain. *Acta Neuropathol* (Berl) **80:** 432–38.

Geier DA, *et al*. (2015) Thimerosal: clinical, epidemiologic and biochemical studies. *Clin Chim Acta* **444:** 212–20. [doi: 10.1016/j.cca.2015.02.030]

Gorski D. (2015) Say it ain't so, Mickey! A holiday measles outbreak makes the happiest place in the world sad. *Science-Based Medicine.* Accessed: 3/25/2015.

Gorski D. (2015) The Disneyland measles outbreak continues apace, and a woman refuses quarantine. Respectful Insolence. *ScienceBlogs* LLC. Accessed: 3/25/2015.

Grandjean P, *et al*. (1999) Methylmercury neurotoxicity in Amazonian children downstream from goldmining. *Environ Health Perspect* **107:** 587–92.

Healy B, Atkisson S. (2008) CBS News Interview for "Open Questions on Vaccines and Autism." http://www.cbsnews.com/news/the-open-question-on-vaccines-and-autism/

Hooker BS. (2014, retracted) Measles-mumps-rubella vaccination timing and autism among young African American boys: a reanalysis of CDC data. *Transl Neurodegener* **3:** 16. [doi: 10.1186/2047-9158-3-16]

Hornig M, Chian D, Lipkin WI. (2004) Neurotoxic effects of postnatal thimerosal are mouse strain dependent. *Mol Psychiatry* **9(9):** 833–45.

Immunization Safety Review Committee. (2004) *Immunization Safety Review: Vaccine and Autism.* National Academy Press, ISBN 0-309-53275-2 www.ncbi.nlm.nih.gov/books/NBK25344/pdf/Bookshelf_NBK25344.pdf

Johnson CL. (2004) In the environment: sources, toxicities, and prevention of exposure. *Pediatr Ann* **33:** 437–42.

Kennedy RF Jr. (2014) *Thimerosal: Let the Science Speak: The Evidence Supporting the Immediate Removal of Mercury — a Known Neurotoxin — from Vaccines.* Skyhorse Publishing, New York.

Li X, *et al*. (2014) Transcriptomic analyses of neurotoxic effects in mouse brain after intermittent neonatal administration of thimerosal. *Toxicol Sci* **139(2):** 452–65. [doi: 10.1093/toxsci/kfu049]

Madsen KM, *et al*. (2002) A population-based study of measles, mumps, and rubella vaccination and autism. *N Engl J Med* **347(19):** 1477–82.

Markowitz L, *et al*. (2013) Reduction in human papillomavirus (HPV) prevalence among young women following HPV vaccine introduction in the United States, National Health and Nutrition Examination Surveys, 2003–2010. *J Infect Dis* **208(3):** 385–93. [doi: 10.1093/infdis/jit192]

Marsh DO, Turner MD. (1995) Foetal methylmercury studying Peruvian fish eating population. *Neurotoxicology* **16:** 717–26.

Murata K, *et al.* (2004) Delayed brainstem auditory evoked potential latencies in 14-year-old children exposed to methylmercury. *J Pediatr* **144:** 177–83.

Omer SB, *et al.* (2009) Vaccine refusal, mandatory immunization, and the risks of vaccine-preventable diseases. *N Engl J Med* **360(19):** 1981–88. [doi: 10.1056/NEJMsa0806477]

Ratajczak HV. (2011) Theoretical aspects of autism: causes — a review. *J Immunotoxicol* **8(1):** 68–79. [doi: 10.3109/1547691X.2010.545086]

Seither, *et al.* (2014) Vaccination coverage among children in kindergarten — United States, 2013–14 School Year. *MMWR* **63(41):** 913–20. [www.cdc.gov/mmwr/preview/mmwrhtml/mm6341a1.htm]

Shandley K, Austin DW. (2011) Ancestry of pink disease (infantile acrodynia) identified as a risk factor for autism spectrum disorders. *J Toxicol Environ Health A* **74(18):** 1185–94. [doi: 10.1080/15287394.2011.590097]

Sharpe MA, Gist TL, Baskin DS. (2013) B-lymphocytes from a population of children with autism spectrum disorder and their unaffected siblings exhibit hypersensitivity to thimerosal. *J Toxicol* 2013: 801517. [doi: 10.1155/2013/801517]

Snyder RD. (1971) Congenital mercury poisoning. *N Engl J Med* **284:** 1014–16.

Takahashi S, *et al.* (2015) Reduced vaccination and the risk of measles and other childhood infections post-Ebola. *Science* **347(6227):** 1240–42. [doi: 10.1126/science.aaa3438]

Verstraeten T, *et al.* (2003) Safety of thimerosal-containing vaccines: a two-phased study of computerized health maintenance organization databases. *Pediatrics* **112(5):** 1039–48.

Verstraeten explained the discrepancies between his initial reported findings in meetings of a positive association of thimerosal-containing vaccines and autism and the final results in a letter to the editor of the journal *Pediatrics*, the next year, (Verstraeten, 2014), saying.

Verstraeten T. (2004) Thimerosal, the Centers for Disease Control and Prevention, and GlaxoSmithKline. *Pediatrics* **113(4):** 932.

Wakefield A, *et al.* (1998) Ileal-lymphoid-nodular hyperplasia, non-specific colitis, and pervasive developmental disorder in children. *The Lancet* **351:** 637–41. RETRACTED.

Whitney CG, *et al*. (2014) Benefits from immunization during the Vaccines for Children Program Era — United States, 1994–2013. *MMWR* **63(16):** 352–55. www.cdc.gov/mmwr/preview/mmwrhtml/mm6316a4.htm

WHO. (2011) Child mortality: Millenium Development Goal (MDG) 4. September 2011. www.who.int/pmnch/media/press_materials/fs/fs_mdg4_childmortality/en/

Zipprich J. (2015) Measles outbreak — California, December 2014–February 2015. *MMWR* 2015. **64(Early Release):** 1–2.

8 Chemosensitivity and Chemoresistance Assays in Cancer

When Claire received her diagnosis, she felt relieved. At least now, she knew. The unknown is often worse than the known. She could set her priorities, begin to focus on increasing her odds of survival and, if necessary, try to prepare for the worst.

When my mother developed breast cancer, treatment options were few and far between. Halsted radical mastectomy was falling out of favor in the late 1960s, due in large part to improved understanding of the mechanisms of spread of cancer from the breast to other tissues thanks to research by Dr. Bernard Fisher, at the University of Pittsburgh. At the time, the prevailing view was that lymph nodes "trapped" breast cancer cells, and that the spread of cancer to other organs was primarily via the lymphatic system. Breast cancer is now known to be a more loco-regional disease, involving many types of tissue near a tumor. Fisher's work revolutionized our understanding and paved the way for many new areas of study in breast cancer metastasis. Even so, for my mom, it was still an option: Once it was observed that the chemo failed to shrink the tumor, she had them take one breast. Her sister, my aunt, recounts how she begged my mother to have the doctors remove both breasts. Mastectomy at the time was seen as a type of female castration, so she opted for breast-sparing lumpectomy when a tumor appeared in her remaining breast.

Given that the rest of the breast cancers in the family thus far appear to be triple negative (ER, PR and Her-2 negative), and that there is a correlation between BRCA1 status and hormone receptor expression, it seems likely that radical mastectomy was the only chance of a curative treatment for her at the time. Treatment with chemotherapy was still in its infancy in the early 1970 — the most important discoveries of hormone-receptor mediated treatment had not yet been fully realized. The idea of using combinations of therapies was introduced in the mid-1970s by Dr. Richard Cooper at the University of Rochester. This advance resulted in shrinkage of tumors in 70% of cases — up from 50% on single treatments. A relatively new class of drugs was being developed, like taxol and tamoxifen — and she was determined to give her family, especially my sisters and I — the very best shot of having her around for a long time.

At the height of her illness, my mother traveled from Ogdensburg, NY to Rochester, NY to visit with specialists researching new options of treatments. I am uncertain of which treatment she endured, but given the research trends in the early to late 1970s, in all likelihood, her doctor's efforts were in vain due to her likely hormone receptor status. I like to think that the doctors learned something from her case.

For women like Claire, options today are much improved: With knowledge of the receptor status, she and her doctors would never waste time trying drugs that seem likely to be ineffective. Today, they might turn to a series of combinations of treatments that work via different mechanisms. If Claire is lucky, she might learn about ways to reduce the guessing game to an exact, precise science.

Near the waterfront in a region near Pittsburgh sits an industrial-looking building. Inside the building, offices churn with people busy filing state regulatory submissions, answering phone calls, talking to doctors, trying to get the word out about the numerous benefits of the ChemoFx® assay for studying and testing cancer cells outside the patient's body. In the lab, other people in lab coats are busy growing cells in culture, treating the cells in plates, scanning and counting nuclei of cancer cells to determine kill rates. The ChemoFx® assay is brilliant in its elegant simplicity. During a biopsy, or during a surgery (e.g., lumpectomy), the surgeon saves a bit of a patient's tumor, and it is handled via a special protocol. Rather than killing the tumor cells outright, some of the cells are harvested and placed in optimized media that promotes survival of human cells. Once harvested and seeded, the tubes are shipped back to Pittsburgh, where they are grown. There, laboratory personnel at Helomics Corporations then try their best to study many biological aspects of the tumor cells, and then using that information, test various types of chemotherapy to determine which might be most likely to kill the tumor cells in the patient. The results are recorded, and effective treatments proven to kill a specific patient's tumor cells are communicated back to the oncologist.

Helomics® (formerly Precision Therapeutics) has conducted world-class leading-edge research demonstrating the utility of their assays' ability to predict the efficacy of specific chemotherapy agents against patients' tumors. One assay in particular, ChemoFx®, appears extremely versatile. In years past, the ChemoFx® assay was used to test many different types of human primary tumors. For the last several years, Helomics® has exclusively tested only gynecological tumors — ovarian, endometrial, and cervical — using the test.

The test can be used to predict overall survival in primary ovarian cancer patients (Herzog *et al.*, 2010), recurrence in ovarian cancer (Tian *et al.*), the outcome of pemetrexed for treatment of mesothelioma (Suchy *et al.*, 2013), treatment response in endometrial carcinoma (Huh *et al.*, 2011), and may be useful in predicting the response of breast cancer to sunitinib (Suchy *et al.*, 2011) and colorectal and lung carcinoma response to cetuximab (Rice *et al.*, 2011).

In reading these papers, I found a reference to an old mentor of mine, Dr. Sam Wieand. Sam worked at the University of Pittsburgh Cancer Institute and directed their Biostatistics division when I started there as an Assistant Professor in the Department of Pathology. I relocated to Pittsburgh help cancer researchers in the then-new Hillman Cancer Center with their data analysis needs in newer, more complex data sources such as whole genome expression arrays, mass-spec proteomic assays, and mutational (SNP) assays. These newer platforms required specialized knowledge of high-dimensional data analysis, for which no standard protocols for interpretive analysis existed. Sam immediately and quickly took me under his wing to help me navigate my way through the nuances of working with high-powered clinical researchers. He regularly advised me on the need to keep the clinical researchers' regulatory needs in mind. In large group meetings I would occasionally propose the use of computational matching algorithms to reduce the possibility of confounding in both prospective and retrospective clinical trials. Sam would invite me to coffee and explain to me how, in spite of the fact that these were excellent ideas, the clinical researchers would be wary of implementing them because they might cause problems with regulatory review by the FDA who, at the time at least, were stoic in their requirement of (purely) randomized clinical trials. I knew that the approaches I was suggesting were harmless to the study in the ways that they FDA might be concerned with; moreover, I knew that if implemented properly, they would actually help bring out findings that might otherwise be masked by accidental biases in the study that can result from pure randomization. Deferring to wisdom over youthful exuberance, we nearly always ended up agreeing that the time for such studies would come "some day."

Sam certainly did his part to help bring about change in the practice of study design. And the research done at Helomics® to date has benefited greatly from his thinking in study design. However, the FDA has yet to approve these simple, brilliant, elegant tests. Moreover, medical doctors sometime fail to see the benefit of predictive assays — all too often, the test results match the chemotherapy regime they were already likely to use on a given patient. Or they don't see the value in saving the patient from treatments that will not work because, they reason, they have selected the treatment using criteria they have used for years. However, their thinking must change. It is not the assay results that match their expectations that matter most, and the assay augments, and does not replace, their existing criteria. The results that matter most are the assay results that do not match their expectations. If my mother had had the ChemoFx® assay in the early 1970s, she could have escaped the negative side effects of the completely ineffective drugs she was given, and perhaps, just perhaps, she would have been able to use that time to find another trial. Or perhaps she simply could have spent more quality time with her family and less time sick from the ineffective treatments.

Because ChemoFx®, and other assays like it, are classified by the FDA as "Laboratory Derived Tests" (LDTs), they fall under the CLIA guidelines of the Centers for Medicare and Medicaid Services (CMS). The FDA and the CMS are currently working to determine how this class of test should be regulated. Patients are reimbursed by some but not all insurance companies. Regulatory specialists at Helomics® submit applications to various state Departments of Health for licenses to test patient samples from their states, and the clinical laboratories at Helomics® are CLIA-certified.

Flaws in the Rationale for Non-Coverage/Non-Reimbursement

The bar is set very high for CSAs, as it should be. Any test that is to be used on patients for diagnosis or therapy selection should be demonstrated to be safe and efficacious. However, if the rationale for non-payment for CSAs were to be applied to drugs for the treatment of diseases, it is unlikely that any progress could be made in the treatment of diseases in humans.

Take, for example, the Blue Cross Blue Shield 2015 statement on their rationale for non-coverage of CSAs:

There are only a few comparative studies that evaluate use of a chemosensitivity assay to select chemotherapy versus standard care, and these studies do not report significant differences in outcomes between groups. A larger number of studies have used correlational designs that evaluate the association between assay results and already known patient outcomes. These studies report that results of chemosensitivity and chemoresistance assays are predictive of outcomes. However, these studies do not evaluate whether these assays lead changes in management and whether any changes in management lead to improved outcomes. In addition, interpretation of these studies is limited by het-erogeneity in test methodology, tumor type, patient population, and chemotherapeutic agents. As a result, the clinical utility of chemoresis-tance and chemosensitivity assays has not been determined, and data are insufficient to determine whether use of the test to select chemo-therapy regimens for individual patients will improve In Vitro Che-moresistance and Chemosensitivity Assays outcomes. Therefore, this testing is considered investigational. (Blue Cross and Blue Shield of North Carolina. 2015. Corporate Medical Policy. In Vitro Chemoresis-tance and Chemosensitivity Assays.)

Let's look at this in more detail:

There are only a few comparative studies that evaluate use of a che-mosensitivity assay to select chemotherapy versus standard care, and these studies do not report significant differences in outcomes between groups.

The number of studies performed does not necessarily correlate with clinical efficacy; in fact, some drugs have been approved with two to three studies. Helomics® has published numerous papers and abstracts supporting their assays. With respect to safety, there are no risks to the patient who opts for ChemoFx® beyond those associated with biopsy, and this is often avoided as the tissue used in the CSA is often taken from a resected tumor.

The Blue Cross Blue Shield statement is misleading as well, as it portrays the field as data poor.

In nearly every one of the published studies, patients treated with drugs predicted by the assays had a higher response rate than patients whose treatment was not informed by a CSA. Many studies have been published now that demonstrate that assay-informed treatments are more likely to show a response.

Further, conducting *"chemotherapy versus standard care"* does not really exist in many clinical setting for cancer, where chemotherapy is routine. The clinical question is not "chemotherapy vs. standard care," rather, it is "chemotherapy with *a priori* information on likely efficacy vs. chemotherapy without such information." Consideration of this difference is immensely important, as it sets the proper context in which a productive discussion of efficacy can go forward.

And at the crux of the issue is survival:

> *...and these studies do not report significant differences in outcomes between groups.*

The focus of ChemoFx® is to better inform patient treatment decisions by the physician, and numerous studies have been done that demonstrate its utility in this respect. However, the statement overall reveals an overarching view in which all chemosensitivity assays are treated as one entity. This is a logic flaw that is harming patients. There are vast differences in strategy and meristics (measurement science) among the various approaches proposed to date and, more importantly, the studies of one technology do not inform on each other. The FDA would never, and should not, consider all drugs of the same category for approval or non-approval based on an arbitrary categorization, or even one based on function. Different mechanisms require independent evidence.

The statement continues:

> *A larger number of studies have used correlational designs that evaluate the association between assay results and already known patient outcomes. These studies report that results of chemosensitivity and chemoresistance assays are predictive of outcomes. However, these studies do not evaluate whether these assays lead (to) changes in management and whether any changes in management lead to improved outcomes.*

Here we see the overgeneralization again in the discussion of these types of assays. Each technology will naturally begin with studies to determine whether there is any correlation between results of use of the assay and patient outcomes. These studies are, by definition, retrospective, and highly informative, as they provide a critical test: The companies would not proceed with assays that did not demonstrate significant correlation.

However, these studies do not evaluate whether these assays lead (to) changes in management and whether any changes in management lead to improved outcomes.

This is convoluted thinking, as it brings in the question of whether an assay is adopted by the clinical community as a criterion for approval by the FDA or for re-imbursement by insurance companies. Again, this is not how a surgical technology or drug would be evaluated. The correlation studies, in fact, do show that an improved outcome is expected. Thus, measures of survival such as progression-free survival, overall survival, etc. would be useful, even in a retrospective study. And companies like Helomics® have reported improved outcomes.

That's where my late mentor Sam Wieand comes in. He introduced and promoted the use of match/mismatch analysis in cases where randomized trials were not possible.

Clinical researchers use the concept of "levels of evidence" in their consideration of adoption of clinical options in their practice. The FDA's gold standard is a randomized, prospective clinical trial — and yet after years of use of these techniques, we still have insufficient tools for assigning chemotherapy treatment to individual patients. Chemosensitivity assays like ChemoFx® can fill this niche.

The FDA's ideal of a prospective clinical trial is not only intractable in this setting — it would be highly unethical. Imagine randomly assigning chemotherapy to patients, given that we know that a better match could be found. Even though a "standard of care" (i.e., no ChemoFx®) vs. ChemoFx® arm study would (and has) determined superior care with ChemoFx®, no one would know whether ChemoFx® is better than "choosing" chemo "by chance." So we see here a scientific and logical Catch-22, and the match/mismatch analysis method should be seen as sufficiently and completely accommodating this level of evidence.

Let us look at just one of the studies, conducted at Yale University:

A *prospective study evaluating the clinical relevance of a chemore-sponse assay for treatment of patients with persistent or recurrent ovarian cancer.* (Rutherford T *et al.*, 2013)

This study demonstrated significant improvement in progression-free and overall survival in cancer patients when patients were treated with agents identified as sensitive by ChemoFx®. The patients in this study had a particularly hard-to-treat ovarian cancer; both platinum-sensitive and platinum-resistant recurrent ovarian cancer patients were included.

ChemoFx®-informed treatment was associated with a 14 month (65%) increase in mean overall survival compared to no ChemoFx® selection, and a 50% improvement in progression-free survival in patients with either platinum-sensitive and platinum-resistant tumors (analyzed together and separately).

Given these impressive results, I called Donald Very, Vice President of Research and Commercial Development at Helomics®. He runs two research laboratories and one clinical laboratory. I asked him how many patients had been tested by ChemoFx® and other tests at Helomics®, and I asked him how things were going with translational success in getting more doctors to see the test as useful for their patients.

"Like most clinical laboratories, we are continually caught in a squeeze between increasing costs and decreasing re-imbursement."

I knew that Helomics®, like many companies, was recruiting medical science liasons (MSLs) to help translate the significance of the clinical findings for practitioners, both in terms of clinical and economic utility. He said that they were working out fairly well.

The MSLs are getting better at communicating the advantages, but at times it can be a task to convince the physician of the clinical utility for his/her patient. It's not really the doctors that are the rate-limiting factor. It's the payers — health insurance providers. Some provide coverage, but some do not. And it's the same battle over, and over again with some payers.

I asked him what he wanted payers to know.
He said:

I want to tell them: "Don't take our word for it: Look at the results of the peer-reviewed publications that show that the assay is scientifically and clinically valid." Patients do better; they have increased progression free survival and overall survival compared to patients who were no treated on the basis of a ChemoFx® result. I want them to know it is far less expensive for the payers because with ChemoFx®, the patients get the right drugs first. Without the test, a patient may receive an ineffective drug.

He said that there have been 16 peer-reviewed publications demonstrating the clinical validity and benefit of treating patients on the basis of a ChemoFx® result over the last few years.

I asked him why the FDA has not yet jumped on the significance of the match/mismatch analysis and the bulk of the published results, and whether they realized non-approval could harm patients.

Don provided a major clarification that should help payers. He pointed out that the FDA does not regulate and approve LDTs, and that there is an ongoing dialog between the FDA, the CMS, clinical laboratories, and lab advocacy groups as to how to best monitor the development, performance qualification, and administration of LDTs.

LDTs do not necessarily fall under the jurisdiction of FDA for regulation, and there are concerns over duplicative and excessive regulation in an area of development that has benefit by the process of continuous improvement. Many major medical institutions have LDTs, which are more akin to clinical services. Unlike medical devices, which can be subjected to manufacturing protocols that insure reproducibility, LDTs are often highly specialized services that have been optimized via years of research and are not available as a process in labs other than those in which they were developed.

He described the ChemoFx® test as a drug response marker, whose clinical use is associated with a significant improvement in a cancer patient's progression-free survival and overall survival. He cited a total of 16 publications, in peer-reviewed journals, that describe the multi-center, prospective and retrospective clinical studies that, combined, provide strong evidence for both the clinical utility, validity, and the cost effectiveness of treating patients on the basis of a ChemoFx® result. Since 2010, the ChemoFx® laboratory has tested over 85,000 tumor samples and over 50,000 gynecological tumor samples. He told me that at least 70% of the physician members of the Society for Gynecological Oncology (SGO) have ordered ChemoFx®, and that an astounding 92.5% (25 out of 27) of the member institutions of the National Comprehensive Cancer Network (NCCN) have submitted specimens for ChemoFx® testing.

I was impressed. So I met with Don and was given a tour of the Helomics® clinical facilities in Pittsburgh, PA. I was shown a thoroughly modern, well-oiled, sophisticated clinical laboratory where regulatory compliance was built into the processes from step 1. They have learned from the experience of 10 years the value of doing things right the first time. From the moment the samples arrive, records are made and filed (electronic and hard copy). Samples left over that are saved for future research are de-identified. Positive controls are put through the entire process of enculturation, growth, and challenged with chemo. They use a dosage-response curve generating workflow, with robotic dosing (for accuracy and reproducibility), and each sample is run at each dose in triplicate for each drug. The automated scanning is verified manually for each sample. Any questionable results are verified by a clinical pathologist. The entire workflow was carefully constructed to insure against contamination.

Currently, as a laboratory-developed test, ChemoFx® is available only at the Helomics® CLIA-certified, NYSDOH-approved clinical reference laboratory located in Pittsburgh, PA. I brought up the FDA issue again during my tour of their labs.

> *Right now, we're in a sort of grey zone — the FDA has labeled our test a "Laboratory-Developed Test," and they (they FDA) are still wrestling with how to best regulate LDTs. They published a Draft Guidance, which, in my opinion, will prove to be onerous on clinical laboratories, if implemented. Not just for our test — for many labeled as LDTs. If the FDA were to regulate LDTs as they currently do for Class I, II, and III medical devices, I believe it would significantly and adversely impact the quality of patient care. LDTs fill a necessary and important role in patient care. Treating clinical laboratories such as ours that develop and perform LDTs like device manufacturers (that develop and sell Class I, II, and III medical devices) would place an unfair and unnecessary financial burden on clinical laboratories and would lead to fewer tests being available for patient care. No one disputes the fact that LDTs must be well-designed, performance qualified, and performed in a rigorously controlled environment to insure patient safety. The debate involves how the development and performance of these tests should be monitored and which government agency should be responsible for the oversight.*

Because ChemoFx® is already conducted as a service in a CLIA-certified laboratory and is subject annually to reproducibility testing via the NYDOH, and other states that require it, the test as a clinical service is repeatedly proven to be up to snuff. For companies like Helomics®, who have done the extensive and successful studies that *can* be done, general acceptance of the ChemoFx® test by oncologists and payers would facilitate the wider acceptance of the test. Doctors, patients, and payers want to know whether the test will work medically and economically — it is clear that wasting time and dollars on ineffective treatments is in no one's interest.

I told Don that it was easy for me to choose ChemoFx® as a success — after all, I had seen the test change my sister's mind about accepting *any* chemo — a clinical outcome that cannot be studied in the context of a clinical trial. I have also seen the data — and my old mentor Sam Wieand's hope for acceptance of results from mismatch/match-type analyses certainly had appeal. I mentioned to him some of the more difficult stories I was running into in my search for successes in translational research — the long-awaited admission of ADHD overdiagnosis, for example, and other unfortunate examples of apparent "profits before people." I told him that I could see how Helomics® fills a niche in which the profit motive and clinical successes were mutually aligned. I expressed concern that readers might find my selection of Helomics® biased.

> *Jim, what's special about this place is just about everyone here has been touched by cancer — many of our employees are cancer survivors themselves. It's great to have the opportunity to come to work every day and have the chance to help patients achieve better outcomes. For many of us, it's way to pay forward the beneficence in our lives made possible by other types of advances in cancer care.*

If I were biased prior to speaking with Don by the published data in support of their assay, I was even more biased toward Helomics® after the interview.

As if being directed toward chemotherapeutic treatments that are likely to be effective is not enough, an additional benefit is that patients whose treatment regimens are planned using ChemoFx® will avoid the pain and suffering due to toxicity and adverse events associated with treatments that would not likely be effective in their case anyway.

Primum non nocere — the Latin phrase meaning "Above all, do no harm!" — is worth contemplation in this context. Helomic's® ChemoFx® is a clear-cut example of translational success. The medical community does not use all of the information at their disposal for identifying treatment that will not likely be effective on an individual patient. Or, at least, they are slow to adjust their approach. Examples include the doctor who wanted to treat my sister's triple-negative breast cancer with long-term low-dose tamoxifen to prevent breast cancer recurrence, knowing the hormone receptor status of her tumor. When, acting as her patient advocate, I inquired whether he knew of any study that demonstrated long-term protection in triple-negative patients, he got upset with me, told me to go back to being my sister's brother, and stop trying to be her doctor. Then he hung up.

Other examples of low expected efficacy associated with biomarkers are being found by the oncology research community, and I hope their peers take heed. Examples include the following:

- Anthracyclines (such as Adriamycin) tend to be effective only with breast cancer patients that are positive for the HER2 receptor (Slamon and Press, 2009);
- CMF chemotherapy (cyclophosphamide, methotrexate and fluorouracil) tends to be ineffective as a follow-up treatment in addition to hormone therapy for hormone-positive breast cancers (Ejlertsen *et al.*, 2006).

These assays pinpoint patients in which treatments will be efficacious, but their "ruling out" of treatment options is of high value: It lends patients the means to avoid wasting time, unnecessary costs and harmful side effects that are the result of an inappropriate chemotherapy regimen, which can be invaluable as well.

ChemoFx® is of high value. I was glad to learn that Helomics® has new products forthcoming: genetic-based tests in colon and lung cancer. Thanks to companies like Helomics®, women now have many more options to ensure that their attempts to be treated are not a waste of their time. In my opinion, insurance companies should clamor for results from tests like the ChemoFx® assay. They won't be wasting money on treatments that are ineffective and, odds are, the patient will have a much better outcome from treatment with chemotherapy agents that are much more likely to be effective for specific patients.

As they progress, cancers evolve. They can develop resistance to previously effective treatments. Further, if the cancer stops responding to a given treatment, the search for still-effective treatments can be guided by a renewed study of the cells harvested from metastatic sites, such as the brain, lung, or liver, taking the guesswork out of the equation. Thus, the clinical utility of ChemoFx® extends into the realm of chemoresistance — and anyone who has fought the battle knows that a round of ineffective chemotherapy is a big deal.

Like cancer, Helomics® is evolving, too. Don told me that they are expanding in services, including high-volume cell culture services, research, including biomarker-informed chemotherapy selection, and expanding the menu of clinical tests offered. They are growing their team, hiring technical staff, and have recently hired additional full-time medical staff (pathologists).

ChemoFx® and assays like it are wonderful examples of the future of personalized medicine. In January 2015, President Obama requested $215 million for personalized, or as he called it "precision" medicine. Reports of successful indicators that can be used to predict outcomes of treatment have been published since the earliest days of hormone status in breast cancer and, more generally, since the mid-2000s (e.g., Hess *et al.*, 2006). It is time for the FDA to admit the successes in the research and to allow the success in translation to take place. It seems a shame that due to an outdated view on study design, the FDA has missed the boat. I believe the FDA should take a very close second look at their publications as well, and try to better understand the real significance of match/mismatch analysis. The ChemoFx® assay is available to patients who can pay for the assay themselves, and to those lucky enough to have their insurance companies recognize the clinical and economic benefits of the test. Helomics®, like many companies, have a compassion care policy for patients in need. I am sure that Helomics® and other companies will continue to run trials that better match the FDA's outdated needs, and that, as Sam and I used to end our conversations, "some day" insurance companies will be in a better position to pay for this quantum leap forward in the quality of care. In the meantime, I hope that lawmakers see this as a high priority to ensure public health, and that patients ask doctors, and their insurance companies, to see the real clinical and economic benefits inherent to the assays.

Note that the surgeon, as well as the oncologist, should both ideally be involved for the assay to work. My sister's tumor was only tested with ChemoFx® after Dr. Nadaraja at the University of Rochester took me up on the challenge of learning the tissue harvesting protocol over a short weekend. My sister was first diagnosed with breast cancer eight years ago, and is still going strong. I encourage gynecological cancer patients to be quite aggressive in requesting the ChemoFx® test and tests like it from their surgeons and oncologists simultaneously to ensure continuity of care.

References

Ejlertsen B, *et al.* (2006) Ovarian ablation compared with cyclophosphamide, methotrexate, and fluorouracil: Similar efficacy from a randomized comparison in premenopausal patients with node-positive, hormone receptor-positive breast cancer. *J Clin Oncol* **24:** 4956–62.

Hess KR, *et al.* (2006) Pharmacogenomic predictor of sensitivity to preoperative chemotherapy with paclitaxel and fluorouracil, doxorubicin, and cyclophosphamide in breast cancer. *J Clin Oncol* **24(26):** 4236–44.

Herzog TJ, *et al.* (2010) Chemosensitivity testing with ChemoFx and overall survival in primary ovarian cancer. *Am J Obstet Gynecol* **203(1):** 68.e1–6. [doi: 10.1016/j.ajog.2010.01.059]

Huh WK, *et al.* (2011) Consistency of *in vitro* chemoresponse assay results and population clinical response rates among women with endometrial carcinoma. *Int J Gynecol Cancer* **21(3):** 494–99. [doi: 10.1097/IGC.0b013e31820c4cb5]

Rice SD, *et al.* (2010) Analysis of chemotherapeutic response heterogeneity and drug clustering based on mechanism of action using an *in vitro* assay. *Anticancer Res* **30(7):** 2805–11.

Rice SD, *et al.* (2011) An *in vitro* chemoresponse assay defines a subset of colorectal and lung carcinomas responsive to cetuximab. *Cancer Biol Ther* **11(2):** 196–203.

Rutherford T, *et al.* (2013) A prospective study evaluating the clinical relevance of a chemoresponse assay for treatment of patients with persistent or recurrent ovarian cancer. *Gynecol Oncol* **131(2):** 362–67. [doi: 10.1016/j.ygyno.2013.08.009]

Slamon DJ, Press MF. (2009) Alterations in the TOP2A and HER2 genes: association with adjuvant anthracycline sensitivity in human breast cancers. *J Natl Cancer I* **101(9):** 615–18.

Suchy SL, *et al.* (2011) Chemoresponse assay for evaluating response to sunitinib in primary cultures of breast cancer. *Cancer Biol Ther* **11(12):** 1059–64.

Suchy SL, *et al.* (2013) Adaptation of a chemosensitivity assay to accurately assess pemetrexed in ex vivo cultures of lung cancer. *Cancer Biol Ther* **14(1):** 39–44. [doi: 10.4161/cbt.22622]

Tian C, *et al.* (2014) Evaluation of a chemoresponse assay as a predictive marker in the treatment of recurrent ovarian cancer: further analysis of a prospective study. *Br J Cancer* **111(5):** 843–50. [doi: 10.1038/bjc.2014.375]

9 Chapter

A Very Special Kind of Brain Cancer Surgery

When I was a boy growing up on the shores of the St. Lawrence River, the public library was my escape. There, I could spend hours studying books on all sorts of topics. I recall in the late 1970s finding books about cancer. I read how interferon was a promising new discovery in immunology, and that experimental treatments in cancer might benefit from its study. I do not recall the exact reference; it seemed like a highly technical source at the time. One book that I checked out that did stick with me, and still affects me to this day, was a paperback published in 1949 by John Gunther. The title was *Death be Not Proud*. This book told the true story of John Gunther's son, Johnny, who was diagnosed with a glioblastoma multiforme. The book spared no detail in the suffering of Johnny, his family, nor in the joys of receiving a reply letter from none other than Albert Einstein as Johnny inquired on a Unified Theory of General Relativity. Johnny's brain tumor was inoperable; it was located at the right parietal part of the brain, deep enough inside where no surgeon could ever hope to succeed in relieve the teen of the certain fate that awaited him. The combination of my own loss in life (mom to breast cancer) and this book helped set me on a path toward biology, then to helping medical researchers with bioinformatics and, ultimately, to express my passion for successes in translational research via this book.

While working at the University of Pittsburgh Cancer Institute, about eight years ago, I had the pleasure of sitting in on one of many presentations designed to update and educate those involved in research on clinical options available to patients. Dr. Ron Herberman, Director of UPCI, had a research interest and focus on immunological approaches to cancer treatment. Some cancers, are outside of the reach of the immune system, and I often wondered what advances existed for inoperable brain tumors such as Johnny Gunther's.

The presentation I saw was on Endoscopic Endonasal Approach (EEA) to brain tumors located deep within in the skull, many times right at the base of the brain stem. The presenter showed video of an actual surgery. I sat, amazed, as I listened to the description of the breaking of the thin bone at the base of the skull, through the nose (or, less commonly, through the cheek) to access the area at the base of the skull. The surgery I saw was of a glioblastoma — a fatty tumor — that had grown to be about the size of an apricot. The tumor had wrapped itself around the base of the brain, and enveloped the brain stem — clearly a sensitive area for any surgeon, and clearly inaccessible from any other angle. And yet the endoscope's light showed the tumor, readily accessible. I wondered how safe any cutting might be in the region. And then the video showed a tube, inserted alongside, sometimes attached to the endoscope, vacuum suctioning the fatty tissue, elegantly, and rather neatly, cleanly, and quickly, removing the tumor, globule by globule, until the tumor was gone.

Tears came to my eyes as I recalled Johnny Gunther's struggle and counted the innumerable children and adults who, in the past, had died needlessly from so-called inoperable brain tumors. I quickly recovered, however, when I realized the beauty and elegance of the approach meant success beyond that imaginable during the 1940s. It reminded me that we sometimes take far too much for granted in modern medicine. Unbelievably, I learned that the hole in the back of the nasopharyngeal area was patched up with skin, sometimes from a cadaver, which performed suitably in most cases for life, without further complications. I learned that infection was rare, as was cerebral spinal fluid leakage.

EEA options exist for over 40 otherwise difficult-to-treat conditions; the doctors at UPCI specialize in naso-septal flap reconstruction. To know where we are today, compared to where we were in the middle of the last century, in terms of advances in the treatment and in many cases curing of what previously had been inoperable brain tumors, is breathtaking, and is cause for celebration. Johnny's brain tumor was not located at the base of the skull, and the outcome for patients with parietal glioblastoma multiforme is still not good, but is improving. In 2007, only 3–5% of patients survived more than five years; in 2010, it was around 8% (SEER). To mitigate risks, MRIs are used to map the tendrils to guide the surgeons as they seek to remove as much of the tumor as possible. Brain stimulation is used to identify key areas that should be avoided to provide as high a quality of life post-surgery as possible. Our friend Avastin, the less expensive drug that can be used to save the eyesight of people with age-related macular degeneration (Chapter 1), was approved for treating glioblastoma by the US FDA in 2009. A case study of the use of high intensity, short pulse electricity in Na Homolce Hospital, Prague, in the Czech Republic reported that four patients out of 20 survived at least seven years post-treatment with no sign of recurrence (Rulseh *et al.*, 2012).

As a card-carrying evolutionary biologist, I look back at my experience in that library, reading of John Gunther, Jr.'s bravery, his lack of complaint about his worsening condition, his intellectual curiosity about his treatments, his repeated attempts to get the truth of the direness of his situation out of his doctors. I marvel at his will to live, and to be, in spite of the struggle.

And I recall, with special fondness, one of John's lasting legacies, his alluring, almost prescriptive poem. I doubt that I have recognized until now the role that this poem has played in my life's choices.

References

Gunther J. (1965) *Death Be Not Proud.* Harper & Row Perennial Library Edition.

Rulseh AM, *et al.* (2012) Long-term survival of patients suffering from glioblastoma multiforme treated with tumor-treating fields. *World J Surg Oncol* **10:** 220. [doi: 10.1186/1477-7819-10-220]

The Unbeliever's Prayer

John Gunther, Junior (1929–1947)

Almighty God

Forgive me for my agnosticism;

For I shall try to keep it gentle, not cynical,

Nor a bad influence.

And O!

If thou art truly in the heavens,

Accept my gratitude

For all thy gifts

And I shall try

To fight the good fight. Amen.

10 Genomics and Personalized Medicine

Since the advent of molecular biology, a bewildering amount of knowledge at various levels of detail has been published about the cellular, protein, genetic, and epigenetic basis of life's function. There is a correspondingly large number of studies at various levels of inquiry on the dysfunction of life we call disease. Commercial enterprises have emerged to provide individual customers with their nearly complete genome sequence. More and more information is becoming available, and increasingly sophisticated ways of using that information are constantly being developed. Society is coming to terms culturally with what it means to have genetic indicators of risk, especially with the passing of the Genetic Information Nondiscrimination Act (GINA) in the US in 2008.

Sorting out which results are most compelling for making progress in medicine is challenging, but there are certain notable examples of findings that we can look back on that are either fundamentally important as base examples of clear-cut applications of existing knowledge in molecular biology with expected effects on human health, or that represent surprising, new findings that were either not predicted by the central tenets of human and molecular biology or, in some cases, have overturned such tenets.

Important Stepwise Advances from Molecular Biology to Genomic Medicine

In the 1980s an era of molecular biology emerged in which it was typical of researchers in all walks of biology to begin to use laboratory techniques to interrogate the DNA sequences of individual genes.

Techniques were invented to be able to visualize the location of specific genes on proteins and to identify the location of specific proteins in the cell. A boon in developmental biology occurred in which it became easy to insert a marker — usually green fluorescent protein — into an animal's genome and have it co-express as a reporter of which tissues a protein was expressed in. Thousands of studies later, we have a fairly sophisticated understanding of the function of just over half of the genes encoded in the human genome.

This "individual gene" era led to a few changes in clinical practice. In 2001, when the human genome was sequenced, there were around 400 genetic tests for diseases. Our understanding of pathways involved in cancer was improving in many ways; we began to understand how tumors could evade immune surveillance; how they used growth factors to recruit blood vessels; how they could signal nearby cells in the matrix and induce a pre-cancerous field response.

The drub imatinib was developed, targeting the *bcr-acl* gene fusion product in chronic myeloid leukemia (Druker *et al.*, 2001). Prior to the development of imatinib (aka Gleevec), no treatment was available to slow the progression of CML. The efficacy of the drug provided an example of the potential of gene sequencing-informed targeted therapies, and is widely hailed as a classic example of success in molecular medicine.

Gene Discovery Era

Gene mapping studies became common in the 1990s–2000s. The goal of these studies was to determine the locus, or loci, of genetic variants involved in disease. They used the association of the inheritance of known genome landmarks with the occurrence of disease among individuals, often in a genealogy. These "gene association studies" would lead investigators to regions of a specific chromosome in which a number of individual genes might exist. Investigators might do some fine-scale mapping to narrow down regions of association until they were small enough (in terms of DNA base pairs) to tackle with Sanger DNA sequencing. The DNA sequences would be determined for those in individuals in the association study, and based pair differences located there would be considered evidence for a pathogenic role of the genes in which they were found.

A great deal of potentially actionable functional knowledge came from these studies. Progress in the knowledge of genes involved in diseases was dramatically advanced in cancer, which led to genetic tests for hereditary colon cancer, breast and ovarian cancer, retinoblastoma, and many others. There are now over 4,000 genetics tests available to help the medical community understand the specific causal genetic and genomic underpinnings of an individual's disease.

Whole Genome Sequencing

The full human genome was sequenced via a competition that became a collaboration between the National Institutes of Health and J. Craig Venter. Although it was expensive and time-consuming to sequence entire genomes, an era of genomic medicine was heralded. Since the first human genome was sequenced, a technological race was on to make genome sequencing faster and less expensive.

Sequence information can be critical to precision medicine. Advances have been made in understanding up to seven molecular subtypes of diabetes (Murphy *et al.*, 2008), each with a potentially different optimal routine treatment. Around 90% of patients with neonatal diabetes that qualify for the shift in the treatment respond medically better to a pill than to regular insulin shots. A small study of infants showed that treatment with sulphonylurea may be safe and effective in infants over six months old prior to genetic testing (Carmody *et al.*, 2014). The shift in oral sulphonylurea treatment, including the cost of sequencing, is recovered after 10 years (Naylor *et al.*, 2014).

This was the result of the discovery of the link mutations in proteins of the KATP channels in many affected individuals (Fournet and

Junien, 2004). KATP forms complexes with other proteins to regulate cross-membrane transfer of molecules involved in glucose metabolism. In β-cells, KATP complexes control the flow of insulin in response to blood glucose concentrations. Diabetes patients with mutations altering KATP channel proteins respond better to oral sulphonylurea therapy than to insulin, with improved control and less frequent hypoglycaemia, and long-term neuroprotection is anticipated (Soundarapandian *et al.*, 2007). Taking a pill for diabetes regulation is better tolerated than constant insulin injections, and thus there is added value beyond the medicinal treatments. There are now over 20 genes that have been causally linked to a growing variety of molecular subtypes (Greeley *et al.*, 2010; 2011), including genetic diagnosis and risk assessment of maturity onset diabetes of the young (MODY). Certain patients with every classically recognized type of diabetes may have their treatment refined via genetic testing. There are concerns, however, that the high degree of heterogeneity, the large number of contributing mutations and the early stage of development of genetic prediction models will lead to overtesting and non-specific testing (Lyssenko and Laakso, 2013). The immense and growing diabetes clinical population means that overtesting and low precision of prediction models could lead to massive profits with relatively few overall clinical benefits and therefore, as for all genetic testing, large, prospective multi-center clinical studies will be needed to measure generalizability of the accuracy, sensitivity and specificity of these tests.

Functional Genomics

Sequencing patients was only one of a myriad of ways in which the knowledge of the human genome sequenced impacted, and continues to impact, medicine and medical research. Due to the public availability of the genomic sequences, companies like Affymetrix and Codelink brought forward platforms that could interrogate the gene expression in thousands, and then tens of thousands of genes in a tissue sample. These platforms held an array of probes that would, with high specificity, bind to parts of RNA (ribonucleic acid) from genes expressed in a tissue.

The first studies were in breast cancer; tumor tissue could be compared to normal breast cancer tissue to identify which genes were turned on/off, up/down in malignancies. The techniques in functional genomics could also be used to study subtypes of cancers and other diseases. The field was greatly aided by the field of bioinformatics, a discipline in its own right.

Some examples of current DNA microarray-based clinical applications include diagnostic virology, including the use of DNA microarrays to detect HIV mutations associated with resistance to antiretroviral drugs (Kozal *et al.*, 1996), detection of respiratory viruses (Coiras *et al.*, 2005), hepatitis C virus (Xu *et al.*, 2005) and CNS viral infection (Leveque *et al.*, 2011).

Gene expression microarrays have not been as widely adopted, in large part due to low reproducibility of the prediction and diagnostic algorithms over time. Instead, more robust "gold-standard" multiplex PCR assays developed using genes discovered using RNA microarrays have been developed for clinical infectious agent (microbial) surveillance and discovery, including tests for a wide diversity of organisms including influenza, venereal diseases, potential bioweapons (e.g., anthrax; Elnifro *et al.*, 2000), coronaviruses, HIV-1 and HIV-2, and emerging infectious tropical diseases such as Ebolaviruses and Lassa Fever Virus (Drosten *et al.*, 2002). Some quantitative PCR tests measure a baseline of viral load, such as Roche's test for Hepatitis C. The movement in the field of molecular diagnostics of microbes is toward tests that can detect hundreds or thousands of organisms in a single sample.

PCR is widely used in genetic tests of many types. Quantitative RT-PCR tests of gene expression are also used clinically to diagnose and detect residual disease in chronic myeloid leukemia by detecting the bcr/abl gene fusion. It has been found to be useful for her-2 gene amplification detection (Mendoza *et al.*, 2013), important in breast cancer treatment considerations.

One of the most exciting developments in cancer genomics was the development of the Pathwork® Tissue of Origin Test, which used expression scores of 2,000 genes to match a tumor of unknown primary origin to 15 different possible tissues of origin. The test had been approved by the FDA twice, once in 2008 for fresh frozen tissue, and again in 2010 for tissues fixed in paraffin. Following the FDA's lead, Medicare indicated positive intention for reimbursement; QALY based cost effectiveness estimated $47,000 however, inconsistent and low reimbursement rates (PGx Reporter 6/20/2012) were thought to have doomed the company, and the test (Ray, 2013).

This option was a potentially serious threat to the long-established and embedded immunohistochemistry assays. Studies had shown much high accuracy of the Pathwork® Tissue of Origin Test (Dumur *et al.*, 2011), with the results showing >95% agreement with classical diagnostic techniques, including clinical correlations and immunohistochemistry (IHC) staining. The authors called for the use of the test to augment existing clinical workflows, especially due to the potential for tumors originating from tissues not included in the initial panel of tissues characterized. It was possible due to the non-inclusion of all tissue types that some tumors could be misidentified, leading to unproven clinical treatment conclusions. The study set-up was called "artificial" by defenders of IHC testing in a Letter to the Editor of *the Journal of Clinical Pathology* (Parkash *et al.*, 2012). The authors of the Letter also claimed equivalence of immunohistochemistry (IHC) testing, and reported a case study (without peer review) of two hard-to-diagnose cases that were also difficult to diagnose with classical methods. The test was considered defunct (Ray *et al.*, 2013), in spite of a study that showed improved survival in patients whose treatments were changed due to tissue of origin identification (Nystrom *et al.*, 2012).

A large multi-center study confirmed the earlier findings of superior primary site identification compared to IHC (Handorf *et al.*, 2013), and the test is now offered by Response Genetics (as the ResponseDX test). An independent study considering neuroendocrine metastasis further confirmed the superiority of the ResponseDX test over IHC (Maxwell, 2014).

Biomarker Era

These two areas of technological development enabled clinical researchers to begin to think about developing multi-marker indicators of disease risk, biomarkers for diagnosis, as well as biomarkers for prognosis. Retrospective clinical studies were conducted after clinical treatment trial outcomes were known to see if a biomarker panel could be discovered that could have been used to predict which patients would have responded to particular treatments. Controversies occurred over the reproducibility of results from an early study in ovarian cancer, in which then-FDA employees developed a mass-spectrometry-based diagnostic test for ovarian cancer (OvaCheck™). Unfortunately, study design issues identified by biostatisticians determined that the results were likely due to differences in the time of processing of the ovarian cancer patient samples and the normal individual samples. Whole-profile analysis in which the identity of proteins and peptides are not known may have held great promise at one time, and in principle could be used for clinical applications in a variety of settings. However, due to an oversight by those involved in the study, an important source of variation that affected whole profile serum proteomic profile was overlooked, and the field developed a consensus that the assays were not reproducible. They can be made quantitative, and ventures in this area are being made increasingly quantitative (Lehmann *et al.*, 2013). Caprion, Inc. (www.caprion.com) is actively pursuing proteomics-based biomarker development in oncology, infectious diseases, and diabetes.

The use of machine learning techniques to identify putative biomarkers from genomic and proteomic data led the field to a rather standard type of study design, in which samples from hundreds of patients were collected and processed. The data from these samples are split (at random) into a training set and a test set each containing representatives of each clinical group reflecting the aims of the study (e.g., treatment vs. control; case vs. control; survivors vs. non-survivors, etc.). The training set was typically composed of roughly half cases (tumors) and half control (e.g., normal tissue). The training set is used to identify a subset of potentially informative markers and to optimize a decision rule, i.e., how to use the combination of markers. The test set was reserved for use to measure the accuracy, sensitivity, and specificity of the biomarker set combined with an optimized decision rule. The optimal split for such studies is around 66%:33%, training:test set.

Putative biomarkers in this setting can be identified either using a univariate or multivariate feature selector (t-test, J5 score) or the apparent clinical utility of each individual marker (AUC; area under the ROC curve). Importantly, the feature selection step should be wrapped within the training loop and combined with assessment of the overall prediction model algorithm (e.g., SVM, logistic regression, Random Forests, etc.). Modelers often split the training set multiple times during feature selection and model evaluation so the performance can be assessed on part of the training set. This is called internal cross-validation and can be used to study many combinations of feature selection + model type + model parameters. The best models may then be used to predict on the test set sample to ensure generalizable estimates of the performance evaluation measures such as Sensitivity, Specificity and overall accuracy.

An important consideration during these steps is class imbalance in which there are unequal numbers of patients in each of the two clinical classes (e.g., cases vs. controls, etc.). Training a model iteratively to maximize accuracy (identically to minimize overall classification error, or *min_ACE*), for example, can lead these machine learning optimized approaches to absurd models, such as predicting all controls correctly but predicting all cases as controls. The global optimum of *min_ACE* assumes that the cost of error in the diagnosis of a case (false negative) is the same as the cost of an error in the diagnosis of a control (false positive). There is no universal rule for establishing the costs for these errors (consider the cost of a false negative of Ebola compared to a false negative for warts).

All else being equal (which it never is), I invented a very simple mathematical function to use during machine learning model optimization that drives models toward SP = 1, SN = 1 even in cases of extreme imbalance. In 2005, colleagues and I created a statistical test to assess the significance of the accuracy achieved during model optimization over a range of feature selection space. The method, called PACE (Lyons-Weiler *et al.*, 2005), uses class label randomization to derive null distributions for the achieved classification error over any range of parameter space, and a lower-end confidence limit to determine whether a model's performance is statistically significant (better than chance).

In the event of imbalance, I (and Haiwen Shi, now at the FDA) invented a simple method called weighted ACE.

If accuracy = ACC, then

$$ACE = 1 - ACC$$

When the study design is highly imbalanced, the model optimization and methods evaluation can result in a distorted outcome, where the goal of finding a modeling method, or a collection of parameter values, or model coefficient values at *min_ACE* leads to a model with perfect accuracy in the larger class (e.g., SN = 1, SP = 0, or SN = 0, SP = 1).

To avoid this outcome during prediction modeling with unequal classes, the errors of common class can be weighted by the inverse of the size of the (relatively) rare class (smaller N).

For case/control studies, define N_- as the number of patients without disease, and $N+$ as the number of patients with the disease. Define N_{+wrong} as the number of test-positive patients who do not have disease (false positives), and N_{-wrong} as the number of test-negative patients who in fact have the disease (misses). We can define the weighted ACE as

$$ACE_w = \frac{\dfrac{N_-}{N_+} * N_{+wrong} + N_{-wrong}}{\dfrac{N_-}{N_+} * N_+ + N_-}.$$

This of simplifies to

$$ACE_w = \frac{\dfrac{N_-}{N_+} * N_{+wrong} + N_{-wrong}}{2 * N_-}.$$

The criterion *min_ACEw* can be incorporated into any machine learning optimization scheme and will avoid biased models. Model optimization and model selection performed to minimize *ACEw* will not suffer from the idiosyncrasies in models due to sample number imbalance (skew). Researchers who perform multiple methods of analysis and prefer more accurate results should select the method based on *ACEw*. Additional knowledge of cost reflecting preference of types of clinical errors can be incorporated in *ACEw* by introducing a cost adjustment factor $+\alpha$ to the cases diagnosed correctly, and $-\beta$ to the cases diagnosed incorrectly. The terms α and β are defined as costs relative to the cost of the corresponding errors in the controls, thus allowing a fully cognizant machine learning optimization scheme.

All past multiplex biomarker studies with imbalanced sample numbers that optimized on *min_ACE* would benefit from being re-optimized using *ACEw*. To date, there are only 13 FDA-approved pharmaceutical drug treatments that have companion single biomarker tests. Seven of these are in cancer. There has recently been a major increase in the number of biomarker publications. Diversification in the care of treatments like diabetes, ADHD, schizophrenia and many other diseases can be expected in the near future. Numerous cause-specific treatments will be seen, but long-term benefits and risks of these novel treatments will require study.

Multiplex biomarker panels approved for use in breast cancer include the OncoType DX® test, the MammaPrint® test, the Mammostrat® test and the Prosigna® test. The Prosigna® test provides an indication that a post-menopausal breast cancer patient will experience distant recurrence-free survival of 10 years or more.

The Oncotype DX® test, using 21 genes, provides a great deal of information. First, it estimates a woman's risk of recurrence of early-stage, hormone-receptor-positive breast cancer. Second, it also predicts how likely she is to benefit from chemotherapy after breast cancer surgery. Third, it is used to estimate a woman's recurrence risk of DCIS (ductal carcinoma *in situ*) or a new invasive cancer developing in the same breast. Fourth, it is used to estimate how likely a woman is to benefit from radiation therapy after DCIS surgery. The MammaPrint® test, using 70 genes, is used to estimate a patient's risk of recurrence for early-stage breast cancer. Chemotherapy may be indicated as a means to reduce recurrence risk. The Mammostrat® test, using five genes, provides an estimate of a woman's risk of recurrence of early-stage, hormone-receptor-positive breast cancer.

Additional multiplex tests have been developed, and the FDA intends to allow the use of archived data with known outcomes as independent validation tests of new biomarker signatures and algorithms to facilitate translation.

New Knowledge on the Regulation of Gene Expression

An entire book series could be written on the knowledge gleaned over the last two decades on gene regulation in eukaryotes. Extensive knowledge on protein–protein interactions, regulatory networks, pathways are available in archived searchable resources such as those hosted at the National Center for Biotechnology and Information (NCBI). A suite of interesting regulatory mechanisms, including gene methylation and the role of microRNAs (miRNAs), knowledge of coordinated gene expression patterns during development and tissue-specific gene expression patterns have been elucidated. The timing of expression of genes that regulate cell cycles is known, as are numerous pathways for various types of programmed cell death (apoptosis). A good course in the natural history of genome biology would be a shot in the arm for any undergraduate biology degree granting curriculum.

Gene expression patterns can be modulated by specific factors, and studies that have demonstrated direct and precise control over certain pathways hold promise for modulation of diseased tissue. However, the trend in medicine it to attempt to focus on an identifiable, unique (patentable) treatment (drug), and thus much of the existing knowledge has not been translated into medicines.

Some surprising results, however, can be found just by looking. Gene expression patterns differ when lungs are transplanted in mice using hydrogen as opposed to nitrogen, and a lung surfactant protein seems to be controlled by this environmental factor (Tanaka *et al.*, 2012). This could lead to shifts in the practice of lung transplants in humans.

Exome Sequencing

Instead of sequencing the entire genome, one option is to sequence just the part of the genome that is expressed, or the "Exome." Thus far, important mutations have been found to be associated with many diseases. It appears that rare variants may confer additional risk in complexes diseases.

Exome sequencing has revealed genes that contribute to the hereditary nature of some relatively rare diseases such as Miller syndrome (Ng *et al.*, 2009), hypolipidemia (Musunuru *et al.*, 2010), mental retardation (Krawitz *et al.*, 2010), among others. Exome sequencing studies have also revealed the identity of genes with high frequency mutations in cancers, including melanoma (Wei *at al.*, 2011), head and neck squamous cell carcinoma (Agrawal *et al.*, 2011), and renal cell carcinoma (Varela *et al.*, 2011).

RNA Sequencing — Transcriptomics

In addition to being able to interrogate panels of specific genes in parallel using probes, next generation sequencing allows one to sequence the entire transcriptome — that is, all of the RNA molecules that are produced in tissue from the DNA in route to being translated into protein sequences (Lister *et al.*, 2008; Mortazavi *et al.*, 2008; Nagalakshmi *et al.*, 2008; Wilhelm *et al.*, 2008). The abundance of each species of RNA molecule in the cell is estimated, expressed as a function of coverage (roughly, the number of copies present in the sequencing project). The idea is that RNA molecules with higher abundance will result in larger numbers of copies during the amplification step using polymerase chain reaction.

Various platforms exist for doing RNASeq, and numerous methods for the analysis of RNASeq data also exist. However, some of the measures of expression intensity for each gene show a length bias, and the assumption that coverage = expression intensity is a strong assumption not supported by data. The genome sequencing conducted can also show high variation in sequencing coverage among genes and areas of genomes, and there are typically only two copies of each gene. This variation is a function of local sequence characteristics, i.e., the effects of the actual nucleotide sequences on the relative efficiencies of polymerase and the sequencing reaction itself.

The bias in expression intensity is due in part to attempts to correct for the expression. As long as comparisons among genes in terms of expression intensity are desired, then between-sample expression intensity comparisons using a difference score such as a delta $(E_A - E_B)$ will be useful. The commonly used so-called "fold change ratio," i.e., (E_A/E_B), is dreadfully biased when used to identify genes that are differentially expressed. It shows such an intensity bias that researchers are effectively blinded to large portions of their data, especially in highly expressed genes.

Once genes are found that appear to be differentially expressed say, between diseased and normal tissue, the list should be subjected to quantitative RT-PCR validation. Genes that do not survive validation are not likely to be important in the comparison being sought by the study. These techniques can also be used to study disease etiology, mechanisms of treatment responses, to identify molecular subtypes of disease, or to identify biomarkers for treatment efficacy. Many, many other applications exist.

One advantage of RNASeq over microarrays is the ability (in principle) to identify novel transcripts. These can include fused genes that encode fusion proteins (as in leukemia, Lilljebjörn *et al.*, 2014), or alternate splice forms (Ozsolak *et al.*, 2011; Mortazavi *et al.*, 2008). In practice, however, the popular methods for examining alternative splice forms provide a score for known alternative splice forms. Identification of novel transcripts would require *de novo* assembly techniques.

Methylomics

DNA that is methylated is not usually expressed, and thus methylation patterns are also of high interest when it comes to understanding differences among tissues. Most studies that seek to identify differentially methylated DNA sequences are limited in that they analyze only the so-called "peaks" in the data. This is problematic for a number of important reasons, not the least of which being that we are diploid organisms. Methylation-driven gene expression patterns can be expected to vary from person to person in part due to their genetics and in part due to their environment. A second important point is that we do not yet fully understand the dynamics of methylation — partial methylation may be missed by peak-only analyses. Further, the size of region in which peaks are sought is important — one large peak may be the convolved signal from two or more smaller peaks — and important differences in one subregion of a genomic neighborhood may be missed by focusing on the larger more regional signal.

Good correlations between RNASeq expression and differential methylation have been found in studies that analyze the entire methylome, not just the peaks, such as studies of PKU methylation and expression patterns (Dobrowolski *et al.*, 2015).

Large Volumes of Data and Ethics of Medicine

Guaranteeing patient confidentiality is of sufficient importance to society that a law was passed that made it criminal for doctors to share patient data with third parties without explicit consent of the patient. With the ability to sequence thousands of genes, an interesting, and very likely, outcome now exists. While examining the sequence variation interpretation report, the doctor, and/or the patient, may notice some incidental finding for which the sequencing test was not ordered. In the past, the FDA required that any medical test for which a report was generated had to be thought to be relevant to the patient's immediate condition for which testing is sought.

With medical genetics, however, it is highly likely that the report may also contain information about the relative risk of other diseases. At question is not whether such incidental findings can be reported; doctors are obligated to report to the patient if, during a routine exam, they make an incidental discovery of an unusual mole, or a perforated eardrum, or a piece of metal lodged in the body from unknown sources. The question with genetic data is whether the patient has the right *not to know*. If, for example, one has an allele that is a marker of familial early age of onset of breast cancer, should the doctors be compelled to tell the patient of this finding? There are two schools of thought on this. The first is that medical doctors "know best." They deal with hundreds to thousands of patients per year, and over time, they will become experienced enough to navigate the subtle nuances of the significance of these incidental findings. This view would leave the option open to interpretation by the doctor, in the context in which the data were made available, considering the disposition of the patient. The doctor would decide.

The second option is more conservative, and would have doctors and boards making recommendations and decisions about such matters, considering the patients' view. One of my sisters adamantly did not want to know her BRCA1 status. In her view, she preferred the coin, as she put it, to remain "unflipped." She later changed her mind, but her concerns will be common among people — some will want to know, and some will not want the extra "worry." They would rather live their lives not knowing that they have a risk of early age of onset Alzheimer's, for example. This type of patient autonomy is not an easy ethical realm to navigate for many doctors, who feel compelled to provide a "heads-up, you may want to watch this" type of advice for what in the past were considered (mostly) age-related illnesses.

Other circumstances could dictate intervention of some sort — further testing, for example. It would be as simple as the doctor saying that they would like to start ordering annual glucose challenge tests to check for diabetes, or heart stress tests for cardiovascular disease. Or they might, in the future, order Neurotrack's test for early Alzheimer prediction, giving patients three to six years' warning to try to learn about ways to prevent neurodegeneration. Certainly there is a consensus that good counseling is needed before, during and after genetic testing.

Either way, the occasional false positive might also result. This is why whole-body CT scans are a bad idea — nearly everyone has some dense masses somewhere in their body, and superfluous follow-up tests, including biopsies, would overwhelm the system. With genetic testing, two types of false positives are possible. The first is an error in the sequence data itself. The human genome is very large, with 2.3 billion bases. Next generation sequencing does not elucidate accurate base calls for every base in the genome; there are sources of noise, and uncertainty is still only roughly assessed. A woman, for example, might seek interventional, prophylactic mastectomy on the basis of a false positive BRCA1/BRCA2 test. Women with clinical mutations (those accepted by the medical community as risk indicators) have an up to 85% risk of developing breast cancer and up to 55% risk of ovarian cancer. However, companies providing whole genome sequencing have issued health advice direct to consumers that could lead to major life decisions.

GAO 2010 Sting Operation of Direct-to-Consumer Personal Genomic Testing Services

In 2010, a sting operation was conducted by the US Government Accountability Office in which fictional customers (employees of the GAO) called genomics companies with questions about getting their genome sequenced and how they could and could not interpret the results. The GAO also sent companies samples representing fictitious customers.

After comparing risk predictions that the companies made for 15 diseases, GAO made undercover calls to the companies seeking health advice. GAO consulted with genetics experts and experts on privacy and contract policy.

In a stunning report (GAO, 2010), the GAO reported to Congress that the companies, (1) 23andMe, (2) deCODEme, (3) Pathway Genomics and (4) Navigenics, among others not named, offered customers nonsensical statements such as "genes are a symptom, not a biological cause of disease"; allowed customers to send in samples from other people without their consent, and provided overall inconsistent results. One company gave inconsistent results for the same sample. The FDA issued letters to 23andMe to cease and desist in distribution health advice and medical interpretation of variants found in their customer's genomes. Similar letters were sent to at least 14 additional companies.

The FDA took the position in the letters that 23AndMe's assay was a medical device under section 201(h) of the Food, Drug, & Cosmetic Act, 21 U.S.C. 321(h). They also pointed out that it is not a laboratory developed test (LDT). The FDA classifies the 23andMe PGS assay a Class III device under §513(f) of the FDCA. This category of device is considered to have the highest level of risk, not allowed on the market before it has been approved.

Knowing what I know about the fundamentals of the accuracy and reproducibility of the base calls made by next-generation sequencing platforms, the FDA got this one right. The company was distributing the test and offering medical advice. At the same time, inconsistent results of the assay itself are a sign of trouble. The problem of varying results with the same sample sent to two companies was also revealed by Kira Peikoff, in an article in the *New York Times* (Peikoff, 2013), who received confusing and conflict results from three companies. She received a lifetime risk prediction of 20.2% for rheumatoid arthritis from 23andMe, and 8.2% lifetime risk of psiorisis. In her results from Genetic Testing Laboratories, the two diseases were among her lowest risks psoriasis (2%) and rheumatoid arthritis (2.6%).

The issue of inconsistent results from sequencing companies can in part be explained by variation introduced by which algorithms they may have selected for the analysis of the read data that is produced by the sequencers. The analysis involved "mapping" the reads to a reference genome and making a base call determination at each site. As straightforward as this sounds, the result of combining any two algorithms for these two steps can have a profound effect on the resulting sequence.

These distressing facts were revealed in a sobering study by O'Rawe *et al.* (2013), who found unacceptably low concordance among variant calling pipelines while analyzing 15 exome sequences. This inconvenient truth may not be welcome news to those vested, but it cannot be overcome by wishful thinking. Comparing genetic variation found between three variant callers, they reported among method average concordance of 57.5% overall. The amount of coverage (number of reads) at a site is usually considered to confer increased accuracy. However, O'Rawe and colleagues found that at sites with the highest coverage, agreement among methods *decreased* to 32.7%. Concordant sites were not much more likely to validate as correct. Discordance between platforms may be as high as 12%, as found in a study conducted by researchers independent of any sequencer manufacturer (Lam *et al.*, 2012).

Pirooznia *et al.* (2014) at Johns Hopkins University found 90.9% concordance among two variant calling methods (SAMtools and GATK) using data from one NGS sequencing platform; however, they cited over 99% sensitivity and 99% specificity for both methods. They found that that filters matter, and that overall the algorithm suite GATK with variant score recalibration was superior, confirming findings of other comparison studies (e.g., Liu *et al.*, 2013). Such high sensitivity and specificity may seem promising; however, exome sequencing results in hundreds of thousands of variants, and thus any of the potentially clinically important variants in an exome sequencing assay may be inaccurate. A collaboration between the University of Chicago and Vanderbilt University (Trubetskoy *et al.*, 2015) only managed a maximum rediscovery of validated exome variants of 89.3% using a consensus of four variant calling methods.

Due in part to the relatively high discordance observed among methods for rare variants, Wall *et al.* (2014) concluded:

> *caution should be taken in interpreting the results of next-generation sequencing-based association studies, and even more so in clinical application of this technology in the absence of validation by other more robust sequencing or genotyping methods.*

The FDA has since approved 23AndMe's assay for one disease, Bloom syndrome, and 23andMe just recently celebrated its millionth customer.

Even if exome data were extremely accurate, how well would consumers fare at interpreting the results? In 2015, a survey study of consumers of personal genomic testing services was conducted to assess their ability to correctly interpret the results provided (Ostergren *et al.*, 2015). The study authors concluded that most customers could accurately interpret the health implications of test results, but found high variation in comprehension with demographic characteristics, numeracy and genetic knowledge, age, and types and format of the genetic information presented. The average comprehension was 79.1% correct. By test type, customers interpreted statin drug response prediction best (range: 81.1–97.4% correct) but fared worse on some types of test (range: 63.6–74.8% correct) on specific carrier screening results. Customers fared poorer on tests that involved recessive trait inheritance patterns.

This survey study did not examine the clinical accuracy or utility of the tests, only the ability of the consumer to interpret the report. Clearly, given the market abuses of genomic testing companies, medical genetic testing must be done in the context of consultation with a doctor. No consumer should take action given genetic information without having the clinically indicative genetic variants in question validated with an FDA-approved clinical test.

Low Penetrance

In clinical genetics when sequence accuracy is in question, one type of false positive could be understood: low penetrance of the disease. Low penetrance occurs when a person may have an allele associated with a given condition but has never shown any sign of the illness. Association studies do not always lead to full understanding of cause and effect, and while we can sequence genomes, some diseases with inherited risk occur after an often unknown environmental trigger, and some may be multigenic; by no means do we understand the entirety of genome biology.

These issues are actively discussed in forums such as within the American College of Medical Genetics and Genomics (ACMG). The two relative views have been debated in the literature as well (Green *et al.*, 2013; Townsend *et al.*, 2013; Korf *et al.*, 2013). McCormick (2014) provides an overview. The best practices in terms of offering health advice to patients are expected to be reviewed and to evolve annually with input from all stakeholders.

A reasonable middle road may involve filters on the data, at the patients' request, to choose to not learn about specific conditions; however, a further balance is needed to prevent unwarranted billable follow-up tests by rogue doctors who might routinely abuse their patients' curiosity about themselves. Additional issues exist in terms of litigation ("my doctor knew but failed to disclose"), or incidental disclosure by other doctors with access to health care records who are unaware of the patients' desire for no disclosure. Overtesting is another issue: Disclosure of genetic information and offering follow-up testing to the patient as if every mutation were clinically actionable must be avoided, and clear guidelines are needed. Follow-up genetic testing should be encoded and especially audited by practice to prevent this kind of abuse.

Molecular Psychiatry

Most of the cases I have mentioned thus far are in general medicine or oncology. Molecular genetics has a lot to say about psychiatry as well, and is helping to unravel the genomic contributors to understand bipolarity (see extensive review by Kato, 2015), risk-taking and thrill-seeking behaviors, autism (O'Roak *et al.*, 2011), schizophrenia (Xu *et al*, 2011; Fromer *et al.*, 2014; Purcell *et al.*, 2014), and the rare (3–5%) *bona fide* cases of frank ADHD. It does not seem as likely that psychiatrists would order genetic testing for tailored treatments unless and until it was determined how to modify the route to treatment for a given patient; however, the data to date is tending to show that there may be many molecular routes to the same disease. Still, a few key genes may play an important role in differential diagnosis of Mendelian psychiatric disorders with similar and overlapping phenotypes (Sassi *et al.*, 2014).

In addition, identifying a genetic basis for lack of expected efficacy of specific treatments in psychiatric patients would seem very important and helpful in ruling out treatments. Routine molecular diagnosis using sequencing as an aid — not a screen — would seem reasonable. Exome sequencing can be made to target specific regions of the genome, and thus the area of molecular psychiatry is likely to see an increase in utilization for testing as an aid to differential diagnosis and risk prediction. Sequencing may also be expected to review targets for new therapies. The attendant ethical questions on generating large genetic profile data sets apply to psychiatry as well as to other areas in medicine.

Radical Findings Impact Understanding of Human Biology and Disease

Ask anyone in the field of medicine in 2014 if the human brain interacted with the lymphatic system and they would report "No." If you asked them how the brain drains fluids, they would most likely reply "via the nasophargeal lymphatic system," but that even that system does not extend into the brain. A study published in June 2015 (Louveau *et al.*, 2015) found, using molecular techniques, that the dura mater, a tough membrane that encases the brain (one of three), is filled with lymphatics, and that it drains brain interstitial fluid, macromolecules and cerebrospinal fluid into the jugular vein. This overturn of basic human biology "knowledge" was achieved using tissue-specific marker interrogation. The implications for genomics and personalized medicine are manifold; the system may be a conduit for drugs that have classically been unable to reach the brain due to the blood/brain barrier. Moreover, any immune system activity in the brain was typically seen as a sign of disease. This knowledge may have implications for studies of the root causes of progressive neurodegenerative conditions such as Alzheimer's disease.

Cell–Cell Signaling via miRNAs

microRNAs (miRNAs) are endogenous, noncoding, small RNA molecules that modulate gene expression functioning both by suppressing protein translation and by targeting messenger RNA degradation. miRNAs regulate a diversity of cellular activities, including development, differentiation, cellular metabolism, growth and division, and apoptosis. miRNAs have been detected in every tissue studied, including various clinically useful body fluids (e.g., serum, plasma, saliva, urine) routinely examined in patients. They tend to be specific to tumor type, and therefore have been investigated as putative biomarkers of diseases, including cancer.

Individual miRNAs are known to influence the expression of multiple genes, and they are simple to produce. Thousands of genes are known to be regulated by miRNAs. The discovery of miRNA was another major advance in understanding basic vertebrate biology, notably in that they embody a type of very strong intercellular signaling. In the immune system, dendritic cells are known to secrete exosomes which can signal antigen-specific immune responses (Segura *et al.*, 2005). The signal strength of miRNAs is strong enough to prevent scarring of the liver due to carbon tetrachloride exposure (Knabel *et al.*, 2015). While most detected miRNAs are not found in exosomes (Turchinovich *et al.*, 2015), a great deal of evidence exists of intercellular signaling via miRNAs bound by extracellular vesicles (Valadi *et al.*, 2007; Skog *et al.*,

2008; Kosaka *et al.*, 2010; Pegtel *et al.*, 2010; Mittelbrunn *et al.*, 2011; Montecalvo *et al.*, 2012).

The specificity of exosome update is as yet mostly unknown; cell-type specific miRNA uptake via exosomes would be part of the intercellular signaling code that would have to be deciphered, at least in part, before good control of delivery would be possible. Nevertheless, miRNAs represent an extremely promising means of therapeutic biological signaling (e.g., Bresin *et al.*, 2015), and much of the knowledge gleaned is made possible by advances in sequencing technologies.

New Strategies for Clinical Trials in Cancer

MATCH Analysis

The US National Cancer Institute and the National Clinical Trials Network are conducting a large prospective molecular allocation trial call MATCH (Molecular Analysis for Therapy Choice). The general idea of MATCH is simple: Identify eligible patients among those who have progressed after some first line of treatment and assign each patient to numerous possible treatment arms based on a molecular profile (e.g., mutations discovered by whole genome sequencing). The first line of mutation-informed treatment will either lead to remission, or progression. If the cancer progresses, further follow-up molecular profiling will be conducted to see if the progressing disease has undergone evolutionary changes, and in search of additional actionable mutations. The consortium seeks enrollment from patients from up to 2,400 sites nationwide, and the trial will examine the clinical efficacy of over 20 targeted cancer drugs. This will be the first trial of its kind, and will provide key information on the utility of a tailored, personalized approach to cancer treatments.

The approach is unique in that rather than using prior knowledge of treating cancer based on site of origin (e.g., lung, prostate, breast, kidney), the entire approach to follow-up treatment will be based on the molecular profile, which will be taken to indicate which of the 20 types of treatment arms a patient should be placed in. A patient with colon cancer, for example, could be the first (and perhaps only) patient in the trial treated with a drug originally studied only for efficacy in lung cancer if their molecular tumor profile indicates likely response to the drug development for lung cancer.

Comparisons of outcomes will not be made across arms (e.g., compared to placebo, or standard of care). Instead, interim progress-free survival and overall survival endpoints will be used to measure success rates after patients are treated with drugs that have, in patients with the same or different types of cancer, demonstrated efficacy in treating any cancer; success in all targeted therapy allocation will be compared, in some of the arms, to patients randomly assigned to default treatments, or treatments augmented with immunotherapy (Abrams *et al.*, 2014).

Some (most notably Tripathy *et al.*, 2014) have questioned whether next-generation sequencing is ready for prime time (clinical use). While they do not doubt the utility of tumor profiling with currently accepted gold-standard sequencing, they do question the utility of routine tumor genome-wide analysis, pointing out (a) if a molecular targeted therapy is known, entire genome sequencing is not needed; instead, the targeted gene can be more accurately sequenced using available gold-standard techniques; (b) the potential for inappropriate and unproven assignment of patients to treatments with unapproved drugs (each with potentially serious side effects). To this, I would add (c) assigning treatment based on tumor mutational profiles may lead to ineffective treatments as the clinical protocol (dosage, delivery, etc.) is often established and optimized via classical clinical trials, and that (as pointed out by Varghese and Berger, 2014), insurance companies are often reluctant or unwilling to reimburse off-label administration of prescription drugs approved for other diseases.

This is a shame, given that molecular data can be so useful *prima facie*. That is, a tumor with the right molecular profile may be expected to respond, or to not respond, to a given treatment based on molecular, not clinical knowledge. This is where population science (efficacy and safety studies in populations) and individualized medicine (efficacy and safety in individual patients) are at loggerheads. One radical solution is Nick Schork's proposed single-patient, or N-of-1 trials (Schork, 2015) in which the clinician attentively focuses on the response of single patients to drugs based on their molecular profile. This idea is the result of seeing numerous instances in which drugs that are useful for only part of the population are, after the fact, found to be identifiable by a molecular marker or biomarker. When expressed in terms of population science, the problem is one of identifying molecular subtypes. Schork cites as his example the finding that Erbitux (cetuximab) seems indicated for EGFR+, KRAS- colorectal cancer subtypes, but not for EGFR+, KRAS+ patients. Prospective studies of utility of the markers in accurately identifying the subsets will be needed, and then clinical studies of these molecular subtypes of disease. The N-of-1 studies would allow the transference of this type of knowledge into the clinic for specific patients based on their exome sequence; however, the current FDA process of registering trials for individual patients requires time and a large amount of paperwork.

Still, exome sequencing has proven useful in uncovering the identity of cryptic syndromes that are hard to diagnosis. A study of evidently inherited neurological conditions without diagnosis at Children's Mercy in Kansas City (Soden *et al.*, 2014) resulted in a molecular diagnosis in 45% of 100 families, leading to treatments in many cases. A broader study (Yang *et al.*, 2014) at Baylor College of Medicine not restricted to neurological conditions diagnosed 504 of 2,000 families (25.2%), also leading directly to treatment once a diagnosis was made. The clinical status of many people with hard-to-diagnose syndromes can be pulled out of limbo. In some cases, patients were found to have two inherited syndromes, conflating traditional diagnosis. Sequencing parents as well as children in a trio analysis increased the rate of successful diagnosis in these studies.

Costs of Genetic Testing

One of the original single-gene tests made possible by successes in translational medicine was Myriad Genetics' BRCA1/BRCA2 test. Their fee, however, made many balk at its use (originally more than $3,200). The costs of exome sequencing for diseases is best understood in terms of sequencing families; the cost is estimated at less than $8,000, and the time to diagnosis is days. A more rapid diagnosis means earlier effective treatments. This will also save children with hard-to-diagnosis conditions from enduring ineffective and inappropriate treatments.

The clinical benefit of exome sequencing cannot be presumed; outcomes are needed to determine if tested cohorts fare better than untested cohorts. Identifying "populations" and "arms" can be challenging in this respect.

"Total Outcome Awareness"

One of the biggest challenges in medical research is acquiring reliable outcomes data. To facilitate N-of-1 trials, and to determine whether exome sequencing and other means of molecular profiling of diseases adds clinical benefit, a "Total Outcome Awareness" would mandate the aggregate reporting of specific outcome measures from patients and doctors. This would allow payors to assess the economic value of specific outcomes. It would also allow doctors to more quickly understand the apparent impact of specific clinical options, and whether a trend may be indicating molecular subtype efficacy. Patients could be incentivized to participate in bi-annual health status reporting, which could include a collection of treatment compliance data and emerging co-morbidity. The diversified value of such feedback would be immense, and an Act requiring such data collection would force the expenditure for data aggregators and data analysts to provide ongoing feedback to the clinical community. Patient identifier data would be siloized within medical facility; however, de-identified data should be made available for public analysis. As health care options are becoming more autonomous, the public should be able to see these measures and understand the rates of success of specific treatments in use in populations similar to themselves. The rate of identification of superior treatments and procedures would increase dramatically. The data could also be used to identify possible unknown adverse events and drug–drug interactions and provide rapid feedback to doctors on their own individual practice. If made into a national program, doctors could compare their outcomes within each disease class to other clinicians nationwide and look at de-identified physician practice profiles, or aggregate statistics from top performing clinicians and adjust their practice accordingly. There are regional efforts to collect outcome data in this manner, but they are often isolated to particular branches of medical practice. Data standards are usually the most serious impediment to projects aimed at integrating diverse sources of information across institutions, and thus such a system would be most effective if it was built *de novo*, from the top down, with input from all stakeholders, including patient groups.

It is important to recognize that most whole genome and exome sequencing-based medical genetic testing for diagnosis will be "ruling-in" type testing, and that a negative result does not mean the patient will not develop the disease (e.g., no mutations in MSH2 does not rule out colon cancer in the future of a patient). The same is true for neuropsychiatric genetic testing.

Companies that currently offer genome and exome sequencing for patients include: Ambry Genetics, Baylor College of Medicine Laboratories, GENDIA, and GeneDx.

References

Agrawal N, *et al.* (2011) Exome sequencing of head and neck squamous cell carcinoma reveals inactivating mutations in NOTCH1. *Science* **33(6046):** 1154–57. [doi: 10.1126/science.1206923]

Abrams J, *et al.* (2014) National Cancer Institute's Precision Medicine Initiatives for the new National Clinical Trials Network. *Am Soc Clin Oncol Educ Book* 71–76.[doi: 10.14694/EdBook_AM.2014.34.71]

Aspelund A. (2015) A dural lymphatic vascular system that drains brain interstitial fluid and macromolecules. *J Exp Med* **212(7):** 991–99. [doi: 10.1084 http://jem.rupress.org/content/early/2015/06/09/jem.20142290.short?rss=1]

Bamshad MJ, *et al.* (2011) Exome sequencing as a tool for Mendelian disease gene discovery. *Nat Rev Genet* **12:** 745–55.

Bresin A, *et al.* (2015) miR-181b as a therapeutic agent for chronic lymphocytic leukemia in the Eμ-TCL1 mouse model. *Oncotarget.* Retrieved from http://www.impactjournals.com/oncotarget/index.php?journal=oncotarget&page=article&op=view&path%5B%5D=4415&path%5B%5D=10057

Carmody D, *et al.* (2014) Sulfonylurea treatment before genetic testing in neonatal diabetes: pros and cons. *J Clin Endocrinol Metab* **99(12):** E2709–14. [doi: 10.1210/jc.2014-2494]

Coiras MT, *et al.* (2005) Oligonucleotide array for simultaneous detection of respiratory viruses using a reverse-line blot hybridization assay. *J Med Virol* **76:** 256–64.

Dobrowolski SF, *et al.* (2015) Altered DNA methylation in PAH deficient phenylketonuria. *Mol Genet Metab* **115(2–3):** 72–77. [doi: 10.1016/j.ymgme.2015.04.002]

Drosten C, *et al.* (2002) Rapid detection and quantification of RNA of Ebola and Marburg viruses, Lassa virus, Crimean-Congo hemorrhagic fever virus, Rift Valley fever virus, dengue virus, and yellow fever virus by real-time reverse transcription-PCR. *J Clin Microbiol* **40(7):** 2323–30.

Druker BJ, *et al.* (2001) Efficacy and safety of a specific inhibitor of the BCR-ABL tyrosine kinase in chronic myeloid leukemia. *N Engl J Med* **344:** 1031–37.

Dumur CI, *et al.* (2011) Clinical verification of the performance of the pathwork tissue of origin test: utility and limitations. *Am J Clin Pathol* **136(6):** 924–33. [doi: 10.1309/AJCPDQPFO73SSNFR]

Elnifro EM, *et al.* (2000) Multiplex PCR: optimization and application in diagnostic virology. *Clin Microbiol Rev* **13(4):** 559–70.

Fournet JC, Junien C. (2004) Genetics of congenital hyperinsulinism. *Endocr Pathol* **15(3):** 233–40.

Fromer M, *et al.* (2014) De novo mutations in schizophrenia implicate synaptic networks. *Nature* **506(7487):** 179–84. [doi: 10.1038/nature12929]

GAO. (2010) Direct-to-Consumer Genetics Tests: Misleading test results are further complicatied by deceptive marketing and other questionable practices. www.gao.gov/assets/130/125079.pdf

Greeley SA, *et al.* (2010) Neonatal diabetes mellitus: a model for personalized medicine. *Trends Endocrinol Metab* **21(8):** 464–72. [doi: 10.1016/j.tem.2010.03.004]

Greeley SA, *et al.* (2011) Neonatal diabetes: an expanding list of genes allows for improved diagnosis and treatment. *Curr Diab Rep* **11(6):** 519–32. [doi: 10.1007/s11892-011-0234-7]

Green RC, *et al.* (2013) ACMG recommendations for reporting of incidental findings in clinical exome and genome sequencing. *Genet Med* **15(7):** 565–74. [doi: 10.1038/gim.2013.73]

Handorf CR, *et al.* (2013) A multicenter study directly comparing the diagnostic accuracy of gene expression profiling and immunohistochemistry for primary site identification in metastatic tumors. *Am J Surg Pathol* **37(7):** 1067–75. [doi: 10.1097/PAS.0b013e31828309c4]

Kato T. (2014) Whole genome/exome sequencing in mood and psychotic disorders. *Psychiat Clin Neuros* **69:** 65–76. [doi: 10.1111/pcn.12247]

Knabel MK. (2015) Systemic delivery of scAAV8-encoded MiR-29a ameliorates hepatic fibrosis in carbon tetrachloride-treated mice. *PLoS One* **10(4):** e0124411. [doi: 10.1371/journal.pone.0124411]

Korf B. (2013) Response to Townsend *et al.* *Genet Med* **15(9):** 752–53. [doi: 10.1038/gim.2013.106]

Kosaka N, *et al.* (2010) Secretory mechanisms and intercellular transfer of microRNAs in living cells. *J Biol Chem* **285:** 17442–52.

Kozal MJ, *et al.* (1996) Extensive polymorphisms observed in HIV-1 clade B protease gene using high-density oligonucleotide arrays. *Nat Med* **2:** 753–59.

Krawitz PM, *et al.* (2010) Identity-by-descent filtering of exome sequence data identifies PIGV mutations in hyperphosphatasia mental retardation syndrome. *Nature Genetics* **42:** 827–29.

Lam HY. (2011) Performance comparison of whole-genome sequencing platforms. *Nat Biotechnol* **30(1):** 78–82.

Lehmann S. (2013) Quantitative Clinical Chemistry Proteomics (qCCP) using mass spectrometry: general characteristics and application. *Clin Chem Lab Med* **51(5):** 919–35. [doi: 10.1515/cclm-2012-0723]

Leveque N, *et al.* (2011) Rapid virological diagnosis of central nervous system infections by use of a multiplex reverse transcription-PCR DNA microarray. *J Clin Microbiol* **49:** 3874–79.

Lilljebjörn H, *et al.* (2014) RNA-seq identifies clinically relevant fusion genes in leukemia including a novel MEF2D/CSF1R fusion responsive to imatinib. *Leukemia* **28(4):** 977–79. [doi: 10.1038/leu.2013.324]

Lister R, *et al.* (2008) Highly integrated single-base resolution maps of the epigenome in Arabidopsis. *Cell* **133:** 523–36.

Liu X, *et al.* (2013) Variant callers for next-generation sequencing data: a comparison study. *PLoS One* **8(9):** e75619. [doi: 10.1371/journal.pone.0075619]

Louveau A, *et al.* (2015) Structural and functional features of central nervous system lymphatic vessel. *Nature* **523:** 337–41. [doi: 10.1038/nature14432]

Lyons-Weiler J, *et al.* (2005) Assessing the statistical significance of the achieved classification error of classifiers constructed using serum peptide profiles, and a prescription for random sampling repeated studies for massive high-throughput genomic and proteomic studies. *Cancer Inform* **1:** 53–77.

Lyssenko V, Laakso M. (2013) Genetic screening for the risk of type 2 diabetes: worthless or valuable? *Diabetes Care* **36 Suppl 2:** S120–26. [doi: 10.2337/dcS13-2009]

Maxwell JE, *et al.* (2014) A practical method to determine the site of unknown primary in metastatic neuroendocrine tumors. *Surgery* **156(6):** 1359–65; discussion 1365–6. [doi: 10.1016/j.surg.2014.08.008]

McCormick JB. (2014) Genomic medicine and incidental findings: balancing actionability and patient autonomy. *Mayo Clin Proc* **89(6):** 718–21. [doi: 10.1016/j.mayocp.2014.04.008]

Mendoza G, Portillo A, Olmos-Soto J. (2013) Accurate breast cancer diagnosis through real-time PCR her-2 gene quantification using immunohistochemically-identified biopsies. *Oncol Lett* **5(1):** 295–98.

Mittelbrunn M, *et al.* (2011) Unidirectional transfer of microRNA-loaded exosomes from T cells to antigen-presenting cells. *Nat Commun* **2:** 282.

Montecalvo A, *et al.* (2012) Mechanism of transfer of functional microRNAs between mouse dendritic cells via exosomes. *Blood* **119:** 756–66.

Mortazavi A, *et al.* (2008) Mapping and quantifying mammalian transcriptomes by RNA-Seq. *Nat Methods* **5:** 621–28.

Murphy R, *et al.* (2008) Clinical implications of a molecular genetic classification of monogenic beta-cell diabetes. *Nat Clin Pract Endocrinol Metab* **4(4):** 200–13. [doi: 10.1038/ncpendmet0778]

Musunuru K, *et al.* (2010) Exome sequencing, ANGPTL3 mutations, and familial combined hypolipidemia. *New Engl J Med* **363:** 2220–27.

Nagalakshmi U, et al. (2008) The transcriptional landscape of the yeast genome defined by RNA sequencing. *Science* **320:** 1344–49.

Naylor RN, *et al.* (2014) Cost-effectiveness of MODY genetic testing: translating genomic advances into practical health applications. *Diabetes Care* **37(1):** 202–9. [doi: 10.2337/dc13-0410]

Ng SB, *et al.* (2009) Exome sequencing identifies the cause of a mendelian disorder. *Nat Genet* **42(1):** 30–35. [doi: 10.1038/ng.499]

Nystrom SJ, *et al.* (2012) Clinical utility of gene-expression profiling for tumor-site origin in patients with metastatic or poorly differentiated cancer: impact on diagnosis, treatment, and survival. *Oncotarget* **3(6):** 620–28.

O'Roak BJ, *et al.* (2011) Exome sequencing in sporadic autism spectrum disorders identifies severe de novo mutations. *Nature Genetics* **43(6):** 585–89.

Ostergren JE, *et al.* (2015) How well do customers of direct-to-consumer personal genomic testing services comprehend genetic test results? Findings from the impact of personal genomics study. *Public Health Genomics*, June 16, 2015. [Epub ahead of print]

Ozsolak F, Milos PM. (2011) RNA sequencing: advances, challenges and opportunities. *Nat Rev Genet* **12:** 87–98.

Parkash V, Domfeg AB, Cohen PJ. (2012) The Pathwork Tissue of Origin Test. *Am J Clin Pathol* **138:** 165–66. [doi: 10.1309/AJCPEPLDWBD0C4NB]

Pegtel DM, *et al.* (2010) Functional delivery of viral miRNAs via exosomes. *Proc Natl Acad Sci USA* **107:** 6328–33. [doi: 10.1073/pnas.0914843107]

Peikoff K. (2013) I Had My DNA Picture Taken, With Varying Results. *The New York Times*, Dec 30, 2013. [www.nytimes.com/2013/12/31/science/i-had-my-dna-picture-taken-with-varying-results.html]

Pirooznia M, *et al.* (2014) Validation and assessment of variant calling pipelines for next-generation sequencing. *Hum Genomics* **8:** 14. [doi: 10.1186/1479-7364-8-14]

Purcell SM. (2014) A polygenic burden of rare disruptive mutations in schizophrenia. *Nature* **506(7487):** 185–90. [doi: 10.1038/nature12975]

Ray T. (2013) Pathwork Dx defunct; future of Tissue of Origin Test unclear. *GenomeWeb*, April 10, 2013. https://www.genomeweb.com/clinical-genomics/pathwork-dx-defunct-future-tissue-origin-test-unclear

Sassi C, *et al*. (2014) Investigating the role of rare coding variability in Mendelian dementia genes (APP, PSEN1, PSEN2, GRN, MAPT, and PRNP) in late-onset Alzheimer's disease. *Neurobiol Aging* **35(12):** 2881.e1–6. [doi: 10.1016/j.neurobiolaging.2014.06.002.]

Schork NJ. (2015) Personalized medicine: Time for one-person trials. *Nature* **520(7549):** 609–11.

Segura E, *et al*. (2005) Mature dendritic cells secrete exosomes with strong ability to induce antigen-specific effector immune responses. *Blood Cells Mol Dis* **35(2):** 89–93.

Skog J, *et al*. (2008) Glioblastoma microvesicles transport RNA and proteins that promote tumour growth and provide diagnostic biomarkers. *Nat Cell Biol* **10:** 1470–76.

Soden S, *et al*. (2014) Effectiveness of exome and genome sequencing guided by acuity of illness for diagnosis of neurodevelopmental disorders. *Sci Transl Med* **6(265):** 265ra168. [doi: 10.1126/scitranslmed.3010076]

Soundarapandian MM, *et al*. (2007) Role of K(ATP) channels in protection against neuronal excitatory insults. *J Neurochem* **103(5):** 1721–29.

Tanaka Y, *et al*. (2012) Profiling molecular changes induced by hydrogen treatment of lung allografts prior to procurement. *Biochem Biophys Res Commun* **425(4):** 873–79. [doi: 10.1016/j.bbrc.2012.08.005]

Townsend A, *et al*. (2013) Paternalism and the ACMG recommendations on genomic incidental findings: patients seen but not heard. *Genet Med* **15(9):** 751–52. [doi: 10.1038/gim.2013.105]

Tripathy D, *et al*. (2014) Next generation sequencing and tumor mutation profiling: are we ready for routine use in the oncology clinic? *BMC Med* **12:** 140. [doi: 10.1186/s12916-014-0140-3]

Trubetskoy V, *et al*. (2015) Consensus Genotyper for Exome Sequencing (CGES): improving the quality of exome variant genotypes. *Bioinformatics* **31(2):** 187–93. [doi: 10.1093/bioinformatics/btu591]

Turchinovich A, *et al*. (2015) Check and mate to exosomal extracellular miRNA: new lesson from a new approach. *Front Mol Biosci* **2:** 11. [doi: 10.3389/fmolb.2015.00011]

Valadi H, *et al*. (2007) Exosome-mediated transfer of mRNAs and microRNAs is a novel mechanism of genetic exchange between cells. *Nat Cell Biol* **9:** 654–59.

Varela I, *et al.* (2011) Exome sequencing identifies frequent mutation of the SWI/SNF complex gene PBRM1 in renal carcinoma. *Nature* **469:** 539–42.

Wall JD, *et al.* (2014) Estimating genotype error rates from high-coverage next-generation sequence data. *Genome Res* **24(11):** 1734–39. [doi: 10.1101/gr.168393.113]

Wilhelm B, *et al.* (2008) Dynamic repertoire of a eukaryotic transcriptome surveyed at single-nucleotide resolution. *Nature* **453:** 1239–43.

Wei X, *et al.* (2011) Exome sequencing identifies GRIN2A as frequently mutated in melanoma. *Nature Genetics* **43:** 442–46.

Xu B, *et al.* (2011) Exome sequencing supports a de novo mutational paradigm for schizophrenia. *Nature Genetics* **43(9):** 864–68.

Xu X, *et al.* (2005) Changes of ECM and CAM gene expression profile in the cirrhotic liver after HCV infection: analysis by cDNA expression array. *World J Gastroenterol* **14:** 2184–87.

Yang Y. (2014) Molecular findings among patients referred for clinical whole-exome sequencing. *JAMA* **312(18):** 1870–79. [doi: 10.1001/jama.2014.14601]

11 Robot-Guided Surgery

The risks of surgery during cancer are real. Release of cancer cells can spread the tumor to new tissues. Surgery in certain regions of the body is very difficult; the vasculature and innervation is highly complex, making each and every surgery unique. Classically, during open radical prostatectomy, surgeons had to spend up to three hours exploring and operating to ensure sparing nerves and avoiding blood vessels. During classical open prostatectomy, a large opening is made in the abdominal cavity, and with less frequency, through the rectum. With prolonged surgery, blood loss was a serious risk factor, and fatigue can set in. Even the steadiest of surgeons' hands can become imprecise. In open prostatectomy, viewing the prostate was difficult; it is located behind the pubic bone, and direct close-up visualization was difficult. Surgeons would spend hours bent over a patient, trying to work as quickly as possible to reduce blood loss. In many cases, the patient's health, quality of life, and safety were at stake, and thus anything that could be done to increase the accuracy of the surgery represents translational advances.

Information about the location of tissue, including nerves and blood vessels, is incredibly important. One might think that during training, a surgeon learns the anatomy of the body in sufficient detail to perform exacting moves during an operation. And they do. However, some forms of surgery either require extra fine motor skills, or require extreme care during specific steps in the operation. Also, a good deal of variation exists from person to person in the anatomy of the human body, especially with blood vessels and patterns of organ innervation, and thus, precise movements can be critical to proper surgical treatment. Other benefits include that the procedure tends to be less invasive, as in the case of robot-guided prostate cancer surgery, where a few small incisions are made on the abdomen, inducing less trauma to the abdominal wall tissues and musculature and reducing the risk of loss of blood. This can lead to speedier recovery, involve less pain after the operation (and thus reduce narcotic usage), and can reduce the risk of infection.

In between the period of open surgery and robot-guided surgery, laproscopic radical prostatectomy became an option in the early 1990s; however, the procedure was very lengthy. Efforts in Europe to improve the method helped to foster its adoption (Skarecky, 2013). In any type of radical prostatectomy, the surgery is fairly traumatic, leading to weeks of recovery for healing of the opening and intravisceral (within-body) incisions.

This approach added many benefits over open surgery; it was minimally invasive, and the surgeon could view the prostate and surrounding tissues directly, improving the overall accuracy and precision of the surgery. Robotic surgery, being minimally invasive, also offers these, and additional benefits.

Typical robot-guided surgery lasts only around 154 minutes (Badani *et al.*, 2007). In a typical robot-guided surgery session, much of the work is done well before the patient enters the operating room. Various forms of advanced internal imaging, via CT scans, are fed into a 3-D surgery mapping software, and the surgeon maps out the planned sequence of steps for the surgery as a protocol. The surgeon's hand can be guided by the placement of instruments into pre-mapped locations.

Studies have shown that surgery is improved by robotic guidance, especially in the areas of correcting degenerative spinal conditions, removing tumors, and correcting spinal deformities. In spinal surgery, the risk of perforations of nerves by pedicel screw placement is thought to be much higher than previously thought: as high as 90% (Wollowick *et al.*, 2011). Robot guidance can reduce this error rate. In some surgeries, the degree of precision is improved enough to reduce the use of radiation to visualize the patient's structures during surgery.

The risk of perforation can also be cut with the use of PediGuard™ by Spineguard. This handheld, wireless device monitors the electrical conductivity of screws being placed to alert the surgeon when they have passage through bone into soft tissue, with accuracy reports of 97.4% (Chaput *et al.*, 2012).

Reducing radiation exposure during surgery is important for both the patient and for the surgical team. One study (Kantelhardt, 2011), reported a reduction in radiation exposure by 56% when using robot-guided surgery. The same study reported a decrease in the length of hospital stay by 27% and an improvement in overall accuracy of implant placement by 70%. The PediGuard™ produce also reduced the number of fluoroscope shots by as much as 30%.

Another study (Devito *et al.*, 2010) looked at 635 surgeries and found an accuracy of 98.3% in 3,271 spinal implants performed with robot guidance. Adverse events encountered included four cases of neurologic issues without permanent nerve damage, a lower rate than previous studies. A non-randomized prospective clinical trial including the use of robotic guidance in radical prostatectomy (Haglind *et al.*, 2015) reported a reduction in erectile dysfunction but no improvement in urinary leakage.

Complications during spinal surgery tend to be due to poor imaging and "tool skiving" (glancing of the drill bit or trocar off the side of the facet; Hu *et al.*, 2013). However, the surgeon has the option, in difficult cases, to abandon the use of the robot, which occurred in the same study in around 10% of the cases. Stoppage of use of the robot in other settings is rarer (Holländer *et al.*, 2014).

Even when studies show no overall improvement, say in the risk of infection (Bochner *et al.*, 2015), there are benefits in terms of human pain and suffering in the use of robots to guide surgeons. Surgeons are human, too, and they experience stress and fear during complex surgeries. A randomized trial collected measurements of stress (heart rate, and heart rate variability) with, and without the use of the da Vinci robotic guidance system (Heemskerk *et al.*, 2014). This, combined with reduced exposure to radiation, makes robot-guided surgery the humane choice of medical practice.

Two important people in my life have benefited from the advances in prostate surgery for prostate cancer. The controversy over PSA aside, both men's diagnosis began with an alert from PSA screening. Standard digital rectal exam indicated further testing. Biopsy resulted in finding of frank cancer. Both men individually found their own doctors, who were very well known for their skill in prostatectomy due to robot-guided surgery.

In the case of robot-guided surgery, typically incisions are made, two on the left and three on the right of the lower abdomen. Surgical instruments, including those for visualizing (camera), cutting, cauterizing, and extraction of resected tissues are inserted after the initial incisions.

After the urinary tract, nerves and blood vessels are excised, the surgeon cuts a wide margin to ensure sufficient safety in attempting to remove any possible infiltrating tendrils of cancer that may have grown through the fairly thin rind-like membrane around the prostate. Once the prostate is freed, the prostate is placed into a receiving bag introduced into the abdominal cavity, to prevent escape of any incidentally free cancer cells, preventing surgery-induced metastasis. Prior to the end of the surgery, a permanent catheter is used to reconnect the bladder and the urinary tract.

Follow-up of prostatectomy includes annual PSA scans, providing a screen for any remote growth of cells that escaped into the blood stream (before or during surgery). Significant increases in PSA are followed by CT scan seeking the location of possible metastases.

In both of my family members' cases, the surgery went very well; incontinence was a lingering side effect, which is not uncommon, due to the permanent catheter and the overall trauma to the area.

I spoke with Dr. Ingolf Tuerk of St. Elizabeth's Medical Center, part of the Steward Health Care System, about the advantages of

RPP over OPP. In the 1990s, he expertly conducted OPP and also mastered laproscopic prostatectomy. Both of these procedures were laborious. During laproscopic surgery, the instruments are stiff and straight, and their movements are counter intuitive, i.e., moving opposite to the surgeon's hands. Dr. Tuerk said that the ergonomic advantages of robotic surgery are significant: The surgical tools are fully articulate, just like a human hand, and the movements are all intuitive, and visualization is excellent.

Criticisms over Additional Cost

Robotic surgery is sometimes criticism for having an additional cost of around $1,500 per patient. The equipment costs over $1 million, with maintenance costs of over $100,000 per year. Lotan *et al.* (2004) analyzed the relative cost of classical surgery, laproscopy, and robot-guided laproscopy and found that on economic factors alone, the cost savings in the form of shortened duration of the surgery and hospital stays did not recoup the additional costs. Son *et al.* (2013) reported that over 95% of patients receiving robot-assisted prostatectomy were no longer using pads, whereas for surgery without the robot, only about 70% were not using pads.

More importantly, several studies have followed patients after robotic surgery, and five-year survival estimates are between 84% and 87% after robotic surgery.

One study that made a splash in the news was conducted by Dr. James Hu. Published in the *Journal of the American Medical Association* (Hu *et al.*, 2009), the study confirmed that patients who underwent robotic prostate removal enjoyed shorter hospital stays, had lower transfusion rates, respiratory complications and surgical complications. However, the retrospective study found higher rates of incontinence and impotence, although the overall rates for incontinence or impotence after a year and a half were very low.

I asked Dr. Tuerk about the Hu *et al.* study, and the ensuing controversy over additional cost. He said that there had been a "battle" going on between OPP and RPP, and that the answers have not been easy to come by. He pointed out that the literature has been inconsistent, and that the actual degree of benefit of RPP over open surgery is hard to determine. The types of studies needed, he said, are randomized prospective clinical studies at multiple centers, with outcome tracking by a third, independent party. The trouble is that few prostate cancer patients will subject themselves to a randomized treatment protocol. The FDA randomized study done in the early 2000s, he said, was done at time when RPP was relatively new; RPP has a long learning curve, and the study compared long-time OPP experts vs. relative novices to RPP. He also pointed out that the study allowed the surgeons to self-report outcomes, which is not sufficiently objective. He said that he knows, from personal experience, that some post-operative patients will tend to overstate the quality of their progress to their surgeons, a sort of machismo/comradeship.

Now, he said, most centers offering RPP have kept a keen eye on quality control; those performing RPP are much more experienced. Centralization allows quality control, he says, and due to high volume of surgeries, they can have better cost control. However, he says the numbers of direct cost do not tell the entire story. He cites the

- reduced consumption of blood products,
- less use of drugs for pain management,
- shorter hospital stays, including less frequent re-treatment or re-hospitalization due to complications, and the
- lifetime costs in terms of pads and urinary continence aids, which are often met by the patient and not covered by insurance, and
- the patient's ability to return to what he calls "complete social integration" as factors that should be considered in the cost analyses.

Douglas Sutherland, a surgeon in Tacoma, WA, addresses the overall issue on his practice's website, where he provides for his patients all

of the details of the controversy over the additional cost in the prostatectomy setting from the surgeon's viewpoint:

*My job as a surgeon is not to determine if the additional cost is justified,
my job is to bring the best product to the war on cancer and consider
the clinical interests of the patient first — not the financial interests of
the healthcare system.* (Sutherland, 2012)

Due to increased risk associated with the learning curve of surgeons
new to robotic surgery, it is important that surgeons be frank and honest
about their level of experience in the use of robot-guided surgery in communicating risks to patients. The literature has numerous estimates indicating that a 150–250 patient learning curve provides proficiency. Some
surgeons have expressed discomfort in switching to robot-guided surgery, knowing that they might be placing some patients at risk. Dr. Tuerk
understands their concerns; he has had experience with all three types of
surgery, and has performed over 1,000 RPPs. He told me, in his subjective experience, the additional cost is clearly worth the health benefits
to the patients. He points especially to the increase accuracy and precision provided by RPP; however he agrees that the companies initially
(around eight years ago) had an overly aggressive marketing campaign
in which they suggested that nearly any pathologist could perform RPP,
which he says is not true, especially if they only perform 20–30 surgeries
per year. To help the field, he has trained eight fellows, sharing his skills
in RPP, since 2008. He sees intrinsic variation among the fellows in their
proficiency after two years of training; it depends on their overall skill as
a surgeon.

Robotic surgery in other areas has led to controversies and lawsuits. Highly realistic training modules with virtual reality simulation
are available for many applications in surgery (see a full review by
McCloy and Stone, 2001). One US company that specializes in the
development of simulations is Mimic Simulations (www.mimicsimu-
lation.com), with increasing realistic simulated surgeries. Residents

trained using Mimic's simulation platform involved in a randomized prospective trial comparing robotic training to laproscopic training (Borahay *et al.*, 2013) not only showed improvement in timed assessment of performance, but they also enjoyed their training more than those in the laproscopic training group.

In the case of robotic guided surgery, the interface for the surgeon is digital. No basic competency program using these simulations is yet available. Currently da Vinci offer some training modules, but an entirely simulated abdomen with random variations within the range of normally observed variances in vasculature, nerve involvement, etc. could be generated *de novo* for each training/evaluation session. Virtual cases could be provided to doctors at random, with and without prior indication, and proficiency could be demonstrated so the learning curve could involve lowered risk to patients and proficiency could be assessed. Such a program has been proposed for knee arthroscopy (Jacobsen *et al.*, 2015).

"Radical prostatectomy done properly is challenging regardless of technique," Dr. Tuerk said. "Whether surgeons use RPP or OPP, we are all are on the same side of the war on cancer."

References

Badani KK, Kaul S, Menon M. (2007) Evolution of robotic radical prostatectomy: assessment after 2766 procedures. *Cancer* **110(9):** 1951–58.

Bochner BH, *et al.* (2015) Comparing open radical cystectomy and robot-assisted laparoscopic radical cystectomy: a randomized clinical trial. *Eur Urol* **67(6):** 1042–50. [doi: 10.1016/j.eururo.2014.11.043]

Borahay MA, *et al.* (2013) Modular comparison of laparoscopic and robotic simulation platforms in residency training: a randomized trial. *J Minim Invasive Gynecol* **20(6):** 871–89. [doi: 10.1016/j.jmig.2013.06.005]

Chaput CD, *et al.* (2012) Reduction in radiation (fluoroscopy) while maintaining safe placement of pedicle screws during lumbar spine fusion. *Spine (Phila Pa 1976)* **37(21):** E1305–9.

Devito, *et al.* (2010) Clinical acceptance and accuracy assessment of spinal implants guided with SpineAssist surgical robot: retrospective study. *Spine (Phila Pa 1976)* **35(24):** 2109–15. [doi: 10.1097/BRS.0b013e3181d323ab]

Haglind E, *et al.* (2015) Urinary incontinence and erectile dysfunction after robotic versus open radical prostatectomy: a prospective, controlled, non-randomised trial. *Eur Urol* pii: S0302-2838(15)00194-3. [doi: 10.1016/j.eururo.2015.02.029]

Heemskerk J, *et al.* (2014) Relax, it's just laparoscopy! A prospective randomized trial on heart rate variability of the surgeon in robot-assisted versus conventional laparoscopic cholecystectomy. *Dig Surg* **31(3):** 225–32. [doi: 10.1159/000365580]

Holländer SW, *et al.* (2014) Robotic camera assistance and its benefit in 1033 traditional laparoscopic procedures: prospective clinical trial using a joystick-guided camera holder. *Surg Technol Int* **25:** 19–23.

Hu JC, *et al.* (2009) Comparative effectiveness of minimally invasive vs open radical prostatectomy. *JAMA* **302(14):** 1557–64. [doi: 10.1001/jama.2009.1451]

Hu X, Ohnmeiss DD, Lieberman IH. (2013) Robotic-assisted pedicle screw placement: lessons learned from the first 102 patients. *Eur Spine J* **22(3):** 661–66. [doi: 10.1007/s00586-012-2499-1]

Jacobsen ME, *et al.* (2015) Testing basic competency in knee arthroscopy using a virtual reality simulator: exploring validity and reliability. *J Bone Joint Surg Am* **97(9):** 775–81.

Kantelhardt SR, *et al.* (2011) Perioperative course and accuracy of screw positioning in conventional, open robotic-guided and percutaneous robotic-guided, pedicle screw placement. *Eur Spine J* **20(6):** 860–68. [doi: 10.1007/s00586-011-1729-2]

Lotan Y, Cadeddu JA, Gettman MT. (2004) The new economics of radical prostatectomy: cost comparison of open, laparoscopic and robot assisted techniques. *J Urol* **172(4 Pt 1):** 1431–35.

McCloy R, Stone R. (2001) Virtual reality in surgery. *BMJ* **323(7318):** 912–15.

Skarecky DW. (2013) Robotic-assisted radical prostatectomy after the first decade: surgical evolution or new paradigm. *ISRN Urol* 2013: 157379. [doi: 10.1155/2013/157379]

Son SJ, *et al.* (2013) Comparison of continence recovery between robot-assisted laparoscopic prostatectomy and open radical retropubic prostatectomy: a single surgeon experience. *Korean J Urol* **54(9):** 598–602. [doi: 10.4111/kju.2013.54.9.598]

Sutherland D. (2012) Robotic prostatectomy. http://www.sutherlandurology.com/robotic-prostatectomy-part-2/ (Accessed May 10, 2015).

Wollowick A, *et al.* (2011) Burying one's head in the sand: are we underestimating the significance of pedicle screw misplacement? *The Spine Journal* **11:** 10 (Supplement) S9–S10 http://dx.doi.org/10.1016/j.spinee.2011.08.033

Chapter 12

Hallmarks and Principles of Translational Research Success

In researching the topics for this book and getting into the details of the studies involved that support the important findings, I noticed a common theme to those studies that can be considered the most successful translational successes. While the entire scientific endeavor is laudable, studies that are most notable tend to share the following characteristics.

1. They asked important questions; more specifically, they addressed a problem important to society. Implicit in this, they were able to recognize the value of their findings to society. As a result, they had no difficulty in communicating the relevance of their effort.
2. The investigators were keen observers of events, patterns and trends around them, often looking to nature for inspiration.
3. They spent time thinking about the problem, and were not hesitant to "search for" correlations, and conduct observational studies to help identify plausible, important new research directions. When faced with barriers, they persisted — sometimes for a decade or more.
4. They stated a clearly translational hypothesis.
5. They clearly spelled out the next translational phases in easy-to-comprehend and logical terms.
6. They did more than confirm existing studies. They paid more than "lip service" to the true translational potential; as cognates, they were dedicated to the clinical problem at hand from question to answer.
7. They tended to ensure accuracy and precision of measurements.
8. They relied on the proper calibration of measurements (avoiding biases).

9. They took steps to balance variables across clinical groups, avoiding confounded study designs, and took pains to insure that control groups were appropriate and relevant to the study.
10. They were not afraid to try an alternative approach, counter to mainstream accepted practices.
11. They easily looked at their problem at a variety of scales — molecular to symptoms.
12. They were careful to use proper interpretation of results from trials. They did not over-interpret their results beyond what was supported by the data from their studies.
13. They paid close attention to and adhered to complete diagnostic criteria of the patients involved.
14. They refused to engage in activities that could resemble, or lead to actual conflicts of interest. If they held a financial interest in the outcomes of their science, they worked even harder to protect the validity of their science, as a matter of principle. Thus, the "profit pressure" reinforced their objectivity — they would not imagine jeopardizing their long-term prospects with short cuts or making leaps of faith in interpretation.
15. They prepared themselves with strong observational data first, allowing their experiments to rule out applications where the treatments or procedures seemed ineffective.
16. They remained ethical, at all costs — they never cheated.
17. They were forthright in reporting the complete set of results, including those that may be counter to their current understanding.
18. As a result, they did not mislead themselves, and others, by presenting only the most positive results.
19. They did not abuse their colleagues by having multiple data analysts analyze their data and then "cherry-pick" the results that made their results "look" best.
20. They asked the right types of question(s) at the right stage(s) of translational research and did not confuse, for example, discovery or research and development with commercialization. Compartmentalization of these activities allowed them to conduct properly

focused activities leading to the appropriate types of successes at the appropriate stages.

21. They tended to see barriers to translation as opportunities for well-applied effort.

I am hopeful that communicating the details of the pitfalls of research that are preventing a greater number of successes will motivate people from all walks of life to demand better from the regulatory process, from scientists, from corporations and from themselves. If more people thought to seek to enroll themselves in a clinical trial for new treatments for whatever affliction they suffer, sample sizes would be larger. If people got involved and demanded more money for the NIH budget, a greater number of larger studies could be afforded. Critical follow-up studies could be conducted. But the research community, and the regulatory community, must get their act together before confidence in their enterprise can exist. Headlines are filled with contradictory findings from nearly identical studies, and just recently (Feb 2015) the FDA reversed their decades-long position on the ills of dietary cholesterol. What is the American public supposed to think? How are they supposed to be able to sort this out? Headlines also include tales of academic misconduct and research fraud. Institutions must do all they can do to weed out the cheaters and should not tolerate abuses of conflicts of interest. Responsible conduct on the part of individual research scientists is needed.

Hallmarks of Shamwizardry

There are plenty of doctors, nurses, teachers and people who work for drug companies who are in biomedical research for the right reasons: to reduce human pain and suffering. Medicine is still a noble cause. I started this book project open-minded, with the goal of finding the best examples of successes in translational research I could find. I did it for my family, my friends, and for myself. In writing *Ebola: An Evolving Story*, I discovered that so many things went wrong, and were wrong with the national and international institutions charged with handling epidemics such as Ebola, that I found myself wanting to read about, learn about and share the positive aspects of modern biomedical research. In that search I, inevitably perhaps, found both positives, and negatives.

Just as I learned about the hallmarks of success, I also learned something critical about the source of the negatives. There is a pattern: There are hallmarks of swindlers and cheats who *are* out for profit regardless of, or in some cases oblivious to, increasing human pain & suffering. Together, these attribute fall into a category of behaviors and dispositions that I call "Shamwizardry."

1. **You will like them. At first.** They tend to be highly charismatic, and tend to make you feel as though they are doing you a favor.

2. **Abuse of positions and conflicts of interest.** They tend to have serious conflicts of interest, and have no qualms about acting in ways that place themselves in positions where they can personally benefit from those conflicts. Some tend to be so bold as to joke about their conflicts of interest, as if that provides them with a pass. It does not.

3. **One-sided arguments.** They will be critical of the developments with which their alternative procedure or treatment is in competition, but they will rarely, if ever, discuss or emphasize the limitations of *their* options. They will not cite any literature that does not support their one-sided view. This is not how science works.

4. **Negative appeals to emotion and other distractions.** When there are no data to support their criticisms of their targets, they will ruthlessly resort to *negative* emotional appeals. Or, they will distract with *non-sequitur* information that draws attention away from the main thrust of the benefits of the new technique or treatment. Or, they may create a false dichotomy in a situation when better understanding is had by considering a continuum, or situation-dependence of conditions.

5. **Willingness to resort to spite and condescension.** When data exists that is counter to their biased view, they will resort to

ad hominem (personal) attacks, coming close to or even going far as to draw into question a person's character. Some go so far as to systematically destroy a person's career. My advice to anyone experiencing this kind of treatment? Meet with them, but never alone; ask if it's ok to take notes; get everything they offer in writing and document everything. And talk with your friends and family about their doings, but do not discuss it with colleagues (don't gossip).

6. **When everything is on the line, they will lie.** Actually, shamwizards will lie simply because there is a slight breeze. These individuals are not interest in promoting real understanding. But they can willfully and woefully misrepresent the truth, especially in highly technical areas where they think they can get away with it.

7. **If allowed to fester, the Shamwizard will become a Tyrant.** Researchers and others in the workplace around the Shamwizard will fail to thrive; they will do only the bare minimum to get through their work week; they will not be inspired to do more than they are asked. Many co-workers will appear to want to keep their heads "below the radar" so as to avoid being singled out. Many will also be stressed if they are asked to participate in unethical research practices, and may remain quiet (and thus complicit) for years.

Shamwizardry is a form of tyrannical quackery in which perfectly good and valid options in medicine and medical research are attacked and dismantled by an overexaggeration of the potential limitations. Shamwizards desperately want to control the way you think, so you believe what they want you to believe. As a result, they lead people to erroneous conclusions.

Sooner or later, however, science catches up with them. The physicist Max Planck was an advocate of the truth. He is famously quoted as saying:

Truth never triumphs — its opponents just die out.

I, for one, am not willing to wait for them to pass on to see progressive change in research back toward pure and applied science.

We saw shamwizardry with the promotion of radiation over Coley's toxins; we saw this in the turfing of Dr. Gretchen LaFever Watson's community behavioral counseling program alternative to off-label amphetamine treatment of ADHD; and we saw this in local *ad hominem* attacks on an excellent surgeon by a local competitor who accused him of promoting robotic surgery just to take a bigger share of the available market. What is remarkable to me is that I did not expect to see this common thread emerge. All but one chapter of this book was written before I began to see the common themes, but they are undeniable.

I've spent 20 years optimizing what should have been straightforward options for the analysis of large genomic, proteomic and genetic data streams. I have helped many people, and have met a few detractors. Some big mistakes were made by early adopters; these mistakes caught on, and have been passed on (such as the use of ratio (fold-change) to express differences, the continued use of the log-rank test in survival analysis). Hopefully, the next generation of researchers will benefit from the knowledge that this effort has provided.

Similarly, advances in our knowledge of the effectiveness of clinical trials are being made. A just-so story told long ago about how measuring things twice with the same instrument with a made-up infinite amount of data has misled most of field of biomedicine into thinking that no useful information can exist in within-arm comparisons. This has effected the field immensely in terms of acceptable clinical trial designs, and yet nearly everyone seems to have missed that the power lies in the within-arm comparisons due to paired samples, and that covariates caused by the main effect are relevant to the main null hypothesis and should not be factored out with ANCOVA. Some will deny this vehemently and try to claim that I do not quite understand the principles of ANCOVA, nor how it is used to isolate variances.

I do understand, quite well; what they do not understand is that the prescription in ANCOVA to use the interaction term if it is significant instead of the main term is post-hockery at its finest — it fails to identify the source of the significance, which can exist within one, or the other arm. The default should be within-arm analyses, and ANCOVA if necessary, depending on empirical demonstration of *incidental covariance*. I have had statisticians tell me that they are not interested in the slightest in the outcome to baseline comparisons. The fairy tale originated by Cronbach and Furby (1970) and Lord and Novick (1968) automatically reduces valid within-arm comparisons to ashes in an utterly unnecessary manner. Also, the mere possibility of a confounding variable does not establish its existence, and if appropriate care has been used to ensure no baseline differences (by multivariate matching, or by combining baseline groups), studies will be made more powerful for the cross-group comparison as well, and such studies should be considered to be more appropriately designed.

In spite of the numerous negatives revealed in my research for this book, I found a number of extremely exciting findings and ongoing studies that are not quite at the "translational stage" of development. The progress being made by researchers at all levels — basic, translational, and clinical — is impressive.

We can only expect to "get there" with such studies if we cast off the binds that tie us to old practices that are known to be flawed. Even promising results from studies are ignored by the FDA unless they are "double blinded, placebo controlled, randomized, prospective" clinical trials. They weighed in on the need for placebo control arms in tests of drugs to help fight Ebola during the 2014 epidemic before any trials were even conducted (Cox *et al.*, 2014) under the idea that patients in Guinea, Sierra Leone, and Liberia enroled in the trials would receive best available care, and the results of any drug trials would therefore be confounded with changes to care for patients who received the treatment with no proper control arm. Doctors Without Borders (MSF) proceeded to evaluate drugs without placebo control arm under the idea that the drugs may help turn the tide of the epidemic, and there were already plenty of people around dying without the new drugs. The need for placebo may be evident when best care is, in fact, available, but it was not realistic of the FDA to think that best available care for Ebola would be available to the larger clinical population upon which the drugs would be used, and therefore even providing best available care could make the outcome of those drug trials irrelevant to the general population.

There are some fairly simple fixes to numerous stages of biomedical research that cost nothing. I'm an expert in complex data analysis, and on my journey through over a hundred research studies, I discovered a few years ago that an extremely commonly used measure of differences between two groups (say, treatment vs. control) is so biased that its use is the equivalent of throwing away a large proportion of the data collected. This particular bias has hindered success in translational research in a most insidious way: Those involved find it hard to believe that using a ratio of two measurements (treatment/control) is in any way misleading because that ratio is used so widely that it cannot be true. Here we see the failure in the understanding of how science works. A philosopher of science once portrayed truth as the consensus belief of scientists, and that change in science occurs via scientific revolutions. The changes in general understanding occurs, under this Kuhnian model of science, as a paradigm shift. This social aspect of science is widely appreciated as fact; however, consensus cannot replace objective, accurate assessments of specific knowledge claims, which is determined by our ability to measure what we hope to understand, and our ability to construct critical tests of hypotheses. We often fail in the area of constructing the right test, which requires (among other things) an understanding of the impact of our decisions on how to represent the data. There are numerous serious biases that result in the use of some methods of analysis, such as so-called "fold change" ratios instead of differences. If we represent the data in a biased manner (say, ignore all numeric measurements that start with "6" or "8"), how can we expect to see a full representation of the data and understand that which we have selected to study?

References

Cox E, Borio L, Temple R. (2014) Evaluating Ebola therapies — the case for RCTs. *N Engl J Med* **371(25):** 2350–51. [doi: 10.1056/NEJMp1414145]

Chapter 13

Future Medicine 1: Early Detection and Cures for Alzheimer's Disease

Think of all of the people you have in your life, your family, friends, neighbors, and your co-workers, the other regulars in your life — your favorite waitress, your priest, your extended family. Now think of all of the places you are familiar with — your home, your neighborhood, your city or town, the roads you know. Think of your favorite places to visit — maybe a park, a diner, your favorite watering hole.

Now imagine waking up, completely removed from your life. You don't recognize anyone; everyone seems a stranger. You don't know where you are — nothing seems familiar to you. You don't know where you're going, or how to get there. You can't remember how to feed yourself. You can't remember how to groom yourself.

That is the eventual world of a person with advanced stage Alzheimer's disease. A person develops Alzheimer's disease every six seconds. There are 5.4 million cases added every year. There are 31 million cases worldwide. By 2050, 50 million, and by 2100, 300 million people worldwide may be afflicted. The cost of Alzheimer's disease is around $600 billion dollars per year.

Now imagine a world in which people over 40 visit a website once a year and take a simple, passive 4 ½ minute vision test. After viewing a few images, they are given instructions after taking the test to visit their GP to sign up for preventative treatment, potentially a prescription for a drug that will clear the disease from their brains, or perhaps an ultrasound scan that clears the brain of the damaging plaques that prevent proper cognitive functioning. Imagine a world in which no one develops Alzheimer's disease.

This is the possible future of a preventative cure of Alzheimer's disease. This is the world that Elli Kaplan imagines, and wants to help build.

Kaplan is the founding CEO of Neurotrack, an early start-up company that exists to bring to market a test that can diagnose Alzheimer's years before any symptoms appear. The test, designed by researchers at Emory University, is a computer-based memory recognition study of a patient's visual information processing skills. It studies how people look at images on a computer screen.

A patient being diagnosed is simply asked to look at the screen and watch a series of images. Their eyes are being tracked by an infrared device. They are presented with a training set of identical pairs of images, one on the left, and one on the right. The patients are then presented with pairs of images, some of which are identical to each other, and some of which are the same as the training set, but paired with a new image not found in the training set. As they examine the pairs of images, the camera captures their eye movements. Neurotrack uses a proprietary algorithm that uses the results of this very simple test to diagnose Alzheimer's, on average, about three to six years before any other symptoms show.

What's happening in the patient's brain is that it is comparing the new images to the array of images stored in short-term memory within the hippocampus. The operation of the hippocampus is among the first parts of the brain affected by Alzheimer's disease. By instinct, almost subconsciously, the human mind automatically seeks novelty in its environment. In the test, the persistence of the gaze on the novel image is higher for healthy, unimpaired individuals. Impaired individuals, by comparison, spend a roughly equal amount of time gazing at the old and new images. Neurotrack's algorithm can sort patients who would otherwise be noticing the novelty in the new images.

There are no highly accurate early methods for diagnosing Alzheimer's. The disease, however, is progressive: It is believed that the build-up of beta amyloid plaque tangles in the brain occurs over 30–40 years before symptoms in most patients. There are also no FDA-approved drugs to treat Alzheimer's disease. Elli hopes that the test will provide drug companies with information they desperately need: an indication of likely Alzheimer's outcome — so they can accrue patients with high risk of developing Alzheimer's disease to their studies.

In a five-year longitudinal study, 100% of the participants who scored 50% or lower went on to develop Alzheimer's disease. In contrast, none of the participants who scored >50% developed Alzheimer's disease (Zola *et al.*, 2013).

I spoke with Elli about her hopes for the future. Her abundant passion for doing something for the greater good is evident. She also has a personal motive for success in translational research in Alzheimer's: She lost both her grandfather, Max, and her grandmother, Vita, to Alzheimer's disease. Her son never got to meet them; in fact, Vita passed on the day her son was born.

I asked Elli what she saw as the advantages of using this type of test. She pointed out that it is short, web-based, education-level and language agnostic and, most importantly, that it is predictive.

"There is no test on the market capable of doing what we can do," she said. "We can help drug companies find patients at exactly the time they are needed — three to six years ahead of dementia."

Elli foresees a time when the ravages of Alzheimer's disease are a thing of the past. She knows of lifestyle factors that have been shown to prevent, and in some cases, reverse cognitive decline due to Alzheimer's: physical exercise, cognitive exercise (learning a new language, learning to play a new musical instrument, crossword puzzles), and diet (Mediterranean diet, Omega 3 fatty acids, coconut oil, and reducing both sugar and carbohydrates). She is excited that these options exist.

But she is also realistic. People don't want to exercise, and even people who know they are likely to develop Alzheimer's may suffer from decision-making impairments. Her company will be launching a large internet-based study, the scale of which has not been seen in medical history. Participants will be able to log in to a website and, just by sitting at their home computer or laptop, be able to have their data logged and included in a longitudinal study to determine their risk of Alzheimer's disease. Alzheimer's may have more than one biological basis, and thus her database will be a treasure trove for data miners and models. Are there undiscovered subtypes of Alzheimer's disease? If participants provide outcomes data on other types of dementia, can the vision test be used for differential diagnosis? Are there patterns, say, that can pick up Parkinson's disease?

I am of the opinion that a new generation of observational studies, powered by the web — in which many people participate — will be of immense use for the clinical diagnosis of many types of neurological defects using high innovative techniques like those in place at Neurotrack. That's why I asked Elli to tell me about her company's investment model.

Neurotrack is an early-stage start-up. In today's funding environment, it competes with companies and foundations that focus on diseases like cancer, and diabetes. As important as those diseases are, Ellie says 2014 was a good year for Alzheimer's disease. The public now understands that age-related dementia need not be accepted as a "normal" part of aging. The next step is for the public to become aware of the sheer scale of the impending pandemic. So, she and her colleagues are taking the funding issue to the public. They are using crowd-sourced funding. She has also called for public outcry — to demand funding priorities for research on Alzheimer's disease treatments, and to demand fast-tracking of treatments and methods of early diagnosis by the FDA.

EP2 and EP2 Receptor Research

In 2005, a group of researchers at Johns Hopkins University found that deletion of a receptor protein alleviated many of the symptoms of Alzheimer's in a mouse model of the disease. In the mouse model, amyloid plaques build up, just like in humans. The full name of the protein they deleted is a mouthful: "prostaglandin E2 (PGE2) E prostanoid sub-type 2 (EP2) receptor," or "PGE2 EP2." PGE2 EP2 had been shown to be important in the development of the innate immune response in brain. They found that the deletion of the PGE2 EP2 receptor in the APPSwe-PS1DeltaE9 model of familial AD resulted in remark-able reductions in lipid peroxidation as the mice aged. This reduction in oxidative stress was associated with significant decreases in levels of amyloid-beta (Abeta) 40 and 42 peptides and amyloid deposition. They also found lower levels of beta C-terminal fragments, the prod-uct of beta-site APP cleaving enzyme (BACE1) processing of amyloid precursor protein.

In January 2015, a group of researchers at the Stanford University School of Medicine reported (Johansson *et al.*, 2015) that they had found that blocking EP2 on microglial cells in these mice had the effect of protecting the mouse brain from amyloid beta. Microglial cells are con-sidered to be the immune surveillance cells of the brain. Importantly, they found that the mice did not lose their memories of mazes learned when they were young.

Aducanumab (BIIB037) Biogen, Inc. (Cambridge)

The two most promising areas for treatment of Alzheimer's disease are a drug, being developed by Biogen (Boston), and an ultrasound scan, being developed by a team in Australia. The drug, called aducanumab (aka BIIB037), a monoclonal antibody, helps trigger an immune system response via microglial cell Fc-receptor–mediated phagocytosis. Its effects were studied in a 166 patient Phase IB trial. Aducanumab was found to reduce both the rate of cognitive decline and showed signs of reducing amyloid plaque in six cortical regions of early-stage Alzheimer's disease brain, measured by MRI scans. The study tested four doses of aducanumab, ranging from 1 mg/kg to 10 mg/kg, against patients taking a placebo. The most exciting news from Biogen is that both the degree of reduction in cognitive decline and the amount of clearing of the plaques tracked the dose — higher doses showed more improvement in both types of measures. Both types of measurements also showed continued improvement as the treatments progressed in time.

Side effects such as microhemmorhaging are known to occur at high doses of aducanumab in animal models. Minor adjustments to dose may be needed to avoid edema in some patients (such as those with the well-known APOE4 genotype), however, the enthusiasm for this drug is very high given the dose response in both outcome variables. Other side effects include headache, diarrhea, and confusion in about one-third of the cases (ALZ Forum, 2015). Aducanumab targets the full amyloid complex, not subunits. They are moving into Phase 3 trials this year. Biogen's FDA-approved offerings to date include five drugs for multiple sclerosis, and two for hemophilia.

High-Frequency Ultrasound, Microglial Cell Activation Cure?

The third promising area is the use of high-frequency ultrasound (Leinenga and Götz, 2015). Researchers in Australia have cleared amyloid plaques from recombinant Alzheimer's model mice. They trained the mice on circuitous mazes for reward and took a number of other measures from cognitive tests when the mice were young. As they aged, the cognitive abilities of the Alzheimer's model mice declined. MRI scans showed clear signs of amyloid plaque. Then, centimeter by centimeter, each mouse's brain was subjected to high-frequency ultrasound scans. These frequencies open up the blood-brain barrier, allowing microglial cells to work on clearing out the plaques. After treatment, the mice were found to have recovered their lost memories — a clear sign of great hope for improvement in the quality of life for survivors of Alzheimer's disease.

I asked Dr. Gerhard Leinenga about the next phases of research; he said they are focusing on transgenic mice to study the precise mechanism of amyloid plaque clearance, and to study ways in which the treatment with ultrasound would be most successful. They are also developing a prototype for opening the blood-brain barrier in a large animal with a thick skull, providing a model for use in humans.

Combined Approach?

It is straightforward but exciting to imagine a combined approach. For progressive cases especially, high-frequency ultrasound could be used to gently coax open the blood-brain barrier not only to allow important microglial cells to work but also to allow entry of promising drugs such as Aducanumab™, or even drugs that showed promise in animal or cell line trials but have not made it to or past Phase I clinical trials (e.g., Eli Lilly & Co.'s drugs solanezumab and bapineuzumab). Thanks to Neurotrack, these patients could consent before dementia set in.

Neurotrack's paired visual diagnostic and Biogen's Aducanumab have both been shown to be effective at the earliest stages of Alzheimer's disease. While there clearly more research to be conducted, the combination of the three technologies seems a promising next stage in the translation of this knowledge into effective reversals — and cures — of existing cases.

People with Alzheimer's disease can still recognize and react very positively to music from many years ago. The long-term storage of music experiences — and accessing that information — has long been thought to involve the temporal lobes. It is critical to understand how this information is stored and, perhaps equally important, how access to this information is preserved. The MRI study (Jacobsen *et al.*, 2015) found instead that music experiences are stored in the regions of the brain associated with complex motor skills — a region called the supplementary motor cerebral cortex. The study found that the deposition of amyloid plaques and loss of neurons in the supplementary motor cerebral cortex was similar to that of other areas of the brain, and thus the mystery of different mechanisms for the access and storage persists.

Each of these areas of development would benefit from large-scale, long-term humanitarian investment. Perhaps they could be listed as options in an Intellectual Property Share Market, so the public could aggregate investment funds and power this research forward.

Additional Information

Neurotrack's website: www.neurotrack.com

References

ALZ Forum. (2015) Aducanumab. ALZ Forum Therapeutics. www.alzforum. org/therapeutics/aducanumab

Crutcher MD, *et al*. (2009) Eye tracking during a visual paired comparison task as a predictor of early dementia. *American Journal of Alzheimer's Disease and Other Dementias* **24(3)**: 258–66.

Jacobsen JH, *et al*. (2015) Why musical memory can be preserved in advanced Alzheimer's disease. *Brain* pii: awv135. http://dx.doi.org/10.1093/brain/awv135

Johansson JU, *et al*. (2014) Prostaglandin signaling suppresses beneficial microglial function in Alzheimer's disease models. *J Clin Invest* **125(1)**: 350–64. doi: 10.1172/JCI77487.

Leinenga G, Götz J. (2014) Scanning ultrasound removes amyloid-β and restores memory in an Alzheimer's disease mouse model. *Sci Transl Med* **7**: 278ra33. [doi: 10.1126/scitranslmed.aaa2512]

Liang X, *et al*. (2005) Deletion of the prostaglandin E2 EP2 receptor reduces oxidative damage and amyloid burden in a model of Alzheimer's disease. *J Neurosci* **25(44)**: 10180–87.

Zola SM, *et al*. (2013) A behavioral task predicts conversion to mild cognitive impairment and Alzheimer's disease. *Am J Alzheimers Dis Other Demen* **28(2)**: 179–84. [doi: 10.1177/1533317512470484]

14 Future Medicine 2: Cancer Vaccines

Immunological research in cancer has led to strides in understanding how tissues progress from benign tumors towards advanced metastatic disease. Our immune systems constantly monitor our bodies for enemies — foreign and domestic. Specialized cells in the thymus called medullary thymic epithelial cells (mTECs) express every normal protein encoding gene in the genome. By presenting normal proteins — normal for each individual, that is — to our immune systems, we constantly drill to be able to tell self- vs. non-self, i.e., friend vs. potential foe.

Certain pathological microscopic organisms such as viruses and bacteria can cause tissue damage, and some kinds of viruses can wreak havoc with our genomes. The link between sexual contact and cervical cancer goes as far back as 1842 when Rigoni-Stern noticed a difference in the rates of cervical cancer deaths in virgins and nuns compared to married women, widows and prostitutes. In the early 1970s, observational studies of the transformation of genital warts (condylomata acuminata) into squamous cell carcinomas led zur Hausen to formulate a hypothesis that cervical cancer may arise from infections with the virus found in the warts. Various and new HPV types were eventually isolated from genital warts. The most direct evidence then came when HPV DNA was isolated from human tumors; zur Hausen (2009) provides a more complete description of this history.

Classical Vaccines Against Infectious Agents that Cause Cancer (Prophylactic Vaccines)

The HPV virus is an infectious agent, and vaccinology against infectious agents was already well-established by the time the link between HPV and cancers was confirmed. Thus, the idea that cancer could be prevented with vaccines that help us defeat viruses that cause cancer was a natural extension of ongoing vaccine research. Translational success was found in Gardasil in 2006 (Merck) and GSK's Cervarix HPV vaccines in terms of bringing the vaccine to market. In countries achieving 50% vaccination, HPV infection rates decreased by 68% in girls aged 13–19 (Drolet *et al.*, 2015). Major decreases in strain-specific infection rates have been seen in the US since the introduction of HPV vaccination programs (Hariri *et al.*, 2015). Herd effects are seen in countries that achieve high enough immunization rates; to date, no such herd effect benefit has been reported in the US.

Adherence rates to the full-dose regimen, however, has been low in the US. Still, the vaccines may be regarded to be the world's first successful cancer vaccine. The HPV vaccines protect against cervical cancer by preventing infection by human papilloma virus spread by sexual contact with an infected person. This overall approach can be considered "xenoergenic" vaccine development because they prime the immune system to respond to foreign proteins.

Therapeutic, Autologous Vaccines

The ideas of developing inoculations to protect against endogenous cancers had what now seems to be a dangerous start. Dr. James Nooth was Surgeon to the Duke of Kent in the 1770s. Due to fears that cancer might be contagious, in 1777, he repeatedly implanted cancer tissue taken from his patients and implanted it under his own skin. The cancer cells, luckily for Dr. Nooth, did not grow. He experienced "pulsation" and inflammation, scabbing and by day four, the symptoms subsided. Similarly, Dr. Jean Louis Ailbert, physician to King Louis XVIII, subsequently injected himself with breast cancer tissue in 1808. While neither men developed cancer, reports are that they experienced inflammation and minor pain (Murphy, 2004). The next example came in 1901 when Dr. Nicholas Senn, at Rush Medical College in Chicago, inserted tissue from a lip carcinoma into his arm. His observations included that the tumor tissue was subsequently absorbed, and disappeared within four weeks.

These early self-experimentations in science, where doctors used themselves as subjects, continued into the 1970s. No one knew whether cancer could be transmitted. Addition details on such studies are available in *Who Goes First? The Story of Self-Experimentation in Medicine* (Altman, 1998). Each experiment led each of the men to conclude that cancer was not contagious. A moment's reflection on HPV, Epstein–Barr and hepatitis virus-induced cancers makes it seem likely that there was genuine cause for concern for transmissible risk. Moreover, the observations that the cancer cells did not grow might have suggested, at least to Dr. Senn and colleagues, that the human body is capable of removing cancer cells via an immune response. This is in part due to the generation of unusual proteins. The immune system does not merely provide surveillance against foreign invaders; it also can protect against enemies from within by removing unusual, potentially harmful proteins that might be produced after mutations change the code for specific proteins. Cancers undergo large numbers of mutations, and any unusual, aberrant proteins they express are called tumor-specific antigens.

Indeed, in the 1970s, the field of immunotherapy was fast developing. Many noted that tumors were observed expressing unusual forms of proteins, or proteins not usually expressed by the tissue from which the cancer evolved. The best review of the early development of an autologous cancer vaccine paradigm time is provided by Kelly and Cole (1998); the best review available of the development of the field of cancer immunotherapy is Miller *et al.*, (2013). What follows is a brief synopsis that does not do the last 30 years of extensive research and knowledge gained justice.

Modern Immunotherapies

The field of immunotherapy has advanced to the point where treatment involves immunomodulation — turning on key protein production in specific cells, and turning them off. Experts speak of "suppressing immune check point inhibitors," i.e., "pulling out the brakes" of the immune response. Overall their understanding appears extremely fine-tuned.

The mammalian immune system is very complex. Thus, the number of approaches to immunotherapy grows as researchers find new ways to educate, augment, and activate the immune system. The majority of the successful effort in cancer immunotherapy has been to develop drugs that help elicit or amplify an immune response. Since 1997, over 20 drugs have been developed, beginning with Rituximab, a monoclonal antibody developed for the treatment of leukemias and lymphomas. Unlike vaccines that protect against infectious agents, the focus of these treatments is not the prevention of first-time cancers; it is usually for the prevention of recurrence, or for use as a treatment to allow the body to rid itself of cancer cells.

Early treatments designed to provoke an immune response such as IL-2 and interferon, although showing lasting responses, are associated with poor side effect profiles. Research to identify compounds that could target mutations in the mitogen-activated protein kinase (MAPK) pathway (including BRAF and MEK inhibitors) showed improved survival and better side effect profiles compared to traditional chemotherapy.

Checkpoint Inhibitors

At the same time, research on the importance of escape of immune surveillance and the importance of immune activation leading to regression of melanoma highlighted the role of immune checkpoint inhibitors. Ipilimumab is a monoclonal antibody that binds the negative regulatory checkpoint molecule cytotoxic T-lymphocyte protein 4 (CTLA-4), and was the first drug to confer a survival benefit in patients with malignant melanoma. In 2011, the FDA approved ipilimumab (Yervoy™, Bristol-Myers Squibb) as a therapy for unresectable or metastatic melanoma that has shown a significant improvement in overall survival (10 months with Yervoy vs. 6.4 months with control; Hodi *et al.*, 2010). It works by "releasing the brakes" of the immune system by preventing the downregulation of T-cell activation. This is accomplished by blocking CTLA-4. Unfortunately, treatment with Yervoy is complicated by grade 3 and 4 immune-related adverse events and, in most patients, unsustained response (~15% durable response). Serious side effects, including deaths due to perforations in the gastrointestinal tract, are possible. Close monitoring of side effects for up to 10 weeks is recommended so additional treatments to alleviate the side effects can be quickly rendered.

Cellular Therapy

A second type of immunotherapy is cellular therapy, in which the cells of the immune system are isolated from a patient, enriched or augmented in culture, and then returned to the patient's body to bolster the immune fight against the tumor. Provenge™ (Sipuleucel-T), which is the first autologous vaccine approved in the US to prevent recurrences of metastatic hormone-refractory prostate cancer, is an example of cellular immunotherapy. Antigen presenting cells expressing the protein CD54 are isolated from the patient. A gene is added that partly encodes an antigen for a prostate-specific protein (PAP), thus informing the immune system of which cells to target. Patients treated with Sipuleucel-T can expect, on average, about four months additional survival.

Other cellular therapy approaches involve the activation of T cells via antigen-presenting dendritic cells with compounds such as Toll-like receptor agonists. There is a wide diversity of methods for administering this therapy, and efficacy varies with the route of administration varies (Fong *et al.*, 2001). A group working at Stanford University under the direction of Dr. Edgar Engleman found a way to induce the activation of dendritic cells *in vivo* in mice. They administered a DC growth factor called "FMS-like tyrosine kinase 3 Ligand" (Flt3L) to mice with B16 melanoma tumors. They then injected oligodeoxynucleotides containing unmethylated CG motifs (CpG) together with a defined tumor antigen. They saw significant anti-tumor responses in the mice due to accumulation of large numbers of mobilized dendritic cells. The Flt3L treatment made the dendritic cells accessible, and a local injection of a mixture of tumor antigen and CpG facilitated their loading, informing the T-cells of the appropriate target. More recently, the same group found a combination of the proteins TNF-alpha and the CD40 binding protein that kick starts the dendritic cells (Cardi *et al.*, 2015) in numerous tumors, including melanoma, with tumors loaded with T-cells hours after the treatment.

Cytokine Immunotherapy

A third broad category is Cytokine Immunotherapy, where the treatment is a general stimulatory one, focused on the induction of stimulatory cytokines (such as IFN-alpha, TNF-alpha and IL-12) and man-made cytokines, such as interferon-α and interleukin-2 (IL-2).

Direct Antibody Immunization

The last category can be called direct antibody immunization, and is similar to classical vaccinations. Nivolumab, a fully human monoclonal antibody against a protein named "programmed cell death protein 1" (PD-1), was found to provide survival benefit in a Phase II trial. Its striking efficacy caused it to be widely accepted, including in tumor types not considered responsive to immunotherapy (e.g. non-small cell lung cancer).

Oncolytic and Non-Cancer Vaccines

Defining the most logical clinical trials is important; rather than, say baseline of care vs. vaccine, it would seem natural to test therapeutic vaccines an augmented form of therapy. In fact, trials now involve the use of pox viruses and tetanus virus both as "primers" of the immune system and as vehicles for the delivery of cancer-specific antigens (e.g., the Poxvirus-based vector ProstVac™). T-VEC, an Herpes simplex virus-based oncolytic treatment, is now approved in melanoma.

Immunomodulation in the 1890s

Many of these approaches are attempting to replicate results from a technique developed way back in the 1890s. Early in cancer immunology, it was observed that kick-starting the immune system overall in ways not related to specific cancers might help the body develop a stronger immune response to the cancer vaccine components.

In 1891, a bone sarcoma surgeon named William B. Coley had the idea that the immune system might be tricked into attacking cancer cells if it were somehow activated. Moving on this idea, he began injecting streptococcal microbes into patients with incurable cancer. His goal was to induce fever in his patients, which was unheard of in his time. The prevailing medical view at the time was that fever was bad for patients. His positive results with live bacteria, and then with their toxins, were very encouraging, and he ended up treating over 1,200 cancer patients (especially bone and soft tissue sarcomas, and lymphomas) with a heat-killed strain of streptococcus. The overall category of treatments became known as "Coley's toxins," and they became a standard option for the treatment of many types of cancer until the 1930s. Coley's contemporary, Dr. James Stephen Ewing, became his supervisor at Memorial Hospital in New York City. Ewing (for whom Ewing's sarcoma is named) did not approve of his treatment. Ewing had ties to a mining company that mined radium (Phelps Dodge) and advocated the new field of radiation treatments. Phelps Dodge offered Memorial about half the world's supply of radium on the condition that they put Ewing in the director's seat at Memorial Hospital. As he promoted radiation therapy over Coley's treatment, Ewing did all he could to shut down Coley's treatments; he criticized them as having potential unpredictable, negative effects on people already weakened with cancer — in spite of the relative past successes, and in spite of similar inconsistencies in the performance of radiation therapy at the time.

Coley was something of an easy target — he held the belief that cancer was caused by infectious agents longer than his peers, and he did vary in his treatment of patients over time. His treatment required the attentive care of a physician over many treatments — and he would modulate the dose in response to each personal's individualized response. This was necessary, as patients showed high variability in the fever response. Coley had found success in sarcomas of the bone and soft tissue, and lymphomas, but little success with other cancers. Some doctors simply refused to believe his results, and when medicine became more standardized, due in part to the outspoken criticisms from his supervisor, Coley's toxins were left out of accepted treatment options, for a time being made illegal to use. Most at the time saw options like fever induction and radiation as competing, and not complementary, options for care. The American Medical Association published a letter concluding that Coley's toxins were not effective in the treatment of cancer, and it was dropped as an approved treatment. It was later re-instated into available practice options as a New Drug, however, radiation and chemotherapy options became the norm, and Coley's toxins were all but abandoned.

Given the reported success rates, the dismissal of Coley's treatments was clearly not deserved. Prior to developing his treatment, Coley had carefully tracked down some 47 anecdotes in the literature supporting the idea that infections and fever might help cancers. He had lost his first patient, a 17-year old girl, to a particularly rapid and aggressive sarcoma. He combed the cases in the hospital for possible curative treatments. He learned of a patient who had complete regression of an inoperable malignancy in his neck after developing an acute skin rash (erysipelas), and he personally tracked the patient down to confirm he was still disease-free. He had also learned of past regression of malignancies associated with erysipelas by a German doctor named Busch. The skin rash had been determined to be caused by streptococcus in 1881. Busch, now enlightened by this advance in basic science, reported tumor shrinkage after injection of patient with malignancy with streptococcus in 1888. Both Coley's son and daughter worked on their treatment value as part of their own research. His daughter, Helen Coley Nauts, worked especially hard to set the record straight; in a review of his meticulous records and letters, she counted 896 patients treated and about 500 cured (>5 year survival). This was as effective or better than any of the contemporaneous treatments for these types of cancers during Dr. Coley's practice, and much, much better than rates for many other kinds of cancer. Helen founded The Cancer Research Institute, became its executive director, and Coley's legacy lives on in the research conducted at that Institute.

Coley's curative rates ranged from 20% to 50%, depending on the type of treatment and the type of cancer (sarcoma vs lymphoma). Why Coley's toxins have not been further studied for use as first line or adjuvant therapy is said to be due to a number of reasons. Coley's toxins are available for use in the US, but only through a lengthy application process to the FDA. It is still listed as a "new drug." Numerous clinical trials have demonstrated efficacy (Kienle, 2012). Descriptions of cost of preparation have it at around $75 per injection. However, Good Laboratory Practices make the production of the toxins expensive, and the actual treatment procedure used by Coley (repeated injections of increasing doses to induce and maintain a fever over weeks) is frowned upon by the IRB (Institutional Review Boards) responsible for ethical conduct of research. In all likelihood, however, the issue is indeed one of recouping costs — exactly how Coley's concoction could be patented and made profitable for viable large-scale and long-term production is unclear. Recombinant Listeria for use in HPV-induced cervical cancer (Cory and Chu, 2014) has excellent results and is now in Phase III trials (Advaxis, Inc. and Aduro Biotech, Inc).

It is now known that dendritic cells are released with high body temperature (Knippertz *et al.*, 2011). This may be one of the factors that made Coley's treatment effective. His original goal was to induce fever. Temperature increase-related activation of dendritic cells may also be why hyperthermia treatments have been shown to help with many different treatment approaches, including directly after radiation, with immunotherapy, and with chemotherapy (Wust *et al.*, 2002; van der Zee, 2002).

Oncologists and patients should find van der Zee's summary rather compelling:

The use of hyperthermia alone has resulted in complete overall response rates of 13%. The clinical value of hyperthermia in addition to other treatment modalities has been shown in randomised trials. Sig-nificant improvement in clinical outcome has been demonstrated for tumours of the head and neck, breast, brain, bladder, cervix, rectum, lung, oesophagus, vulva and vagina, and also for melanoma. Additional hyperthermia resulted in remarkably higher (complete) response rates, accompanied by improved local tumour control rates, better palliative effects and/or better overall survival rates

There is even a Society for Thermal Medicine, with their own journal: the *International Journal of Hyperthermia*. A large number of studies have been conducted on the efficacy of various modalities of hyperthermia (local vs. whole body). Research on hyperthermia indeed continues to show efficacy in many cancer types (e.g., Feyerabend *et al.*, 2001), and the mechanisms for the effects on dendritic cell stimulation are being elucidated (Srivastava, 2001; Knippertz *et al.*, 2011; Matsu-moto *et al.*, 2011). Whole body delivery systems include ultrasound, microwave radiation, thermal baths, and pre-heated chemotherapy. Local methods include heat lamps, ultrasound, direct contact heating elements, and others. There has even been a study in breast cancer to attempt to identify genomic mechanisms of hyperthermia resistance in breast cancer (Amaya *et al.*, 2014). They found that heat disrupts mitotic regulators and G2/M phase progression in breast cancers.

Fever-induced release of dendritic cells and additional effects on Coley's concoctions may also well be reflected in the more specific approaches now being studied. An approach similar to Coley's is still used today in the normative treatment of superficial bladder cancer with live *Mycobacterium bovis* bacillus Calmette-Guerin (BCG). It is also some-times injected directly into Stage III melanoma. In fact, of all of the vaccine treatments to date, BCG-based vaccines are the only one in routine clinical use. A number of recombinant strains exist; of these, the most promising appear to be made to express Th1 cytokines (e.g., Luo *et al.*, 2011).

A more comprehensive review of this interesting history is provided by McCarthy (2006). MbVax, a company in Hamilton, Ontario (Canada) prepares "Coley's Fluid" preparations for compassionate use in countries that allow this route and has published directions for its preparation. Many in immunological approaches to cancer treatments look to Coley for inspiration. Researchers have studied viruses and bacteria as vectors to simultaneously introduce tumor-associated antigen into the bloodstream and activate an immune response (Shahabi *et al.*, 2010).

A Need for Rational, Collaborative Vaccine Design

Studies of karyotypes (pictures of chromosomes) had long revealed that in most chronic myelogenous leukemia (CML) patients, a chromosomal abnormality led to a fusion of chromosomes 9 and 22. This chromosomal event also involves the fusion of two genes. *bcr and abl.* As a result, most CML patients also have an unusual protein, made from pieces of the two unrelated proteins. Researchers at a company called Ciba-Geigy sought a compound that had an inhibitory effect on the *bcr-abl* protein, which had showed increase tyrosine kinase activity and was considered an "oncogene." The researchers search for compounds that would show activity against the aberrant protein involved luck and skill. First, their screen resulted in the finding of good inhibition of *bcr-abl* by 2-phenylaminopyrimidine. They then added 2-phenylaminopyrimidine to the compound to increase the binding efficiency. The modified product was called Imatinib.

The commercialized fruit of those labors was Gleevec, which directly targets an aberrant protein. Historically, CML was known to be associated with a Philadelphia chromosome (Druker *et al.*, 2000). Gleevec targets the *bcr-abl* chimeric protein, the product of the transcription of the fusion of the *abl1* gene (normally located on chromosome 9) to a location in the *bcr* ("breakpoint cluster region") gene (normally located on chromosome 22). The fusion of the two chromosomes does not always involve the same regions, and other diseases can result. However, >95% of CML patients have the *bcr-abl* translocation. CML patients now enjoy close to normal lifespans (Gambacorti-Passerini *et al.*, 2011).

In a stand against costs, in 2013, a large group of physicians published a white paper noting that the cost of Gleevec was prohibitive, even to US consumers. With 119 cancer specialists as co-authors, the white paper (Experts in Chronic Myeloid Leukemia, 2013) found that the cost was so high as to be "immoral," and that no company should raise prices for sheer profit. They said that Novartis has recouped their investment costs at $30,000 (which was based on the cost of the then state-of-the-art treatments for CML) in two years. Yin *et al.* (2012), funded by Bristol-Myers Squibb, conducted an economic analysis and claimed that the economic value of the quality of life years afforded to the patients (nearly always >17.5 years, vs. <9 months survival) vastly outweighed the cost of the drug. Their estimated value to society was $143 billion, compared to the cost of $14.2 billion. Then, in an added twist, the Indian Supreme court rejected Novartis' two bids to stop the production of a generic form of the drug. Generic Gleevec (Imatinib) is now available at cost of a few dollars a pill.

Gleevec was shown in 2002 to be effective against gastrointestinal tumors (Demetri *et al.*, 2002). Follow-up studies have also been successful, and its use has revolutionized the approach to treating gastrointestinal tumors. To date, a minimum of 3.6 million people are expected to have their lives due to the use of Gleevec or its generic form to treat, and cure, what used to be an incurable disease.

When people make the claim "Doctors don't want cures, they want treatments," a common claim I hear from "laypeople" not involved in biomedical research, I politely caution them from making generalizations and point to the 119 doctors who made the case that human lives are priceless, but pricing drugs so high that society cannot realize the benefits must be avoided. I also point to the egregious cases of unethical behavior on the part of some clinicians. In some ways, we have it right. In other areas, such as ADHD overdiagnosis, we have a long way to go. The development of Gleevec is universally hailed as a success in rational drug design: thinking one, or two steps ahead, and engineering the next phase of the compound for treatment.

The wide diversity of approaches ongoing for cancer vaccines could be a net benefit to society if a rational approach to vaccine development is undertaken. The history of vaccines against infectious diseases has shown that, due to evolution, the use of a monovalent vaccine nearly always gives way, via translational research, to multivalent vaccines (e.g., influenza vaccines, Gardisil-9, etc.). A forward-thinking approach by the NCI would be to gather cancer vaccinologists by cancer type and promote the funding of, and development of, multivalent vaccines and multipronged approaches to immunotherapeutic treatments for each cancer type right from the start. These ideas already exist in the form of questions on the combined use and order of use of immunomodulators in melanoma (Sullivan and Flaherty, 2015). Pembrolizumab works on the immune response via a different pathway than ipilimumab, although both are immune checkpoint inhibitors. Others inspired by Coley's approach are studying the utility of using attenuated bacteria in combination with chemotherapies (Grille *et al.*, 2014), and some have called for clinical trials of the procedure itself (Maletzki *et al.*, 2012).

The degree to which personalization of the vaccine might be possible, or required, should be considered an added-value variable — and to a measure of degree — not either/or. Vaccine development is also consistent with a future of personalized medicine. Vaccines could potentially be tailored to target specific arrays of proteins or peptides for each patient, based on what is known of the cancer(s) that tends to occur in their families, depending on the molecular subtypes and the proteins that are known to be expressed.

Proponents of capitalism often cite the honing effects of competition as a justification of the paradigm. They believe that competition has the effect of improving a product or a service and, in many instances, that may be true. However, there is often an unmeasured "decay" effect of competition. In an arena where few of the players can survive, the "losers," when lost, may be lost forever. Cancer vaccines that are abandoned may hold the promise of being a component in a much more effective vaccine than any one of the players on the field. Two vaccine programs have already been abandoned: CancerVax (Canvaxin) and the MyVax program (of the Genitope Corporation). Physicians could already be losing important tools in their vaccinology toolbox due to the erosive cost of competition. This could delay or prevent the development of vaccines for some types of cancer, and thus, competition should be avoided, and national and international collaborations should be encouraged and funded.

For those who might feel this position is not realistic, or naïve, I'd like to point to the international effort to fight Ebola. As late as it was, it is a testimony to our humanity. Deaths due to Ebola virus disease are horrific, in part because the illness progresses so fast, death comes as a surprise. Deaths come so fast that they often occurred in public — at the height of the epidemic, people were dying several feet away from the door of a clinic. Bodies were piling up in remote hospitals whose staff had been decimated by the virus. Doctors from nearly every country in the world came to work in Sierra Leone, Guinea, and in Liberia, to help squelch the threat of a global pandemic. Clearly a vaccine is needed for emerging diseases like Ebola that have high mortality and high rates of spread. Death and suffering due to cancer is no less horrific, it's just often more private, and by the time the patient is terminal, death is rarely, if ever, a surprise. Cancer is still, however, a public health issue, as well as a private battle.

Witnessing my own family members suffer the pain of end-stage cancer first hand, and seeing its effects on family structure, has made the issue of cancer especially real for me. I challenge my clinical and business colleagues to set up an IP Share Market for cancer vaccine components. I believe the public will invest massively in the search for cancer vaccines. This third arm of funding would also prevent those with financial conflicts of interest (vested in the *status quo* of non-vaccinology oncology) from accusations that they do not want to prevent cancer because their livelihood depends on it.

Melanoma Vaccine Development as a Promising Example

The reported long-term survival of Coley's toxins dramatically outpaces those gained by other headline-winning immunomodulators

(Provenge™, 4 months; ipilimumab, 3.6 months). A side-by-side clinical trial comparison of, say, ipilimumab, to Coley's toxins might sound
reasonable, but it should be realized that some of the treatment options
one might like to compare are descendants (in some cases indirectly)
of Coley's toxins. That said, the area in which I would expect Coley's to
be effective would be Melanoma (skin cancer originating from mela-
nocytes, the cells that produce melanonin, a pigment which, ironically,
protects against skin cancer). The study of immunological strategies
in melanoma is a crash-course in modern collaborative science, and in
immunology itself.

In modern immunology, the field is focused various components
of immunomodulation (making some change in the immune system).
Some parts of the immune system might have to be kept in check
(inhibited) and others stimulated (immunostimulation). Immunologists
learned that the immune system has specific "checkpoints," parts of the
system that work, for example, to prevent positive feedback loops on
processes that might get carried away and damage tissues in the body.

They therefore focused on releasing the brakes, with treatments
called "checkpoint inhibitors." Shut down a checkpoint, and the immune
system can become more activated, or stimulated.

Underneath those complex signaling controls are the active attacking agents of the immune system. Most people will be familiar with
white blood cells (macrophages); these are by activated T-cells to attack
foreign or unusual antigens, and thus identify and attack signs of danger
in the body (foreign and endogenous). Without information from the
T-cells, the macrophages do not detect abnormal cells. There are also
B-cells, dendritic cells, eosinophils, and a host of other smaller cousins
of white blood cells. These white blood cells respond to areas of damage
and danger and release toxins (e.g., peroxide) and host of their own signaling molecules, i.e., interleukins and cytokines, including TNF alpha
(tumor necrosis factor alpha). Some of the effects of TNF alpha are to
induce fever, cause cell death (apoptosis), and local inflammation. It is
also known to inhibit tumorigenesis and viral replication.

The interplay among all of these variables is complex; nudge the right variables, the patient survives melanoma. Nudge the wrong variables, the patient can undergo severe, life-threatening conditions, such systemic inflammation and autoimmune disease of the gastrointestinal tract.

The history of modern immunological approaches to melanoma begins with the original idea to identify tumor antigens (aberrant proteins expressed by tumor cells) and somehow coax or, more appropriately, teach the immune system to specifically attack the malignant cells, leaving healthy cells throughout the body intact. Melanoma vaccines are experimental, and thus to be ethical and considerate of the treatment needs of patients, clinical studies are usually conducted in the context of current clinical care. Thus, questions such as "Does this method of stimulating the immune response outperform standard care?" are not usually asked. Instead, studies focus on the effect of, say, a vaccine in addition to the standard care. This is called "the adjuvant setting," and is, in many ways, "unfair" to the late-comer treatment. It can be more difficult to isolate the primary effect of immune stimulation and, for example, determine whether a second treatment has added to the survival of patients or, say, to tumor shrinkage, caused by a vaccine compared to a chemotherapeutic agent when the chemo treatment has already had an effect. It may be that chemo may be more effective after the immune system has ravaged a tumor. Treatment order sensitivity is a variable of continuing interest in oncology.

To date, the advances in immunology have been mostly considered adjuvant to a primary treatment. ipilimumab (Yervoy) is a human monoclonal antibody to CTLA-4 that has shown long-term survival in Phase III clinical trials (Hodi *et al.*, 2010; Robert *et al.*, 2011). Patients who experienced a complete response (14/15) were found to be disease-free at 54–99 months after treatment (Prieto *et al.*, 2012).

Coley Revisited

Some might challenge the cancer immunological communities to acquire renewed interest in the further study of the mechanisms of

Coley's toxins and other so-called "unproven" non-specific immuno-stimulatory treatments. It takes a historical perspective to see that the assumptions behind this inference are partially correct. Two studies in melanoma come to mind; these are usually downplayed because they use historical data as a comparator, and not a concurrent randomized control group. I reproduce the abstract here to demonstrate the non-trivial, advanced thinking in the mid 1970s:

MacGregor AB, Falk RE, Landi S, Ambus U, Samuel ES, Langer B. (1977) Adjuvant immunostimulation in malignant melanoma with oral Bacille Calmette-Guérin. *Can J Surg* 20(1): 25–30.

Results of the administration of oral bacille Calmette-Guérin (BCG) as an adjunct to standard treatment in 62 patients with malignant melanoma indicate that this drug is of value in preventing distant spread of the disease when it is limited to one region and in its early stages. BCG increases survival in patients with visceral metastases. In those in whom these metastases are surgically resectable, it inhibits the development of further metastases. Oral BCG treatment does not affect the course of the disease in patients with massive hepatic or intracranial metastases.

Gutterman JU, Mavligit G, Gottlieb JA, Burgess MA, McBride CE, Einhorn L, Freireich EJ, Hersh EM. (1974) Chemoimmunotherapy of disseminated malignant melanoma with dimethyl triazeno imidazole carboxamide and Bacillus Calmette-Guérin. *N Engl J Med* 291(12): 592–7.

Eighty-nine patients with disseminated malignant melanoma were treated with combination of dimethyl trizeno imidazole caboximide (DTIC) administered intravenously and Bacillus Calmette-Guérin (BCG) administered by scarification. The results were compared to those in a comparable retrospective group of 111 patients treated with DTIC alone. Metastatic areas regional to BCG immunization showed an augmented response to chemotherapy. Thus, chemoimmunotherapy-treated patients with lymph-node metastasis had a remission rate of 55 percent compared to one of 18 percent for patients treated with

chemotherapy alone (p = 0.0025). The duration of remissions and sur-
vival was significantly longer for patients (both nonvisceral and vis-
ceral metastases) treated with chemoimmunotherapy than for those
treated with chemotherapy alone (p = 0.05, 0.001, respectively). A good
prognosis was associated with immunocompetence before treatment or
an increase in immunocompetence during treatment. Chemoimmuno-
therapy was well tolerated without serious morbidity. Further trials
of chemoimmunotherapy are indicated in patients with disseminated
malignant melanoma as well as disseminated solid tumors.

In the first study, the response is readily seen as important. In the second study, the responses are extremely impressive, and besides the use of a historical (recent, I'm sure) non-concurrent control group, the BCG treatment was impressive. A small prospective randomized trial published the next year reported higher remission rates in patients treated with BCG and chemo than with chemo alone (Ramseur *et al.*, 1978). While the sample sizes were small, the issue of statistical power is non-sequitur once a significant result has been found.

In fact, there have been many small relatively modern studies that repeatedly find positive responses with Coley's toxins. The prevailing paradigm for clinical translation requires large, multi-center prospective studies. Accumulating evidence across multiple studies is called "meta-analysis." Many repeated confirming instances, at some point in a clinical treatment, is considered sufficient impetus to move to large-scale trials.

Multiple such studies have been conducted demonstrating the clinical efficacy of BCG in superficial bladder cancer (e.g., Pan *et al.*, 2014; Houghton *et al.*, 2013), including evidence of its use in preventing of recurrence. The most significant and more recent study of BCG was the Morton *et al.* (2007) study of the use of BCG in melanoma after resection of up to five regional or distant sites, and its use in combination with a vaccine. Due to the lack of additional benefit of the vaccine in the BCG+ vaccine study group, the study was halted and all patients moved to the BCG alone study group. This is impressive, as it meant that resection plus attenuated BCG was sufficiently good as far as the positive outcomes achievable at the time. For the study overall, 42.3% of stage IV and 63.4% of stage III patients were expected to survive to five years. In 2001, Stewart and Levine called for further study of BCG alone after resection.

Other studies of BCG in melanoma continue to show efficacy (e.g., 56% regression when used in combination with imiquimod, with no patient deaths due to melanoma; Kidner, 2012).

Current research on BCG as a first-order treatment for melanoma is rare; only eight clinical trials listed at NCI.gov list BCG as a component of treatment for melanoma. At the time of this writing (June 2015), the Ludwig Institute for Cancer Research is still recruiting patients with advanced metastatic melanoma for a Phase I study of intralesional BCG followed by ipilimumab therapy (NCI trial NCT01838200).

To a degree, almost all modern immunological approaches in cancer can be seen as derivative of Coley's initial studies, especially the approaches that try to induce the immune response overall (cytokine approach). They can be thought of, as least in part, as more refined and granular approaches to achieve the successes reported with Coley's toxins. If the effect of fever is to induce dendritic cells, there may be safer medical means to induce fever. Perhaps the use of non-cancer vaccines as adjuvants may be sufficient. Why not utilize the benefit of the original approach? It is not enough to palliate that modern immunomodulator research is the descendent, in many ways, of Coley's research. What if the mechanisms of stimulation are distinct? For example, there may be cytotoxic effects of his treatment as well (Lundin and Checkoway, 2009). According to one study, the active molecule in Coley's toxin is interleukin-12 (IL-12), rather than tumor necrosis factor (TNF) or endotoxin (LPS). Others (Kienle, 2012), considering the breadth of published evidence, have concluded that Coley's toxins activate a variety of immunological responses simultaneously, i.e., a "cytokine storm," and that current immunological focus on activating individual components of the immune system may be relatively ineffective because they induce only a partial response. Whatever the mechanism(s) behind the efficacy of Coley's treatment, modern researchers may be missing an important "baseline" of sorts, and some drugs that have been rejected by the FDA may have been approved if they had been shown to be curative when used in combination with Coley's toxins.

The success rates of all of their exploratory treatments may very well be enhanced, or may do not better than his treatment; they may even make drugs that appear marginally promising into blockbusters. Moreover, Coley's successes with the types of cancers he studied is matched by high performance in many, many other types of cancers (see review by Kienle, 2012). Citations of high cost of including the treatment in studies (due to best laboratory practice preparation) should be compared to the cost of excluding the potential added value to the treatment and should include precise calculations of the cost of the latest partial immunomodulator being studied. For the field to move forward rapidly, the competitive model should be replaced by the collaborative, and the lawyers must allow the best lead combinations to drive forward. They should promote easy and rapid licensure across companies.

Radiation was not subjected to the same level of scrutiny that Coley's toxins were — the standard to tie mechanism to efficacy was much higher. Oncologists knew of the effects of radiation on cells, and on chromosomes; however, the intensely detailed efforts to understand the complexities of the immune system now have researchers studying various aspects of the treatment, one at a time. Much more is now known about the mechanisms of non-specific treatments. For example, the effects of fever and elevated temperature on the host response, immune cells, cytokines, antimicrobial defense, antitumor activity, and immune surveillance are better known. Fever activates a heat-shock response, resulting in the expression of heat-shock proteins (HSP). One response to HSP is dendritic cell activation and transformation into mature antigen-presenting cells, leading to immune recognition of antigens. NK-cell and T-cell activation, tumor cell necrosis and apoptosis (programmed cell death), and dendritic cells maturation and migration into lymph nodes are all enhanced by increased temperature (Basu and Srivastava, 2003).

The accumulated reported clinical results for non-specific immunomodulations should be taken seriously, allowing new questions to be asked in more effective ways. It seems that the history of cancer treatments certainly would have been very different if Ewing and others could have recognized the potential combined utility in radiation and Coley's treatments. One might wonder now, for example, if Coley's and radiation were to be used in tandem, for a few weeks' time, and then perhaps followed by chemotherapy, if the number of tumor antigens released by the damage to the cells from the radiation would enhance the immune response. If Coley's results are replicated in large-scale trials as a first-order treatment for many cancer types, chemotherapy could become a second line of defense for many patients. How many patients could see the side effects of chemotherapy, including severe toxicity and death, reduced, or avoided altogether?

Since the 1990s, high-dose interferon (HDI) treatment has predominated treatment of melanoma in the US. An exceptionally good predictor of the efficacy of HDI (time to progression and overall survival) is the presence of an autoimmune response (Gogas *et al.*, 2006; Krauze *et al.*, 2011). Patients who fail to show autoimmunity could be switched to adjuvant non-specific bioimmune induction, moving them into immunological overdrive, and improving the outcome for more patients.

This is the direction that the field is going, says Dr. Lisa Butterfield, from the UPCI Immunologic Monitoring and Cellular Products Laboratory at the University of Pittsburgh Cancer Institute. I spoke with her, and she emphasized how important it is to realize that the ongoing efforts reflect attempts to understand the entirety of the immune system to define rational, targeted treatments: individualized medicine. She was familiar with the folklore aspect of the rumors that doctors want treatments, not cures — she said she has heard similar things from a couple of members of her family. Lisa, and other researchers like her, support and work with oncologists like Dr. Kirkwood. She says that in melanoma, in particular, research has brought about a level of understanding of molecular changes tumors, and has reveal a host of different types of immunological responses occurring in patients. This knowledge then allows more detailed studies of immunological targets that are more likely to lead to increases in overall survival and remission, because different immunological stimuli are needed for different patients.

The results of this added layer of knowledge are complex immunotherapy clinical trials in which the researchers attempt to induce more potent anti-tumor responses.

"When we look at tumors in different patients," she said, "Some tumors are already infiltrated with CD8+ cells, and some are not. We know that the outcome is better for patients with these kinds of immune cells already present in their tumors at the time of diagnosis. In the best cases, it's an inflamed tumor, or what we call an 'active infiltrated tumor.' The immune system is already activated."

"Wow, Lisa, that sounds like important, basic information," I replied. "Do the assays exist for the many different kinds of cells in the immune system?"

"Oh, yes, we have many antibody tests, and H+E stains, which stain with antibodies for CD8+ (killer T-cells), CD3 (T-cells), and CD45RO cells. The CD45RO cells are memory cells, which show that the immune system has reacted to target tumor antigens."

"Are these assays available for every melanoma patient?"

"Not yet," she said. "For patients with inactive, non-infiltrated tumors, we are working to develop vaccines to support cap T on T-cells. This is so important to outcome I think they should include the immune score as a standard part of the pathology report in colorectal cancer. It's too early for that in melanoma, however."

I asked her of additional challenges that might exist, and what barriers exist to making this a more routine part of clinical practice.

Patients should try to get involved in clinical trials, and insurance companies should support this. Recruitment for clinical trials is too low. Also, researchers are losing access to tissues from diagnosed

melanomas: The support for a centralized, shared tissue bank is dwin-
dling. Also, the tumor can change it immunological status. We need to
find out if the usefulness of the immunological assays changes over time.
Does it matter when it is run? Perhaps it should be re-checked later.

She went on to say that there a myriad of vaccines under development aimed at CD8+ activation; there are no treatments yet to specifically activate only CD45R0 cells, but it is downstream. She described
other techniques, such as "adoptive transfer," in which the clinician takes
samples of the patient's blood, enriches and expands CD8+, CD8 and
CD4 helpher or natural killer cells.

It began to seem to me again that they were tweaking different
parts of the same system, and that perhaps the non-specific immune
activation by Coley's really was already potentially more practicable.
So I asked Lisa about the idea of using non-specific immune activators
as the baseline, and other treatments of adjuvant. She described to me
research studies focused on IL-2, which seemed to mostly mimic the
overall effects, and reminded me that the goal is to find out what works
in each patient. I asked her how far off individualized treatments might
be for melanoma.

"In one sense, we are already there, due to mutational screening.
We can predict for certain classes of drugs which one will work, and
which are not likely to work, in specific patient. We also look at each
patient's degree of immune system activation."

She said that some of her colleagues, in particular Mark Davis at
Stanford, are working to define and characterize the normal immune
system, to be able to identify suppressed or deleted autoimmunity.

The trends are summarized well by Topalian *et al.* (2011):

Although clear clinical efficacy has been demonstrated with antitumor
antibodies since the late 1990s, other immunotherapies had not been
shown to be effective until recently, when a spate of successes established
the broad potential of this therapeutic modality. These successes are
based on fundamental scientific advances demonstrating the toleragenic

nature of cancer and the pivotal role of the tumor immune microenvironment in suppressing antitumor immunity. New therapies based on a sophisticated knowledge of immune-suppressive cells, soluble factors, and signaling pathways are designed to break tolerance and reactivate antitumor immunity to induce potent, long-lasting responses. Preclinical models indicate the importance of a complex integrated immune response in eliminating established tumors and validate the exploration of combinatorial treatment regimens, which are anticipated to be far more effective than monotherapies. Unlike conventional cancer therapies, most immunotherapies are active and dynamic, capable of inducing immune memory to propagate a successful rebalancing of the equilibrium between tumor and host.

Breaththough via Combined Treatments

Adverse events from side effects of immunomodulation are not uncommon, especially in treatment with checkpoint inhibitors that unleash a Th1 response. Patients can develop unpredictable, organ-specific autoimmunity, leading, for example, to perforated gastrointestinal tracts, hepatitis, and colitis.

Yervoy (ipilimumab) specifically targets a protein called CTLA4, located on the surface of T-cells. Yervoy appears to activate the immune system's response to tumor antigens. A study in 2011 demonstrated that Yervoy prolonged survival in patients, with 502 patients with Stage III or Stage IV inoperable melanoma (Wolchok *et al.*, 2011). Like the V600E study, the focus was the added effect of Yervoy when used in combination with DTIC for the treatment of advanced melanoma. The result was impressive: Three-year overall survival was 20.8% among patients treated with DTIC plus Yervoy, compared with 12.2% among patients treated with DTIC alone.

One of the most exciting breakthroughs in immunotherapy for melanoma is the combination of Yervoy and a new drug, Opdivo. A Phase I trial of the combination (Postow *et al.*, 2015) had shown the two-year survival rate for all patients receiving both drugs as 79%. The very best

best-responding dose level had a two-year survival rate of 88%. The two-year survival rate of patients receiving conventional chemotherapy for melanoma is about 15%.

A Phase II trial in which tumors "disappeared" in 22% of patients due to the combined use of Yervoy and Opdivo has generated much interest. None of the patients on the single drug arm showed remission. Of the patients receiving the combination therapy (Opdivo+Yervoy), 59% showed marked reduction in tumor size, while only 11% showed response to Yervoy alone. The side effects, however, were fairly common: A full 54% of patients on the combined treatment experienced colitis or diarrhea.

The Phase II trial showed that the combination had a response rate of 61% compared to 11% for Yervoy alone in patients without a BRAF mutation. For patients with a BRAF mutation, the response rate was 52% for the combination compared to 10% for Yervoy alone.

Overall, 53% of patients treated with concurrent Opdivo+Yervoy experienced serious (grade 3 or 4) adverse events, although many were out-of-normal range reports of functions without physiological effects requiring medical intervention (aka asymptomatic laboratory abnormalities). Phase III trial results presented at the American Society of Clinical Oncology (ASCO) on May 28, 2015 showed the results were consistent in a larger cohort of 945 patients. After nine months, the median progression-free survival was 11.5 months for the combination, 6.9 months for Opdivo alone, and 2.9 months for Yervoy alone. Other indicators were consistent with this finding. The response rates for the combination, nivolumab, and ipilimumab groups were 57.6%, 43.7% and 19%, and the average reductions in tumor burden (depth of response) were 52% with the combination and 34% with Opdivo alone. Average tumor burden actually increased in patients receiving Yervoy alone. As in the Phase II trial, the rate of adverse drug-related side effects was the highest in the combination group (55%), a large percentage (36%) of which had to stop the therapy due to side effects. The study authors noted that many patients who discontinued immunotherapy due to adverse events went on to experience prolonged progression-free survival.

The combination of Opdivo and Yervoy is comparable in efficacy to that of Keytruda (pembrolizumab), which was approved by the FDA for the treatment of patients with unresectable or metastatic melanoma and disease progression following Yervoy and, if BRAF V600 mutation positive, a BRAF inhibitor. Keytruda, a monoclonal antibody, binds to the PD-1 receptor and blocks its interaction with PD-L1 and PD-L2, releasing PD-1 pathway-mediated inhibition of the immune response, allowing an anti-tumor immune response. Genentech also has an FDA-granted breakthrough anti-PD1 drug, MPDL3280A.

The Phase III study of the combination of Opdivo+Yervoy also revealed that patients with PD-L1-negative tumors may benefit more from combination treatment than Opdivo alone, whereas patients with PD-L1 positive tumors may do just as well with Opdivo alone. This clearly suggests a trial that combines Keytruda for PD-L1-positive patients followed by the Opdivo+Yervoy treatment compared to Opdivo+Yervoy alone for PDL1-positive patients.

PDL1 and PDL2 attach to PD1 molecules on the surface of tumor, effectively shielding the tumor from the immune system. Studies of Nivolumab (MDX-1106) have demonstrated efficacy in numerous studies, including lung cancer, melanoma, colorectal cancer, renal-cell cancer, ovarian cancer, pancreatic cancer, gastric cancer and breast cancer (Brahmer *et al.*, 2012; Gettinger, *et al.*, 2015; Topalian *et al.*, 2014; McDermott *et al.*, 2015). This drug, which costs around $120,000 per treatment, and any anti-PD1 antibody, comes with its own biomarker: it can be expected to work especially well on tumors expressing PD1. PD1 tumors have shown response. Thus, patients should request the PD1 status of their tumor prior to accepting treatment.

PD1 is an important modulator not only of macrophage activity but also of the innate immune system, and thus it plays an important role in the inflammatory response to sepsis (Huang *et al.*, 2009), most likely via a B-cell mechanism (McKay *et al.*, 2015). These new strategies using anti-PD1 or PD-L1/2 targeting treatments would be a reasonable part of any terminal cancer treatment. Pharmaceutical drug companies should do all that they can do to keep the cost per treatment course to a minimum.

There are two approved PD-1 treatments and numerous others in clinical development. Research on modulating the side effects is needed.

The remission rates being seen with some of these immunomodulation treatments are approaching the reported performance of Coley's toxins. One must also wonder if inducing a fever in these patients might help the combination therapy even further to activate dendritic cells.

Molecular Allocation Trials

Other promising treatments in melanoma show high response rates, in particular in studies that take advantage of the correspondence between a molecular profile of a tumor and the likelihood of it responding to a particular treatment. There is a large consortium of researchers focused on Molecular Allocation: assigning, prospectively, patients to specific treatment arms in a large multi-center clinical trial to assess the utility of the allocating patients to treatment arms based on theranostic biomarkers (biomarkers that indicate specific treatments).

In about half of all melanomas, a gene called BRAF is mutated. BRAF plays a role in cell growth, and mutations in BRAF are common in numerous types of cancer. One specific BRAF mutation often found in melanoma is known as V600E. A trial studying the drug Vemurafenib, which targets V600E, found that overall survival was improved by 63% and progression-free survival by 74% compared to the use of the drug DTIC (dacarbazine; Chapman *et al.*, 2011). The study involved 675 patients with previously untreated Stage IIIC or Stage IV melanomas that could not be removed with surgery. Each patient had the V600E mutation in BRAF. Vemurafenib turns off the pathway, and had previously been found to reduce the size of melanomas. Other examples of mutation-targeting therapies include Tafinlar (dabrafenib) and Mekinist (trametinib).

Neoantigens

Other researchers have recently taken the approach of augmenting immune system activation via vaccines developed with known melanoma tumor antigens with components that are targeted at antigens specifically found in each patient's tumors. Such antigens are called "Neo-antigens," and can be made to target tumor-specific antigens with precision down to individual amino acid differences. In a small, three-patient study (Carreno *et al.*, 2015), information gleaned from exome-sequencing and combining peptide binding *in silico* and *in vitro* peptide recognition analysis revealed various neoantigens in patients that included some non-synonymous substitutions. The immune system is sufficiently precise to detect small differences among normal and altered proteins. Their approach led to a highly accurate list of potential immunogenic tumor peptides for targeting. Because the sequence information comes directly from the patient's tumor, the specificity of the immune response will likely be high.

Their targeting involves re-injection of CD40L+TLR ligand matured, melanoma-peptide pulsed autologous dendritic cells into patients. The result? The much sought-after CD8+ T cell expansion in all three patients. Their success is likely due in part to the use of IL-12p70 producing dendritic cells as a source of cellular vaccine. Each of the three patients in the study had been treated with Yervoy prior to tailored vaccine treatment.

Similarly, Wolchok *et al.* (2015) studied anti-CTLA-4 responders versus non-responders and found a molecular signature of mutations in certain sequences that were similar to sequences found in certain infectious diseases, such as *Streptococcus pyogenes*, yellow fever virus, and tuberculosis. The immune response to tumors may involve a form of convergent selection, whereby specific sequences, if aberrant, activate the immune memory that we will already have in response to common infectious diseases.

Research from members of the same group (Zamarin *et al.*, 2014) found good responses in distant tumors when they combined treatment of melanoma in mice first with melanoma cells, followed by immune activation via the oncolytic Newcastle disease virus (NDV). A local inflammatory response in the injected tumor site also lead to lymphocytic infiltrates, evidenced by the presence of tumor-specific CD4(+) and CD8(+) T cells in tumor present in the mice never injected with the virus. There was no evidence of distant virus spread. Thus, oncolytic viruses seem to be yet another promising method to spark immune responses by bringing forth tumor antigens.

Other studies have also shown improvements in outcomes with combined therapies that do directly target the immune system. For example, Robert *et al.*, (2015) studied the effects of combining dabrafenib (cell growth inhibitor) and trametinib (upstream inhibitor of proliferation, differentiation, and transcription regulation) on patients with BRAF V600 mutations and found improved overall 12-month survival in the combination therapy group. Similarly, Flaherty *et al.* (2012) found that dabrafenib plus trametinib was more effective than dabrafenib alone in terms of progression-free survival. The next natural line of study would be to combine personalized (molecular profile indicated) *combined* approaches of immunotherapy drugs with other approaches that shut down responses to cell growth signals, or target mitotic apparatus.

Financial Means to Foster Cross-Pollination

Projected costs of individual doses of each of these treatments tend to be prohibitively expensive, even as stand-alone prescriptions. Therefore, the approach of combining all available strategies: Yervoy plus Opdivo plus chemotherapy or Keytruda, or perhaps all four, would seem intractable to market due to cost. Such a study would also cross market interests (Yervoy plus Opdivo are products of Bristol-Myers Squibb, while Keytruda is a product of Merck). To accelerate trials that attempt numerous combinations, an appropriate collaborative business model would allow combining intellectual property via funds derived from an IP Share market (Lyons-Weiler, 2009) through which stakeholders could offer their IP specific vaccine components. The economically successful immunological approaches per cancer type would then lead to payments to each of the contributors of the final combined vaccine, and payments to the investors who invest in specific components or combinations. This is the democratization of capitalism. A new era in biomedical research funding is needed that combines the best of capitalism, science, and democratization of decision making so companies move forward in a way that protects the population from the scourge of cancer. Because the upfront costs would be provided specifically for research on individual approaches, the pharmaceutical companies would not have to recoup extensive R&D costs, thus bringing down the cost, making large trials of combination therapies more tractable.

There are many excellent reasons to have confidence that melanoma will soon be treated effectively with a dynamic program tailored for each patient — as long as the funding is there to sustain accurate molecular profiling and to fund combined treatments. As promising as these results are, for now, targeting specific tumors by molecular profile with drugs that are most likely to be effective, and attempting to also induce an immune response will have to suffice, until the fever induced by Coley's toxins (or otherwise) is used as the baseline treatment, and the non-immunological treatments studied as adjuvant.

Caution on Hormone Therapy for Melanoma Patients

A case report of a woman whose melanoma micrometastasis suddenly grew after hormonal therapy (progesterone) indicates that, as in breast cancer, uterine and ovarian cancer, hormonal status of the tumor may be an important variable to consider for targeting therapies (Mordoh *et al.*, 2013).

Additional Biographical and Historical Accounts of Coley's Story

Coley's story is more than a historical footnote. He is considered to be the father of modern cancer immunology. Non-specific immunostimulation may prove to be among the most economical options. Clinical trials are needed that study their effects in combination with numerous other more granular approaches. There are numerous accounts of the history of Coley's toxins. Kienle's account is the most detailed. Reports of the number of patients treated by Coley vary in the modern accounts.

Kienle GS. (2012) Fever in Cancer Treatment: Coley's Therapy and Epidemiologic Observations. *Glob Adv Health Med* **1(1):** 92–100. [doi: 10.7453/gahmj.2012.1.1.016]

Literature Cited

Amaya C, *et al.* (2014) A genomics approach to identify susceptibilities of breast cancer cells to "fever-range" hyperthermia. *BMC Cancer* **14:** 81. [doi: 10.1186/1471-2407-14-81]

Basu S, Srivastava PK. (2003) Fever-like temperature induces maturation of dendritic cells through induction of hsp90. *Int Immunol* **15(9):** 1053–61.

Bolhassani A, Zahedifard F. (2012) Therapeutic live vaccines as a potential anticancer strategy. *Int J Cancer* **131(8):** 1733–43. [doi: 10.1002/ijc.27640]

Brahmer JR, *et al.* (2012) Safety and activity of anti-PD-L1 antibody in patients with advanced cancer. *N Engl J Med* **366(26):** 2455–65. [doi: 10.1056/NEJMoa1200694]

Carmi Y, *et al.* (2015) Allogeneic IgG combined with dendritic cell stimuli induce antitumour T-cell immunity. *Nature* **521(7550):** 99–104. [doi: 10.1038/nature14424]

Carreno BM, *et al.* (2015) Cancer immunotherapy. A dendritic cell vaccine increases the breadth and diversity of melanoma neoantigen-specific T cells. *Science* **348(6236):** 803–808. [doi: 10.1126/science.aaa3828]

Chapman PB, *et al.* (2011) Phase III randomized, open-label, multicenter trial (BRIM3) comparing BRAF inhibitor vemurafenib with dacarbazine (DTIC) in patients with V600E BRAF-mutated melanoma. Paper presented at: 47th Annual Meeting of the American Society of Clinical Oncology; June 3–7, 2011. Chicago, IL. Abstract LBA4.

Cory L, Chu C. (2014) ADXA-HPV: a therapeutic Listeria vaccination targeting cervical cancers expressing the HPV E7 antigen. *Hum Vaccin Immunother* **10(11):** 3190–5.

Demetri GD, *et al.* (2002) Efficacy and safety of imatinib mesylate in advanced gastrointestinal stromal tumors. *N Engl J Med* **347:** 472–80.

Drolet M. (2015) Population-level impact and herd effects following human papillomavirus vaccination programmes: a systematic review and meta-analysis. *Lancet Infect Dis* **15(5):** 565–80. [doi: 10.1016/S1473-3099(14)71073-4]

Druker BJ, Lydon NB. (2000) Lessons learned from the development of an abl tyrosine kinase inhibitor for chronic myelogenous leukemia. *J Clin Invest* **105(1):** 3–7.

Experts in Chronic Myeloid Leukemia (119 authors). (2013) The price of drugs for chronic myeloid leukemia (CML) is a reflection of the unsustainable prices of cancer drugs: from the perspective of a large group of CML experts. *Blood* **121(22):** 4439–42. [doi: 10.1182/blood-2013-03-490003]

Feyerabend T, *et al.* (2001) Local hyperthermia, radiation, and chemotherapy in recurrent breast cancer is feasible and effective except for inflammatory disease. *Int J Radiat Oncol Biol Phys* **49(5):** 1317–25.

Flaherty KT, *et al.* (2012) Combined BRAF and MEK inhibition in melanoma with BRAF V600 mutations. *N Engl J Med* **367(18):** 1694–703. [doi: 10.1056/NEJMoa1210093]

Fong L, *et al.* (2001) Dendritic cells injected via different routes induce immunity in cancer patients. *J Immunol* **166(6):** 4254–59.

Gambacorti-Passerini C, *et al.* (2011) Multicenter independent assessment of outcomes in chronic myeloid leukemia patients treated with Imatinib. *J Natl Cancer Inst* **103(7):** 553–61.

Gettinger SN, *et al.* (2015) Overall survival and long-term safety of Nivolumab (anti-Programmed Death 1 antibody, BMS-936558, ONO-4538) in patients with previously treated advanced non-small-cell lung cancer. *J Clin Oncol* pii: JCO.2014.58.3708.

Gogas H, *et al.* (2006) Prognostic significance of autoimmunity during treatment of melanoma with interferon. *N Engl J Med* **354(7):** 709–18.

Grille S, *et al.* (2014) Salmonella enterica serovar Typhimurium immunotherapy for B-cell lymphoma induces broad anti-tumour immunity with therapeutic effect. *Immunology* **143(3):** 428–37. [doi: 10.1111/imm.12320]

Hariri S, *et al.* (2015) Reduction in HPV 16/18-associated high grade cervical lesions following HPV vaccine introduction in the United States — 2008–2012. *Vaccine* **33(13):** 1608–13. [doi: 10.1016/j.vaccine.2015.01.084]

Hodi FS, *et al.* (2010) Improved survival with ipilimumab in patients with metastatic melanoma. *N Engl J Med* **363:** 711–23.

Houghton BB, *et al.* (2013) Intravesical chemotherapy plus bacille Calmette-Guérin in non-muscle invasive bladder cancer: a systematic review with meta-analysis. *BJU Int* **111(6):** 977–83. [doi: 10.1111/j.1464-410X-.2012.11390.x]

Huang X, *et al.* (2009) PD-1 expression by macrophages plays a pathologic role in altering microbial clearance and the innate inflammatory response to sepsis. *Proc Natl Acad Sci USA* **106(15):** 6303–308. [doi: 10.1073/pnas.0809422106]

Kelly JR, Cole DJ. (1998) Gene therapy strategies utilizing carcinoembryonic antigen as a tumor associated antigen for vaccination against solid malignancies. *Gene Ther Mol Biol* **2:** 14–30.

Kidner TB, *et al.* (2012) Combined intralesional Bacille Calmette-Guérin (BCG) and topical imiquimod for in-transit melanoma. *J Immunother* **35(9):** 716–20. [doi: 10.1097/CJI.0b013e31827457bd]

Kienle GS. (2012) Fever in cancer treatment: Coley's therapy and epidemiologic observations. *Glob Adv Health Med* **1(1):** 92–100. [doi: 10.7453/gahmj.2012.1.1.016]

Knippertz I, *et al.* (2011) Mild hyperthermia enhances human monocyte-derived dendritic cell functions and offers potential for applications in vaccination strategies. *Int J Hyperthermia* **27(6):** 591–603. [doi: 10.3109/02656736.2011.589234]

Krauze MT, *et al.* (2011) Prognostic significance of autoimmunity during treatment of melanoma with interferon. *Semin Immunopathol* **33(4):** 385–91. [doi: 10.1007/s00281-011-0247-y]

Lundin J, Checkoway H. (2009) Endotoxin and cancer. *Environ Health Perspect* **117(9):** 1344–50. [doi: 10.1289/ehp.0800439]

Luo Y, Henning J, O'Donnell MA. (2011) Th1 Cytokine-secreting recombinant *Mycobacterium bovis* bacillus Calmette-Guérin and prospective use in immunotherapy of bladder cancer. *Clinical and Developmental Immunology* Article ID 728930, 1–13.

Lyons-Weiler J. (2009) Time for an IP Share Market? *The Scientist*, Feb 1, 2009. http://www.the-scientist.com/?articles.view/articleNo/27084/title/Time-for-an-IP-Share-Market-/

Maletzki C, *et al.* (2012) Reevaluating the concept of treating experimental tumors with a mixed bacterial vaccine: Coley's Toxin. *Clin Dev Immunol* 2012: 230625. [doi: 10.1155/2012/230625]

Malmström PU, *et al*. (2009) An individual patient data meta-analysis of the long-term outcome of randomised studies comparing intravesical mitomycin C versus bacillus Calmette-Guérin for non-muscle-invasive bladder cancer. *Eur Urol* **56(2)**: 247–56. [doi: 10.1016/j.eururo.2009.04.038]

Matsumoto K, *et al*. (2011) Optimization of hyperthermia and dendritic cell immunotherapy for squamous cell carcinoma. *Oncol Rep* **25(6)**: 1525–32. [doi: 10.3892/or.2011.1232]

McCarthy EF (2006) The toxins of William B. Coley and the treatment of bone and soft-tissue sarcomas. *Iowa Orthop J* **26**: 154–58.

McDermott DF. (2015) Survival, durable response, and long-term safety in patients with previously treated advanced renal cell carcinoma receiving Nivolumab. *J Clin Oncol* pii: JCO.2014.58.1041.

McKay JT, *et al*. (2015) PD-1 suppresses protective immunity to Streptococcus pneumoniae through a B cell-intrinsic mechanism. *J Immunol* **194(5)**: 2289–99. [doi: 10.4049/jimmunol.1401673]

Miller MJ, Foy KC, Kaumaya PTP. (2013) Cancer immunotherapy: present status, future perspective, and a new paradigm of peptide immunotherapeutics. *Discovery Medicine* **5(82)**: 166–76.

Mordoh J, Tapia IJ, Barrio MM. (2013) A word of caution: do not wake sleeping dogs; micrometastases of melanoma suddenly grew after progesterone treatment. *BMC Cancer* **13**: 132. [doi: 10.1186/1471-2407-13-132]

Morton DL, *et al*. (2007) An international, randomized, phase III trial of bacillus Calmette-Guerin (BCG) plus allogeneic melanoma vaccine (MCV) or placebo after complete resection of melanoma metastatic to regional or distant sites. ASCO meeting, Abstract 8508. http://meeting.ascopubs.org/cgi/content/short/25/18_suppl/8508

Murphy T. (2004) Case Studies in Biomedical Research Ethics. Massachusetts Institute of Technology.

Pan J, Liu M, Zhou X. (2014) Can intravesical Bacillus Calmette-Guérin reduce recurrence in patients with non-muscle invasive bladder cancer? An update and cumulative meta-analysis. *Front Med* **8(2)**: 241–49. [doi: 10.1007/s11684-014-0328-0]

Postow MA, *et al*. (2015) Nivolumab and ipilimumab versus ipilimumab in untreated melanoma. *N Engl J Med* **372(21)**: 2006–17. [doi: 10.1056/NEJMoa1414428]

Prieto PA *et al*. 2012. CTLA-4 blockade with ipilimumab: long-term follow-up of 177 patients with metastatic melanoma. *Clin Cancer Res* 2012; **18:** 2039–47. doi: 10.1158/1078-0432.CCR-11-1823.

Ramseur WL, *et al*. (1978) Chemoimmunotherapy for disseminated malignant melanoma: a prospective randomized study. *Cancer Treat Rep* **62(7):** 1085–87.

Robert C, *et al*. (2011) Ipilimumab plus dacarbazine for previously untreated metastatic melanoma. *N Engl J Med* **364:** 2517–26.

Robert C, *et al*. (2015) Improved overall survival in melanoma with combined dabrafenib and trametinib. *N Engl J Med* **372(1):** 30–39. [doi: 10.1056/NEJMoa1412690]

Shahabi V, *et al*. (2010) Live, attenuated strains of Listeria and Salmonella as vaccine vectors in cancer treatment. *Bioeng Bugs* **1(4):** 235–43. [doi: 10.4161/bbug.1.4.11243]

Srivastava P. (2002) Interaction of heat shock proteins with peptides and antigen presenting cells: chaperoning of the innate and adaptive immune responses. *Annu Rev Immunol* **20:** 395–425.

Stewart JH 4th, Levine EA. (2011) Role of bacillus Calmette-Guérin in the treatment of advanced melanoma. *Expert Rev Anticancer Ther* **11(11):** 1671–6. [doi: 10.1586/era.11.163]

Sullivan RJ, Flaherty KT. (2015) Pembrolizumab for treatment of patients with advanced or unresectable melanoma. *Clin Cancer Res* pii: clincanres.3061.2014.

Topalian SL, Weiner GJ, Pardoll DM. (2011) Cancer immunotherapy comes of age. *J Clin Oncol* **29(36):** 4828–36. [doi: 10.1200/JCO.2011.38.0899]

Topalian SL, *et al*. (2014) Survival, durable tumor remission, and long-term safety in patients with advanced melanoma receiving nivolumab. *J Clin Oncol* **32(10):** 1020–30. [doi: 10.1200/JCO.2013.53.0105]

van der Zee J. (2002) Heating the patient: a promising approach? *Ann Oncol* **13(8):** 1173–84.

Weber JS, *et al*. (2013) Patterns of onset and resolution of immune-related adverse events of special interest with ipilimumab. *Cancer* **119(9):** 1675–82.

Wolchok JD, *et al*. (2011) Phase 3 randomized study of ipilimumab (IPI) plus dacarbazine (DTIC) vs. DTIC alone as first line treatment in patients with unresectable Stage III or IV melanoma. Paper presented at: 47th Annual

Meeting of the American Society of Clinical Oncology; June 3–7, 2011. Chicago, IL. Abstract LBA5.

Wust P, *et al*. (2002) Hyperthermia in combined treatment of cancer. *Lancet Oncol* **3(8)**: 487–97.

Yin W, *et al*. (2012) Value of survival gains in chronic myeloid leukemia. *Am J Manag Care* **18(11 Suppl)**: S257–64.

Zamarin D, *et al*. (2014) Localized oncolytic virotherapy overcomes systemic tumor resistance to immune checkpoint blockade immunotherapy. *Sci Transl Med* **6(226)**: 226ra32. [doi: 10.1126/scitranslmed.3008095]

zur Hausen H. (2009) Papillomaviruses in the causation of human cancers — a brief historical account. *Virology* **384**: 260–65.

15 The Future of Translational Research

Having always been a person with an eye firmly planted on the future, with a deep appreciation for the past, this chapter is by far the one I have looked forward to writing the most. Change and reform are both needed on many levels. The people I have interviewed in this book are involved in biomedicine with their priorities in a correct and beautiful order: Reduce human and suffering, and profit will follow as a result of that success. If more people in academic medical research and in corporate medical research were encouraged to put these priorities in the correct order, profit pressure would reduce.

Of course, it would be an understatement to say "Of course, money is important." In my experience, doing things right leads to monetary successes unless that success is interfered with or impeded by those with conflicts of interest. All may be fair in love and war, but all is not fair in science and health care. There are people among us whose selfish actions forestall improvements in health care. They are responsible for the human pain and suffering that ensues, and they should be held responsible when their shamwizardry is revealed. If all involved in biomedical research can learn to recognize and no longer tolerate their shameful actions, we can expect a brighter future.

Funding Science vs. Financing R&D

There is a large difference between funding science and financing R&D. The NIH, and to a lesser extent, the NSF, have begun to act more and more like a financing arm of the government, focused primarily on funding large consortia selected by those with power in the funding agencies on a select few priority studies that may or may not ever provide translational potential needed to learn new and exciting details about human biology and nature. We as a society need to separate, in our minds, the funding of science for the discovery of pure and applied knowledge from the financing of research and development toward marketable goods. We need to see them as equally important, with pure and applied knowledge feeding the biomedical advances. Science for the sake of knowing must return if we are to have clinicians that understand the value of new scientific knowledge.

Commercial science (i.e., R&D) is driven largely by internal prioritization and funding, and for public companies, this means by the quarterly report and Wall Street. This process is driven primarily by investors, and tends to volatile. While that is good for skimmer investors, it is terrible for consistent, long-term research and development. The process is not sufficiently democratic; go/no decisions are based on the next quarter. Long-term investment by the companies need augmentation from a third arm of public funding. The funding could be at various levels: Creative Phase Funding, Phase I, II, III, and Commercialization. The funding could still come from investors, but instead of buying shares of an entire company, investors could purchase shares of specific intellectual property in an IP Share Market. Department budgets would grow with an influx of dedicated funds that must be applied toward the translation of specific IP.

Short-Term Patents and Profit Protection on Novel Applications of Natural Compounds for Medical Benefit

In 2005, I was invited to give a presentation to Pharma at a PharmEd symposium. The theme of my talk was improving how we analyze high-dimensional microarray data using machine learning approaches to quickly evaluate hundreds of competing methods for global gene expression data normalization, transformation, and identification of the correct differentially expressed genes out of the 40,000 or so on a gene chip.

I was very much looking forward to sharing what I had learned with Pharma so they could improve their research for the benefit of all of us. I was also looking forward to the day because my colleague and champion of science Sudhir Srivastava, who was then the Program Director of the Early Detection Research Network at the National Cancer Institute, was scheduled to give the plenary presentation. I was looking forward to congratulating him on the fine job he did in bringing people from across the nation together to work collaboratively on finding new ways to diagnose cancer early. They set up and managed tissue banks, so people studying one type of cancer could have access to a larger number of patients, a critical factor in retrospective studies aimed at identifying molecular biomarkers for cancer.

I arrived in New Jersey the evening before. Sudhir called me at around 8:00 pm. I was excited — perhaps he, too, was in town and we could have dinner. Instead, he told me that he could not make the meeting and wondered if I could do him a favor and give a plenary presentation the next morning (at 8:00 am). I told him how sorry I was that he couldn't make it, but that yes, I had some material on a topic that had been a burning issue for me for some time: My friend, Kunwar Shailubhai's discovery that uroguanylin will likely provide us the ability to prevent colon cancer.

Every day, we shed, as part of normal, healthy functioning, part of our intestinal lining. It is also how we get rid of the old tissue lining our guts. The same is true for mice. There is a mouse used in research that is missing a critical gene. Apc-Min/+ mice develop polyps in the colon, and at in adulthood develop colon cancer. Shailubhai and his colleagues understood the signaling role that a protein, named uroguanylin, played in the regulation of proper programmed cell death in the colon. Uroguanylin is naturally expressed in the healthy gut, and in other tissues in the body. In a landmark study (Kunwar *et al.*, 2000), they fed these mice a normal diet and fed another group of the same kind of mice a diet that contained the protein. Mice fed with uroguanylin developed about half the number of polyps, but these polyps remained small and did not progress to full-blown malignancies. Shailu worked at Monsanto at the time. The company made the decision not pursue colon cancer prevention studies because running prophylactic trials could be long, arduous and extremely expensive. Shailu knew he had a clinically important product. With very mild side effects, the molecule was active at the site where it was needed when included in the diet. Shailu knew that he could reduce pain and suffering in people who were at high risk to get colon cancer. Some people have a high risk, especially those with Lynch syndrome (hereditary non-polyposis colorectal cancer) and those suffering with inflammatory bowel diseases. However, it was determined that uroguanylin peptide might not be a suitable drug candidate for clinical trials due to its inherent instability and cost-prohibitive manufacturing on a large scale. Thus, development of an analog of uroguanylin with superior stability, ease of manufacturing was the only serious option.

Ten years ago, I told this story to the executives, middle managers, and scientist in attendance at PharmEd. In my presentation, I showed a picture of a football stadium which could seat 50,000 people. In the next slide, I showed, one after the other, additional football stadiums until there were 10 on the screen. I reminded them that 50,000 people die in the US from colon cancer every year, and that in 10 years' time, the failure to bring uroguanylin to market — as a pill, a cookie, a milkshake — anything — would cost our society one-half of a million human lives. I told them that they *had to* act on this, that they, and they alone, were in the position to save these lives.

I also told them that if the rules prevented them from reducing pain and suffering, that they had a responsibility to change the rules. I reminded them that their lawyers work for them, not the other way around, and I suggested that they take a trip to Washington, DC, to meet with their Congressional representatives, turn their lawyers into lobbyists, and to ask for patent law reform in the US that would allow short-term monopoly production rights, exclusive rights to grant license, and rights to the profit from the sale of naturally occurring compounds when a company made a discovery as important as uroguanylin. I thanked them for their time.

The room burst into applause. It was not a mere polite applause; the attendees let me know I had struck a chord with deep reverb in their struggles in their own professional lives. I felt that perhaps my message would change things for colon cancer patients.

One by one, after the plenary session, men in suits and ties came to me. Vice Presidents of Research and other executives congratulated me. We stood in a semi-circle.

These were professionals. They knew the position I was coming from: I had told them about my mother's death from breast cancer, and I'm sure they saw me as a naïve idealist. I was satisfied. I had squared my conscience with them; by chance, I had had the opportunity to take the message to the very people I thought could make the largest difference. They all patted me on the back and shook my hand. They really wanted to take me up on the challenge. Some of them hung around to tell me that they, too, had IP that could change the world, but for the same, or very similar reasons, they could not bring it forward.

In the meantime, Shailu left Monsanto and with the help of three of his colleagues and friends founded a new pharmaceutical company, Synergy Pharmaceuticals (NASDAQ:SGYP). Shailu's immediate goal was to discover superior analogs of uroguanylin that are suitable for drug development, and he succeeded in identifying two superior analogs, namely plecanatide and SP-333. Both of these compounds are structurally close to uroguanylin and possess superior stability. Importantly, both analogs mimic biological functions of uroguanylin and are suitable for drug development. Ten years and 500,000 colon cancer deaths later, Shailu's company, Synergy Pharmaceuticals, Inc., is well underway to success in their clinical trials with these analogs of uroguanylin. Plecanatide is being developed by Synergy for the treatment of chronic idiopathic constipation (CIC) and irritable bowel syndrome with constipation

(IBS-C). Plecanatide has fewer side effects than a similar-acting drug, Linaclotide. SP-333 is being developed for opioid-induced constipation (OIC) and ulcerative colitis. Extremely positive Phase II clinical trials found effective dose and minor side effects (diarrhea) for both drugs. These results were followed by results of a large Phase III clinical trial for Plecanatide, reported at the end of June 2015. In this study, 3.0 mg and 6.0 mg doses of Plecanatide met the study's primary endpoint and showed significant improvement over the of durable responders (FDA outcome for CIC) compared to placebo during the 12-week treatment period (21.0% in 3.0 mg and 19.5% in 6.0 mg dose groups compared to 10.2% in placebo; p<0.001 for both doses). Here, too, plecanatide was found to be safe and well tolerated with diarrhea in 5.9% of patients in 3.0 mg and 5.5% of patients in 6.0 mg dose groups, compared to 1.3% of placebo-treated patients. They have reported similarly positive Phase II results for SP-333 for the treatment of OIC and Phase III results are expected at the end of next year.

One might wonder why the focus of Synergy research has been on CIC and IBS-C, if the promise of uroguanylin was to prevent colon cancer. The mechanisms of the activities of Plecanatide and SP-333 are extremely well characterized: Uroguanylin and its analogs are GC-C agonists. They were designed to mimic the normal activities of uroguanylin, GC-C activation results in the cyclic GMP pathway activation, and a host of healthy, normal functions: proper fluid and ion transport through the gut epithelial tissues, reduction in gastrointestinal inflammation and polyp formation, a reduction of visceral hypersensitivity, and proper functioning of the cGMP mediated programmed cell death (apoptosis). The pH ranges of the analogs are also well-characterized.

There are good reasons for SP's strategy of focusing on these diseases first. Clinical development on the drugs' utility in preventing colon cancer would require very long prospective randomized trials, with identification of populations at high risk of colon cancer. People with high risk of colon cancer typically either have familial risk, or are identified by having numerous benign polyps or polyps showing varying degrees of hyperplasia — beyond the time in which the processes lead to eventual colon cancer.

Under FDA criteria, the best trial would be a decades-long prospective trial on all of the high-risk groups. The study would have corresponding control groups — with patients randomized per treatment, or dose (the prophylactic uroguanylin analog) and placebo. The feasibility of such a study is fairly low — and its duration certainly would not satisfy the short attention span of prospecting investors. Hence, prophylactic clinical trials focused on colon cancer prevention could be very challenging and cost-prohibitive.

Thus, a wise and economically feasible strategy for a start-up company like Synergy would be to focus on a "high success low risk" approach. SP's studies have instead focused on functional bowel disorders and GI inflammation — related diseases of the bowel, diseases that have identifiable, short-term, extremely clearly defined clinical outcome measures, such as reversal of constipation, reduction in signs of inflammation, and proper bowel functioning. In Shailu's case, one of the most important, and very specific, outcome measures was complete spontaneous bowel movement (CSBM) frequency with minimal negative side effects. In this regard, Shailu's (and SP's) focus on these other disease first has been brilliant.

The Phase IIB study of plecanatide for IBS-C was a 12-week, double-blind, placebo-controlled, dose-ranging study to assess the safety and efficacy of plecanatide in 424 adult patients with IBS-C. Patients given plecanatide showed an overall responder rate of >40% compared to 24.7% for placebo. Again, side effects were minimal, especially compared to the nearly 20% diarrhea associated with the FDA approved Linzess®, an analog of the *E. coli* enterotoxin responsible for Traveler's diarrhea.

If the FDA approves plecanatide, or SP-333, for the clinical treatment of these very common gastrointestinal diseases, which are very stressful for patients, Shailu will have significantly reduced human pain and suffering. Inflammation is often a precursor to cancer, so simply using these drugs in the care and treatment of these clinical groups will likely reduce the incidence of colon cancer. Then, one can hope that their off-label use in the preventative care for families at risk of colon cancer will be possible, although the drugs cannot be marketed for this purpose. There will almost certainly be incidental protection against colon cancer in patients with chronic constipation and IBD populations as a result of curative treatment of both of the conditions, which often lead to colon cancer.

The best outcome for society would be a smaller clinical trial studying the utility of plecanatide and SP-333 for the prevention of recurrence of colon cancer. Another possibility is a study with smaller number of people — matched between control and treatment groups — with short-term outcomes such as the number of polyps, or progression of polyps from benign to pre-cancerous — measured by gene expression. Such a study might not be necessary for the clinical application toward colon cancer prevention, but that type of study would help high-risk populations and their oncologists realize immense potential gains in the prevention of colon cancer.

A New Gold Standard for Clinical Trials (1–5 Years)

A new gold standard in needed for clinical trials; the old one is inefficient, and wasteful. It is not just that incorrect inferences have been made based on the lack of finding significant differences between outcome groups, while the most pressing information on safety and efficacy lies in the overall consideration of the before-and-after results within arms. It is also that important trials that should be conducted become infeasible, or would be unethical. For Shailu, and SP, they were able to find other diseases involving the same critical pathway leading to the beneficial discovery that can aid patients in numerous conditions. This is a reflection of the rational design behind the initial discoveries by Shailu and his collaborators (Kunwar *et al.*, 2000).

But other diseases exist for which clinical trials are needed that would require decades-long studies (Alzheimer's disease), or unacceptable conditions for patients (randomized robotic vs. open prostatectomy), or unethical treatment strategies for patients (randomized selection of myriad of chemotherapeutic agents to demonstrate efficacy of chemosensitivity assays). For these diseases, there are no corollary clinical conditions, and no intermediate disease states. Such clinical conditions may deserve a separate categorization for submission of studies to the FDA.

I foresee a future in which these principles and requirements for effective clinical research are demonstrated via mathematical proofs of higher power and superior efficiency in the within-arm inferences I advocate. I also foresee a future in which we will know, for each and every clinical trial, the symptoms of *relevant* confounders (beyond multicollinearity), where computational case matching is conducted as a matter of routine; where a more enlightened public learns the importance of their critical role in participating in clinical trials. Improvements in the design of these trials will include specific control-panel-like indicators that a trial result has fallen into specific, predictable zones of performance. Using a standard set of simulation tools, in which the numerical and preliminary data of entire clinical trials beforehand are completely specified, investigators will be able to *learn* fine-tuned, clinically meaningful specific benchmarks, and thus identify, and justify, specific outcome measures.

These improvements will require a better overall understanding of where the power lies in RCTs, and will require reversals, revisions and replacements to outdated and incorrect FDA Guidances. Unless these reforms are adopted, with FDA leadership and encouragement, the FDA can, justifiably, be held as responsible for the human pain and suffering caused by the lack of preventative measures and treatments that they could have approved, but failed to due to their insistence of a decades-old protocols for clinical trial design and analysis.

Those functional and operational considerations aside, the future of medicine looks very bright. Here are some of the advances being made, and some that are forthcoming.

Approval of a larger Number of Natural Compounds with Clinical Efficacy (3–12 Years)

The nutraceutical industry is booming. Care should be taken to provide clinical evidence for health claims that those in the industry truly feel are warranted. It would be very good to know which natural compounds are truly effective, and which are most effective, for their supposed health benefit. I hope readers of this book will consider the immense value in a short-term exclusive profit clause for the commercialization of naturally occurring compounds, and enabling improvements in the operational aspects of clinical trials to allow discoveries like Shailu's to come to fruition faster. Moreover, I hope society acts on this knowledge. In the US, I foresee a Clinical Trials Reform Act that mandates the FDA to study, via mathematics, simulations, and the re-analysis of previously submitted data, the effects of refusing positive results from outcomes-to-baseline. Such an act should require the FDA to revisit past rejection decisions that resulted although promising (significant) results were seen within the treatment arm, due to the increased power, but not found in the across-groupwise comparison, due to the relative lack of power in that comparison. I hope Pharma comes to see nutraceuticals not merely as competitors, but as a gold mine of potential valuable treatments and cures, and begins to partner with them for their most promising products in a manner that leads to clinical trials.

A naïve interpretation of the interactions between Pharma, medical practitioners and alleged "natural cures" underlies much of the myth that "doctors do not want cures, they only want treatments." A good example came to me from a family member who sometimes refers people to me. I often act as a patient advocate, helping them identify the most critical biomarker tests for their type of cancer, and I help people find clinical trials that might be most beneficial to them, especially in difficult, late-stage and aggressive cases. I learned about Graviola, a South American plant that is touted by its advocates as an alleged cure for cancer, and was forwarded some information. The information read (verbatim from their website):

Cancer Killing Dynamo

Advertisement

Indigenous people from the Amazon, Andes and The Carribean (sic) have used the bark, leaves, roots, flowers, fruit and seed from the Graviola Tree for centuries to treat heart disease, asthma, liver problems and arthritis.

It's also used as a natural remedy for infections, fever, digestive problems, high blood pressure and plenty of other uses.

But did you know it is a cancer killing dynamo? Scientific studies show that the leaves of the Graviola plant are effective in destroying malignant cancer cells. The phytochemicals appear especially effective in targeting the cancer cells, leaving healthy cells untouched.

Wow. A natural cure for cancer? So why haven't you heard about this miracle tree? Take a wild guess.

Many people without a scientific background will read this and assume that because "*Scientific studies show that the leaves of the Graviola plant are effective in destroying malignant cancer cells,*" that Pharma and the medical community do not want to bring Graviola forward as a treatment because it kills cancer cells. There are multiple websites selling Graviola as a cure for cancer, and they claim that some unnamed pharmaceutical company killed the funding for the program after they found it was so effective because they could not exclusively profit from it. They cite an unnamed scientist who leaked the "truth" about Graviola after he left the company.

The implied and drawn conclusions are that Pharma has a cure, but that because they cannot find a way to profit, they are hiding the truth. The presumption is that Graviola is safe. This flies in the face of the scientific studies that have been conducted; studies have found that while extracts from Graviola kill cancer cells in cell culture, they also damage nerve cells. Studies in rodents found extensive liver and kidney toxicity. Simply because a compound has been shown to "destroy cancer cells" does not make it a medicine. Many compounds kill cancer cells in culture. I am certain that gasoline would kill cancer cell lines, of any kind. Some compounds, however, also harm normal cells, and therefore until efficacy and safety studies are conducted, it would be irresponsible to advertise such compounds with misleading statements such as those that would play on the hopes and fears of people without sufficient education or knowledge to be able to discern when the data being cited are insufficient to support the implied claims. The use of unwarranted claims to sell Graviola products would prey on the hopes and fears of people facing death and suffering. So let's look at the available data behind the claims.

Some of the animal research on Graviola on safety is compelling, and numerous studies have shown that it kills a variety of types of cancer cell in *in vitro* (in cell lines). It apparently regenerates Beta cells in the pancreas of Wistar rats (a diabetic rat model; Adeyemi *et al.*, 2010), and there is evidence in mice that it can significantly downregulate EGFR mRNA expression, stop the cancer cell cycle in the G0/G1 phase, and induce apoptosis in MDA-MB-468 cells. It also slowed tumor growth by 32% in a xenograft breast cancer mouse model (Dai *et al.*, 2011). It appears to reduce tumorigenesis and metastasis in pancreatic cancer cells *in vitro* (Torres *et al.*, 2012).

These are all promising and compelling results. However, they are not human studies, and each result should be independently replicated before attempting human trials.

Anyone who knows me knows that I am not an apologist for Pharma, and I am intolerant of anyone who stands to profit at the expense of human pain and suffering. However, the translational research needed for any compound — natural or not — is time-consuming. Graviola is no different. The first step after promising animal studies (assuming tolerability and sufficiently low toxicity) is to conduct Phase I dose-escalation trials. These are limited usually to 3 vs. 3 patients at various doses to identify possible side effects and to find the maximum safe and effective dose. The second phase is usually Phase II safety and efficacy trials, with a larger (but still small) number of patients — usually around 20 or 30 per treatment group (arm). Usually, the control group is the standard baseline of care, but this is not always true. If these are successful (sufficiently good outcomes considering any adverse events), a Phase III prospective randomized trial is conducted using much larger numbers of patients per treatment arm. Sometimes, for ethical reasons, the new treatment is found to be so effective at an interim outcome measurement that the patients in the control arm are switched to the treatment arm, effectively terminating the study early. This is conducted with the oversight of an Institutional Review Board. Sometimes, at Phase III, the significance of the adverse events becomes apparent, and the harm of the treatment to the patient is seen to outweigh the benefits, and the trial is terminated and the new treatment abandoned.

There have also been reports of an NIH study in 1976 in which extracts of stems and leaves from Graviola were found to be effective in humans, and the internet rumor mill has it that the results were in an internal report that was never published. Such websites never offer any motive for researchers in 1976 to suppress such an important finding. Others cite a 1976 plant screening program by the National Cancer Institute, in which Graviola leaves and stem showed active toxicity against cancer cells. The study that is cited that purported to show clinical efficacy in *humans* is often cited as:

> "*Anon. Unpublished data, National Cancer Institute. Nat Cancer Inst Central Files (1976). From NAPRALERT Files, University of Illinois, 1995.*"

In spite of extensive searching, I could not locate this report on the web. So I wrote to NAPRALERT, which is a natural products database founded by the late Prof. Norman Farnsworth at the University of Illinois College of Pharmacy in Chicago. I was referred to NAPRALERT, and my query was responded to by Dr. Guido Pauli, a faculty member of the Pharmacognosy graduate program at the University of Chicago. Pharmacognosy is the study of medicinal uses of plants and other natural sources of medicinally useful compounds. He put me in contact with Dr. James Graham, Editor of NAPRALERT. In a series of e-mail exchanges, Dr. Graham assured me that this study, which was an internal communication, was in his words, cell line screening of plant compounds

> *I did a quick check of the database, and the citation information you provided refer back to our (NAPRALERT) citation number X0001.*
>
> *If this is the case, they are unpublished data (internal data between NCI and UIC researchers, most notably Professors Farnsworth, Fong, Cordell, Kinghorn and Soejarto, from our research group), going back probably to the 1950s, up through to the 1976 citation date.*
>
> *The 1995 date is apparently when the database was accessed and this citation was provided. I assume these variable dates are the source of your question?*
>
> *I also assume you are aware of the massive amounts of research done at NCI, including massive screening programs of the anticancer-activity of tens of thousands of chemicals and natural product extracts over the years.*
>
> *The data in NAPRALERT citation X0001 refer to internal correspondence, mainly raw screening data, (from an indeterminate number of plant species on an indeterminate number of unspecified bioassays). Bioassay systems include both Hippocratic screening data of plant extracts and plant chemical isolates on mice, to in vitro screening data using one or more of whatever cell lines were current at the time(s) of sample submission.*
>
> *Hope this helps, and apologies again for the delayed response to your inquiry.*

In a second email, Dr. Graham affirmed that these were not clinical trials.

All activities reported in this "citation" record (screening data on 138 plant species — mostly methanol and aqueous alcoholic extracts) were done on cell lines.

If your anticipation was that these were clinical data, they were not. This is raw extract screening data on cell lines.

The natural products literature is quite a mixed bag, and any interpretation ("oft-cited" reference) of this unpublished data as clinical research is completely unfounded.

I hope this helps? Perhaps if previous authors and editors were as careful as yourself, this kind of stuff (bad references copied and amplified in the literature) would not be clogging up our journal-space. Just a thought.

None of the necessary research for claims of efficacy of Graviola have ever been conducted — and yet the hypothesis that Graviola is effective is reported to have been around since at least 1975. Part of the reason why Graviola and other so-called natural treatments should be avoided, for now, by consumers is because they may harm humans in ways that we do not yet understand. This can include, for example, depletion of the natural bacterial flora in the intestine, unknown side effects with other drugs, liver and kidney toxicity, interactions with FDA-approved drugs, and many other negative effects on health that may, or may not, be balanced by the presumed positive effects on a person's tumors. And these effects are all presumed unless a study has shown effectiveness in humans. There are numerous drugs that have shown promise in animal studies only to fall flat in humans. Our physiology is different (lower body temperature), our genes and pathways are different (evolution), and we are larger. Effective dose-finding is important because if the drug is effective, the dosages that balance any dangerous side effects with any potential benefits will be most clinically useful and best tolerated by patients. Ultimately, anyone convinced to take Graviola *instead of* FDA-approved drugs may be wasting precious time, which is terribly risky for late-stage cancer patients.

The FDA has issued warning letters to companies that make unwarranted claims about Graviola on their websites, and a Montana man was fined $80,000 for being in contempt of court for failing to comply with the FDA's warning to stop making unwarranted claims. The standard for the right to claim medicinal efficacy are high in the US, and they should be. Some compounds in Graviola may or may not help cure some types of cancers safely, but there is no published evidence that supports claims in either direction.

Organ Replacement via Organogenesis

There are over 100,000 people in the US waiting for organ transplant. The controversy over stem cell research and US President George W. Bush's ban on stem cell research severely hampered progress in understanding basic developmental biology for over a decade. The ability to harvest and grow somatic stem cells has renewed that progress. In the future, when a person loses an organ due to chronic illness or trauma, their doctors should be able to harvest cells from the damaged organ (either stem cells or cells from a healthy region of the organ) and grow replacement organs either in their body, or in the lab for a time, and then implant the new organ — derived from their own tissues — and thus replace their organs.

These types of procedures have already replaced a Swedish girl's hepatic vein (Olausson *et al.*, 2014), a trachea in a 30-year old woman with five-year follow-up (Gonfiotti *et al.*, 2014), a trachea in a 36-year-old Eritrean man, who had cancer of the trachea; a 12-year old boy (Elliot *et al.*, 2012), and a two-year old girl (Children's Hospital of

Illinois, 2013). The two-year old girl, who had been born without a trachea, survived an additional three months, and was called a "pioneer" by her doctor after she died at 34 months. Progress is being made in mouse and rat models in the production of organoids from adult human stem cells for thymus, liver, stomachs, kidneys, teeth, retinas, and hearts. Tear duct (Tiwari *et al.*, 2014) and salivary gland regeneration (Ogawa and Tsuji, 2015) are under development.

The typical procedure involves creating an artificial or natural scaffold upon which properly potentiated stem cells are sprinkled. A replacement thymus was created by mixing healthy thymus cells with stem cells, and the organ spontaneously developed. Numerous patients have had urethra replaced by a very similar technique called "cell seeding," in which healthy cells from the patient's organs are used to seed a scaffold (De Filippo *et al.*, 2015).

One of the challenges of these developments is to insure the proper innervation and vasculaturization of new organs, which will be critically important to ensure their function. This could be achieved via involvement of the rest of body (*in vivo* development, as in the case of kidneys, where dialysis could be effective while the organ grows), or by *in vitro* models of the organ's *in vivo* environment (as in the development of hearts, where pumping fluid require a synthetic but realistic circulatory system). Approaches using 3D printing that embed blood vessel-like channels for vascular perfusion look promising (Miller *et al.*, 2012; Zhao *et al.*, 2012; Wang *et al.*, 2014).

This approach will have numerous advantages over organ transplant. First, organs readily available for transplant are rare, and they require a tissue match. Second, they also require immune system suppression — and these drugs are expensive. Some patients pay $8,000–$10,000 per year for anti-rejection drugs. The drugs also increase the risk of infection and autoimmune disease. Beyond these risks, it is now well-appreciated that a weakened immune system is more likely to fail to remove dangerous endogenous cells, and that can progress to cancer. If a person has a progressive disease that will eventually lead to organ failure, the replacement organ will be grown before there is a life-threatening medical crisis; as biomedicine is now focused on being able to predict diseases long before clinical manifestation, this will become more commonplace. Harvesting organ cells in children for use later when their progressive condition worsens may become an option. As the demographic trends in the US see an aging baby boomer population, the need for organs will increase, and thus research in the area of organ replacement should be given high priority.

Artificial Eyes (AEyes) (5–10 Years)

Just as the loss of sight is devastating to a person's life, the acquisition of sight can be powerfully enabling. Neural implant devices and other means of transmitting information into the brain are beginning to show promise in generating visible images. A series of breakthroughs are needed before we have truly effective artificial eyes. Such devices could be, in many ways, vastly superior to human eyes. Not only could they perceive a broader range of the UV spectrum by compressing the entire UV spectrum into a range normally perceivable by our brains, AEyes could also feed recognition information into the human mind, a sort of mental augmentation, in which algorithms designed for Deep Learning for computers could help people recognize things that they have never before seen or learned about. Imagine knowing the name of everyone simply by looking at their face. For some, this would be spooky — a bit Big Brotherish, and certainly it would be technology that could be used for ill-gotten or criminal gains. There is already an artificial cornea for use in the case of damaged cornea and age-related macular degeneration. It has a telescoping lens that allows people to see at farther distances (Tremblay *et al.*, 2013). Ironically, the ultimate future of the loss of eyesight could be augmented vision, just like people with artificial limbs have found that spring-legs provide them with an edge in athletics.

Increasing Use of Brain Scans (EEG) and Visual Tests for Diagnosis and Outcomes Management (5–10 Years)

In Chapter 13, I review the outstanding promise Neurotrack's rapid, simple vision test that could lead to early diagnosis of Alzheimer's disease. The diagnostic rule associated with the test is designed to (hopefully) be specific for Alzheimer's disease. There are many additional types of neurological disorders, including dementias, that may be reflected in the way that the hypothalamus processes short-term visual (or auditory) information. Gaze persistence is just one of many dimensions of information that each subject's eye movements could be studied for diagnostic utility, either for differential diagnosis, or for outright diagnosis. The human eye, for example, experiences micromovements that help us see continuity (a type of eye "jittering" that is thought to cause multiple cones and rods to sample the same part of the image. Poor jittering could reflect some other type of disease. Pupil dilation patterns, blinking patterns, the speed at which the eyes transfer from one image to another are just some of the additional dimensions of information that a data miner could enjoy parsing through to develop machine-learning optimized rules for diagnosis of schizophrenia, evidence of stroke, depression, and many, many other types of neurological disorders.

Better Treatments Using What Works, Not Merely What's Novel (Ongoing)

During the 2014/2015 Ebola epidemic, a team of researchers screened over 2,800 FDA-approved compounds for their ability to inhibit the Ebolaviruses' cellular entry system in one screen. They found 53 promising leads. A number of drugs designed or used for one condition have also been found to have positive clinically important side effects. Low-dose aspirin, for example, is recommended for men over the age of 50 to help prevent colon cancer. The well-known effects of Viagara (Sildenafil) were discovered when the drug was being studied for potential efficacy as cardiovascular drug, and as potential treatment for high blood pressure.

Reducing the Paperwork Burden of IND's for Compassionate Use Terminally Ill Patients (1–2 Years)

A company is needed that specializes in providing a service via which they will, under a signed HIPAA waiver from each patient:

(1) collect all of the relevant information from all of the doctors involved in the care of terminally ill patients;

(2) file all necessary regulatory paperwork needed for successful IND disclosures;

(3) follow up with the FDA with informative letters accurately representing the urgency of the patients' condition as the FDA decision making takes undue time;

(4) follow up with each doctor on the patients' teams with news of the outcome of the FDA's decision, and prospectively collect letters of appeal in the event they are needed.

Reducing Human Pain and Suffering by Making Effective Treatments Available to the Poor (Ongoing)

The scourge of HIV continues to plague the planet, and reducing the number of new infections worldwide is an important part of controlling the disease rate within the global population. An organization called Medicines Patent Pool (MPP) was formed to answer the WHO's call to make certain drugs (antiretrovirals) proven to be effective at keeping HIV titres below transmissible levels. MPP's charter is to facilitate proper licensure of HIV drugs to generic drug manufacturers worldwide to prevent brand-name drugs from being priced out of reach of the populations who need them the most.

This type of effort, and the use of biosimilars, is likely to increase in the future, especially for other deadly emerging diseases.

New Molecular Target Classes for Effective Treatments (Early Stage, Ongoing)

Basic knowledge of genomic biology is growing by leaps and bounds. While the functions of many (nearly half) of the proteins encoded by the genes in our genome are not yet known, we now know, for example, that small, hairpin like RNA structures called miRNAs are among the many natural means the body uses to transmit signals to turn genes on and turn them off. In addition, we know that they can be carried among cells via microcapsules of cell membranes called exosomes. Exosome-mediated, tissue-specific manipulation of gene expression is an important futures medicine concept in part because they would use the body's own signaling mechanism to alter gene expression states and, for example, trick cancer cells and precancerous cells into undergoing programmed cell death (apoptosis) by turning on genes that had been silenced. These molecular mechanism based treatments would barely qualify as "drugs"; they are more analogs to replacing lost blood or serum. Similarly, means of re-patterning methylation could help with everything from Parkinson's disease to healing severed spinal cords.

References

Adeyemi DO, *et al.* (2010) Histomorphological and morphometric studies of the pancreatic islet cells of diabetic rats treated with extracts of *Annona muricata. Folia Morphol (Warsz)* **69(2):** 92–100.

Children's Hospital of Illinois. (2013) Hannah's Story. www.childrenshospitalofillinois.org/trachea-surgery/?lite

Dai Y, *et al.* (2011) Selective growth inhibition of human breast cancer cells by graviola fruit extract *in vitro* and *in vivo* involving down-regulation of EGFR expression. *Nutr Cancer* **63(5):** 795–801. [doi: 10.1080/01635581.2011.563027]

De Filippo RE, *et al.* (2015) Penile urethra replacement with autologous cell-seeded tubularized collagen matrices. *J Tissue Eng Regen Med* **9(3):** 257–64. [doi: 10.1002/term.1647]

Elliott MJ, *et al.* (2012) Stem-cell-based, tissue engineered tracheal replacement in a child: a 2-year follow-up study. *Lancet* **380(9846):** 994–1000. [doi: 10.1016/S0140-6736(12)60737-5]

Gonfiotti A, *et al.* (2014) The first tissue-engineered airway transplantation: 5-year follow-up results. *Lancet* **383(9913):** 238–44. [doi: 10.1016/S0140-6736(13)62033-4]

Miller JS, *et al.* (2012) Rapid casting of patterned vascular networks for perfusable engineered three-dimensional tissues. *Nat Mater* **11(9):** 768–74. [doi: 10.1038/nmat3357]

Ogawa M, Tsuji T. (2015) Fully functional salivary gland regeneration as a next-generation regenerative therapy. *Nihon Rinsho Meneki Gakkai Kaishi* **38(2):** 93–100. [doi: 10.2177/jsci.38.93]

Shailubhai K. (2000) Uroguanylin treatment suppresses polyp formation in the Apc(Min/+) mouse and induces apoptosis in human colon adenocarcinoma cells via cyclic GMP. *Cancer Res* **60(18):** 5151–57.

Tiwari S, *et al.* (2014) Human lacrimal gland regeneration: perspectives and review of literature. *Saudi J Ophthalmol* **28(1):** 12–18. [doi: 10.1016/j.sjopt.2013.09.004]

Torres MP. (2012) Graviola: a novel promising natural-derived drug that inhibits tumorigenicity and metastasis of pancreatic cancer cells *in vitro* and *in vivo* through altering cell metabolism. *Cancer Lett* **323(1):** 29–40. [doi: 10.1016/j.canlet.2012.03.031]

Tremblay EJ, *et al.* (2013) Switchable telescopic contact lens. *Optics Express* **21(13):** 15980–86.

Wang XY, *et al.* (2014) Engineering interconnected 3D vascular networks in hydrogels using molded sodium alginate lattice as the sacrificial template. *Lab Chip* **14(15):** 2709–16. [doi: 10.1039/c4lc00069b]

Zhao L, *et al.* (2012) The integration of 3-D cell printing and mesoscopic fluorescence molecular tomography of vascular constructs within thick hydrogel scaffolds. *Biomaterials* **33(21):** 5325–32. [doi: 10.1016/j.biomaterials.2012.04.004]

Postscript: Is Vaccination a Translational Success Story?

A number of controversies are ongoing at the time of the writing of this book that makes writing a definitive treatise on vaccines as a translational success especially challenging.

Controversy #1. Dr. William Thompson (CDC Senior Scientist Whistleblower)

At the time of this writing, Dr. Thompson stands by his assertions. A book containing the full transcripts of this revelations to Dr. Hooker is now available (CDC Whistleblower, Skyhorse Publisher). In these conversations, Dr. Thompson not only revealed that results were omitted for African American males in the DeStefano *et al.* (2004) study; he also revealed that results from so-called idiopathic autism cases — cases that occur with no other co-morbid condition — were also excluded by the CDC team from the publication. Thompson told Hooker that the exclusion of that group's result was the one that bothered him the most. Hooker's re-analysis of the CDC's data simply recapitulated the results found, but not published by the CDC, and the fact that the journal in which it was published retracted Hooker's paper, but has stood by the DeStefano *et al.* (2004) paper even after the IOM/NAS listed it among the 17 of 22 vaccine safety studies they rejected due to fatal flaws (Institute of Medicine, National Academy of Sciences. 2012) is cause for grave concern over the objectivity of vaccine safety research in general. The withdrawal of Hooker's paper was based on an "expression of concern" over the statistical analysis Hooker used, and an alleged conflict of interest in Hooker's suggested reviewers. I asked Hooker about what conflict of interest the journal thought might have existed. He said:

> *"I have no clue what they were talking about regarding the peer reviewers. They claimed originally that I did not disclose that I was on the board of Focus for Health. However, I was not on the board of Focus for Health when the work was completed for the paper nor when the original grant was made for me to do the work."*

The concern over Hooker's statistical analysis cannot explain why Hooker found the same result that the DeStefano *et al.* team found in their analysis, and excluded from their results.

In 2012, the Institute of Medicine/National Academy of Sciences' report rejected the original DeStefano *et al.* (2004) study as one of 17 out of 22 studies they considered to have fatal flawed. The fact that the CDC still lists those 17 studies, ignoring the National Academy of Sciences' assessment of the quality of the design of the studies draws the CDC into question as a source of reliable, unbiased, scientific information on vaccine safety overall.

In spite of the IOM/NAS's concerns, and in spite of one of the co-authors admitting fraud in the research behind the study, the journal *Pediatrics* has not retracted the DeStefano *et al.* (2004) study.

Controversy #2. Merck Safety Study Trial (Merck Employee Whistleblowers)

Another pair of vaccine whistleblowers — this time Merck employees — claim that Merck falsified data on effectiveness (or efficacy) of their Measles/Mumps/Rubella (MMR) vaccine. In one of their complaints, they allege that Merck added concentrated mouse antigens to the vials containing the blood from vaccinated mice to increase the apparent immune response. They allege that Merck took actions to defraud the United States for over a decade. The vaccine itself may be losing efficacy (waning efficacy) and Merck is alleged to have a systematic program designed to hide this essential fact, including "double bonuses" for work done to conceal the low efficacy. If these allegations bear out, this would clearly amount to attempts by Merck to defraud the US government — and willfully place a significant portion of the US public at risk for developing measles. This has led some to speculate that the 2006 mumps outbreak, and a 2015 Disneyland measles were from waning immunity, not from unvaccinated individuals, as has been alleged. If these two whistleblowers are telling the truth, Merck not only broke federal law — they also deserve to lose the contract as they have demonstrated themselves willing to put people's lives at risk by lying about the effectiveness of their MMR vaccine.

The allegations in United States v. Merck & Co. include that Merck "failed to disclose that its mumps vaccine was not as effective as Merck represented; (ii) used improper testing techniques; (iii) manipulated testing methodology; (iv) abandoned undesirable test results; (v) falsified test data; (vi) failed to adequately investigate and report the diminished efficacy of its mumps vaccine; (vii) falsely verified that each manufacturing lot of mumps vaccine would be as effective as identified in the labeling; (viii) falsely certified the accuracy of applications filed with the FDA; (ix) falsely certified compliance with the terms of the CDC purchase contract; (x) engaged in the fraud and concealment describe herein for the purpose of illegally monopolizing the US market for mumps vaccine; (xi) mislabeled, misbranded, and falsely certified its mumps vaccine; and (xii) engaged in the other acts described herein to conceal the diminished efficacy of the vaccine the government was purchasing."

A second, anti-trust suit (Chatom Primary Care v. Merck & Co.) contains similar allegations, which they filed on behalf of the US government after the FDA failed to provide adequate follow-up due to their statements of concern.

The long-term efficacy of vaccines is not part of the typical study of the effectiveness of vaccines. In September 2015, a judge dismissed Merck's motion to dismiss. This case is still pending at the time of this writing. It is worth noting that former CDC Director Julie Gerberding, was hired into the position of President of Merck's vaccine division, and then moved to the position of Executive Vice President for Strategic Communications, Global Public Policy and Population Health. Gerberding recently sold over 38,000 shares of Merck Stock for $2.3 million. Gerberding was Director of CDC from 1998–2009, and has been quoted as being "bullish on vaccines."

Controversy #3. HPV Vaccine Safety and Utility Questioned

When a vaccine is prescribed for a disease, the research involved should demonstrate that the benefit (reduction of risk of disease) is greater than any potential harm from the treatment (side effects, adverse events). The human papillomavirus is responsible for around 10,000 cancer deaths in the US each year (all cancer types, SEER data). These cancers do not develop at or near the time of infection, but rather years after. Vaccination against HPV is thought to be warranted due to the effect of reducing the spread of HPV in the population, thus reducing cancer risks. Vaccination is recommended for both males and females aged 13 to 26.

Over 70% of women clear the virus within the first year, and over 90% of women clear the virus within two years, and therefore some question the utility of the vaccine. While a persistent HPV infection would be more problematic, however, only about 10% of HPV cases progress into a pre-cancerous lesion. However, an increasing number of reports of serious adverse events are being published, reflecting physician's concerns over the safety of HPV vaccines. Japan has decided against universal vaccination, citing serious adverse event rates around 5%. This is much higher than the rate estimates provided by the CDC.

The types of adverse events include death, migraine headaches, fainting, and autoimmune disorders.

Tomljenovic *et al.* (2014) describes in a full case report the development of a serious autoimmune disorder called POTS/CFS after HPV vaccine booster injection. It is critically important to recognize that many of the safety research studies conducted for HPV vaccine used a placebo that included aluminum adjuvants — thus leaving any adverse reporting to the trial only to those that result from the vaccine itself. Any adverse events due to the adjuvants, or interactions between the vaccine and adjuvants, would be unknown in such a study design, and if the safety research for a specific HPV vaccine, or any vaccine for that matter, involves the wrong type of placebo, those specific vaccines should be relegated to experimental treatment status. Aluminum in the bloodstream has long been recognized as neurotoxin, and various syndromes are attributed to the aluminum adjuvants, including Gulf War syndrome and Autoimmune/inflammatory syndrome induced by adjuvants (ASIA; Perricone *et al.*, 2013); Postural Orthostatic Tachycardia with Chronic Fatigue Syndrome (POT/CFS; Tomljenovic *et al.*, 2014). For a full assessment of the safety of vaccines, the importance of the distinction between studying vaccines with a true placebo and with a partial placebo cannot be overstated. Studies of adjuvant — containing placebo vs. vaccine will miss increases in adverse events due to adjuvant.

Public health policy is usually a much simplified version of the medical reality. But in the case of vaccine safety, the public policy is a cartoon caricature of reality. Adverse events that are reported are usually not carried forward in the CDC's public policy statements. A study of the adverse events reported in the VAERS (Slade *et al.*, 2009) found a rate of 53.9 reports per 100,000 doses distributed. They found a total of 772 reports (6.2% of all reports) describing serious adverse events, including 32 reports of death. The rates (per 100,000 vaccinations) were 8.2 for syncope (fainting); 7.5 for local site reactions; 6.8 for dizziness; 5.0 for nausea; 4.1 for headache; 3.1 for hypersensitivity reactions; 2.6 for urticaria; 0.2 for venous thromboembolic events, autoimmune disorders, and Guillain-Barré syndrome; 0.1 for anaphylaxis and death; 0.04 for transverse myelitis and pancreatitis; and 0.009 for motor neuron disease. There was an overabundance of syncope and venous thromboembolic events compared to other vaccines.

It is worth revisiting whether some the ADHD "overdiagnosis" (discussed at length in Chapter 6) is actually a real epidemic of injury due to the use of neurotoxic adjuvants. There are strong indicators from examinations of the effects of such compounds on methylation pathways (Waly *et al.*, 2004). The Freedom of Information Act led to the release of a 2000 internal CDC report in which a statistically significant increase in the rates of "neurological development disorders with increasing cumulative exposure to thimerosal" in children three months of age. While individual disorders were "nearly significant," when combined (as they are now in ASD), the CDC found increased risk of specific delays (ICD9 code 315), developmental speech disorder (dyslalia, ICD9 code 315.39), autism (ICD9 code 299.0), stuttering (ICD9 code 307.0), and attention deficit disorder (ICD9 code 314.0). The fact that it took a Freedom of Information Act request to secure the report, entitled "Thimerosal VSD Study Phase I," and stamped "CONFIDENTIAL" and "DO NOT COPY OR RELEASE" does not increase one's confidence in the CDC's statements over vaccine safety and their continued denial of any link between neurological disorders and vaccines that include additives like aluminum, a known neurotoxin. The authors of the report were Thomas Verstraeten, Robert Davis, and Frank DeStefano. Verstraeten and DeStefano are currently at the center of attention of the ongoing inquiries resulting from Dr. William Thompson's revelations to Dr. Hooker. This result has been confirmed independently by a number of studies (Geier & Geier (2005), Young *et al.*, (2008)). See Geier *et al.* (2015) for a full review.

While thimerosal has been removed from most of the pediatric vaccination schedule, it is still in the flu vaccine for pregnant mothers, and in three other vaccines (the CDC recently reported in testimony to Congress it was only present in one).

Thompson represented the use of scientific misconduct and fraud as hard-wired, rampant, and enforced by his supervisors. One big question is what other published studies conducted in vaccine safety research have been compromised by the science-compromising tactics and culture at the CDC that have been alleged by Thompson, and found by many others. These include US Senator Tom Coburn, who found widespread waste, abuses and numerous instances of fraud; The Office of the Inspector General (Levinson, 2009), who found nearly 100% non-compliance in the CDC's Special Government Employees on Federal Advisory in reporting conflicts of interest; and David Wright, former director of the US Office of Research Integrity, who issued a letter upon his resignation claiming extensive problems at the CDC, the National Institute of Health, and the Public Health Service. Robert F. Kennedy, Jr. wrote about Poul Thorsen, who published a study claiming that the rise in autism after mercury was removed from vaccines in Denmark demonstrated the safety of Thiomerosal. Thorsen's integrity is in question, as he is alleged to have absconded with $2 million in fraudulently acquired CDC funds. In April, 2011, Thorsen was indicted by a US Attorney in Atlanta, Georgia for embezzlement of funds from a CDC grant to the North Atlantic Neuro-Epidemiology Alliance.

Harro *et al.*, (2001) showed that the efficacy of a HPV 16-L1 virus-like particle with, and without aluminum adjuvant, was 40 times stronger than natural infection. Efficacy was measured for the vaccine with, and without adjuvant via antigen titers as measured by ELISA. A second big question is why are adjuvants like aluminum, known neurotoxins when injected directly into the bloodstream, still being used?

We need reform in vaccine safety research, and we needed it ten years ago.

Additional References

Couette M, Boisse MF, Maison P, *et al.* (2009). Long-term persistence of vaccine-derived aluminum hydroxide is associated with chronic cognitive dysfunction. *J Inorg Biochem* **103**:1571–1578.

Geier DA, Geier MR. (2005). A two-phased population epidemiological study of the safety of thimerosal containing vaccines: a follow-up analysis. *Med Sci Monit* **11**(4): CR160–70.

Geier DA, *et al.*, (2015). Thimerosal: clinical, epidemiologic and biochemical studies. *Clin Chim Acta* **444**:212–20. doi: 10.1016/j.cca.2015.02.030.

Harro CD, *et al.* (2001) Safety and immunogenicity trial in adult volunteers of a human papillomavirus 16 L1 virus-like particle vaccine. *J Natl Cancer Inst* **93**(4):284–92.

Institute of Medicine, National Academy of Sciences. (2012). Adverse Effects of Vaccines: Evidence and Causality. http://www.nap.edu/catalog/13164/adverse-effects-of-vaccines-evidence-and-causality

Kennedy, RF, Jr. 2015. Central Figure in CDC Vaccine Cover-Up Absconds with $2M http://www.huffingtonpost.com/robert-f-kennedy-jr/central-figure-in-cdc-vac_b_494303.html

Levinson, 2009. CDC's Ethics Program for Special Government Employees on Federal Advisory Committees. Dept. Health and Human Services Office of Inspector General http://oig.hhs.gov/oei/reports/oei-04-07-00260.pdf

Passeri E, Villa C, Couette M, *et al.* (2011). Long-term follow-up of cognitive dysfunction in patients with aluminum hydroxideinduced macrophagic myofasciitis (MMF). *J Inorg Biochem* **105**:1457–63.

Perricone C. (2013). Autoimmune/inflammatory syndrome induced by adjuvants (ASIA) 2013: unveiling the pathogenic, clinical and diagnostic aspects. *J Autoimmun* **47**:1–16. doi: 10.1016/j.jaut.2013.10.004.

Slade BA, *et al.* (2009). Postlicensure safety surveillance for quadrivalent human papillomavirus recombinant vaccine. *JAMA* **302**(7):750–57. doi: 10.1001/jama.2009.1201.

Tomljenovic L, Spinosa JP, Shaw CA. (2013). Human papillomavirus (HPV) vaccines as an option for preventing cervical malignancies: (how) effective and safe? *Curr Pharm Des* **19**:1466–87.

Tomljenovic L, *et al.* (2014). Postural orthostatic tachycardia with chronic fatigue after HPV vaccination as part of the "autoimmune/auto-inflammatory syndrome induced by adjuvants": case report and literature review. *J Investig Med High Impact Case Rep* **2**(1):2324709614527812. doi: 10.1177/2324709614527812.

Waly M, *et al.* (2004). Activation of methionine synthase by insulin-like growth factor-1 and dopamine: a target for neurodevelopmental toxins and thimerosal. *Mol Psychiatry* **9**(4):358–70.

Young HA, Geier DA, Geier MR. (2008). Thimerosal exposure in infants and neurodevelopmental disorders: an assessment of computerized medical records in the Vaccine Safety Datalink. *J Neurol Sci* **271**(1–2):110–18.

Index